W0114523

AIDS IN ASIA

AIDS IN ASIA

The Challenge Ahead

Edited by
Jai P. Narain

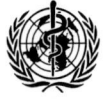

World Health Organization
Regional Office for South-East Asia
New Delhi

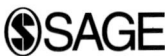

Los Angeles | London | New Delhi
Singapore | Washington DC | Melbourne

Copyright © *Indian Institute of Health Management Research, 2004*

All rights reserved. No part of this book may be reproduced or utilised in any form or by any means, electronic or mechanical, including photocopying, recording or by any information storage or retrieval system, without permission in writing from the publisher.

First published in 2004 by

SAGE Publications India Pvt Ltd
B1/I-1 Mohan Cooperative Industrial Area
Mathura Road, New Delhi 110 044, India
www.sagepub.in

SAGE Publications Inc
2455 Teller Road
Thousand Oaks, California 91320, USA

SAGE Publications Ltd
1 Oliver's Yard, 55 City Road
London EC1Y 1SP, United Kingdom

SAGE Publications Asia-Pacific Pte Ltd
3 Church Street
#10-04 Samsung Hub
Singapore 049483

Published by Vivek Mehra for SAGE Publications India Pvt Ltd, typeset in 10 pt Aldine401BT by Star Compugraphics Private Limited, New Delhi.

Library of Congress Cataloging-in-Publication Data

AIDS in Asia: the challenge ahead/editor, Jai P. Narain.
    p. cm.
Includes index.
    1. AIDS (Disease)—Asia. I. Narain, Jai P. II. Narain, Jai P.

RA643.86.A78A538   362.196'9792'0095—dc22   2004   2004015917

ISBN: 978-07-619-3225-3 (PB)

SAGE Team: Payal Dhar, Praveen Dev, Neeru Handa, Rahul Sharma and Santosh Rawat

CONTENTS

List of Tables

LIST OF FIGURES

LIST OF BOXES

MESSAGE FROM THE DIRECTOR-GENERAL, WHO

The AIDS pandemic poses an unprecedented threat to society globally and calls for concerted action. As we have seen in Thailand and Cambodia, an emergency response is needed in Asia and in other parts of the world. This is not only to ensure prevention activities, but to provide access to life-saving antiretroviral therapy (ART) to those living with HIV/AIDS.

Prevention and care are part of a continuum and reinforce each other. To mitigate the impact of the pandemic on individuals, families and societies, enhanced access and appropriate use of ART are urgently needed.

On 22 September 2003, in response to the many concerns expressed by the World Health Assembly in Geneva, I mentioned that the failure to provide antiretroviral therapy to patients in the developing world was a global health emergency. Together with UNAIDS, the Global Fund and our other partners, we have set a target of providing ART to 3 million people by 2005.

I urge all countries and organisations to do everything necessary to achieve the '3 by 5' objective. The WHO is committed to providing support to achieve this goal.

Lee Jong-wook
Director-General
World Health Organization

MESSAGE FROM THE REGIONAL DIRECTOR, WHO/SEARO

Since 1981, when AIDS was first reported in the United States of America, the disease has spread widely, affecting all continents and all countries of the world, including Asia. From what was called a white plague during the early 1980s, AIDS has come to be known today as the most devastating health and socio-economic problem afflicting the global community since the 14th century.

The HIV/AIDS problem is highly dynamic and a matter of grave concern to Asia, which already has the next highest number of people living with HIV/AIDS after Africa. Home to 50 per cent of the world's population, any small increase in HIV prevalence is translated into large numbers of infections that would severely put the already stretched infrastructure under strain. Poverty, economic disparities, illiteracy, and cultural and gender-related issues all contribute to Asia's vulnerability to HIV and the enormous potential for the epidemic to spin out of control unless the problem is addressed now.

This book is an attempt to put the spotlight on the AIDS problem in Asia, to describe the epidemiological aspects, and the responses mounted over the past two decades. The valuable lessons learnt so far would be helpful in formulating future policies and designing strategies relevant to the Asian context. The AIDS epidemic in Asia is still at an early stage. Hence, while some countries like Thailand have enormous experience in dealing with it, there are many others with relatively recent epidemics and hence with lesser experience. Learning from each other will help the region find solutions relevant to its unique cultural and social milieu.

The book, therefore, makes a valuable contribution to our understanding of the AIDS problem in Asia and the issue to be addressed. It deals with new initiatives and global priorities and their relevance to and implications for Asia.

Uton Muchtar Rafei
Regional Director
WHO Regional Office for South-East Asia

PREFACE

The human immunodeficiency virus (HIV), which causes acquired immunodeficiency syndrome (AIDS), is the leading infectious cause of adult deaths in the world. Experiences in different countries show that HIV can be prevented with high political commitment, adequate human and financial resources, and sustained interventions. It is well recognised that the impact of the HIV/AIDS epidemic in the developed and developing countries differs. Up to 95 per cent of new HIV infections now occur in developing countries, which are unfortunately also the least equipped to respond effectively. With the availability of new drugs, clinical management of HIV has improved remarkably, enabling AIDS patients in developed countries to survive longer. However, these facilities are still beyond the reach of those in the developing world, calling for innovative approaches to enhance access to antiretroviral therapy and their use in Asia and Africa. The new '3 by 5' WHO initiative to enhance HIV treatment access thus assumes great significance. In order to use these new approaches more effectively, rationally and equitably, there is a need for better understanding of the changing epidemiology of HIV infection and the responses to the epidemic at the country level.

This book, focused on Asia, is in recognition of the tremendous importance of HIV/AIDS as an unprecedented health and development threat in the region. It highlights the many advances in HIV research, as well as the new initiatives and their applications throughout the developing world, particularly in the Asian context.

The book describes the situation in Asia, programmatic issues and challenges, and the responses required, both in the area of the national AIDS control programmes and in research and development. The social dimensions and the potential economic toll the epidemic could unleash in Asia is covered in some detail by Nielsen and Melgaard. At present, as the pandemic continues its relentless march, Africa remains the hardest hit, where HIV has devastated families, communities and societies, and reversed the health gains achieved over the past two to three decades.

In view of this, Asia could learn from the African experience not only in terms of the devastating impact of HIV, but, more importantly, how to respond to it. Professor Ahmed Latif, dean of Zimbabwe's Medical School, provides an insight, including some lessons that one could learn from Africa's experience.

This volume also has specific papers on the HIV/AIDS problem and the evolving responses to it from many countries, including Thailand, India, China, Sri Lanka, Nepal and Afghanistan. Some of the lessons learned include the critical need for national commitment and adequate resources, and for scaling up effective prevention and care interventions while at the same time addressing the underlying HIV-related risk behaviours and vulnerabilities. These issues are further elaborated in a paper on behaviour change among young people who are most vulnerable to HIV/AIDS.

The role played by injecting drug users in the AIDS epidemic and the close correlation between STI and HIV are explained comprehensively by Swarup Sarkar et al., and Heiner Grosskurth and Gurumurthy Rangaiyan respectively. The remarkable success achieved by Thailand through its 100 per cent condom use programme is described by Wiwat Rojanapithayakorn, who first pioneered this in the Ratchaburi province in Thailand. The programme has since then demonstrated its effectiveness in Cambodia and is presently being tried in many other countries in Asia.

In the area of care and support, antiretroviral therapy (ART) is now a global priority. While ART is the standard of care in developed countries, in the developing world, unfortunately, particularly in Africa and Asia, where the majority of people with HIV/AIDS live, patients have no access to these life-saving drugs. Increasing access and ensuring appropriate use of ART is now top priority for all stakeholders. In the UN General Assembly in September 2003, WHO's director-general Dr. Lee Jong-wook declared the failure to deliver HIV treatment as a global health emergency and set a target of providing ART to 3 million people in the developing world by 2005. This has come to be known as the '3 by 5' target.

Affordability and accessibility of new drugs is clearly an issue of major concern for developing nations including those in Asia. These are addressed by Professor Ranjit Roy Chaudhury in his paper on enhancing access to drugs and by Dr. Sombat Thanprasertsuk et al. on Thailand's experience. Experiences such as these show that ART is indeed sustainable and the '3 by 5' target achievable provided additional resources are available and national capacity is strengthened.

It is also clear that HIV/AIDS cannot be tackled by the health sector alone; it requires a broad multi-sectoral response. Within this partnership, the civil society and NGOs, particularly those based at the community level, have a crucial role to play. This is highlighted by Teresita Bagasao. Also important is the issue of interaction between HIV and tuberculosis, which is of crucial significance to Asia as it is for countries of Africa. Much progress has already been made in Asia in forging collaborations between the two programmes. Finally, no discussion on HIV/AIDS can be complete without the mention of vaccine development. This is dealt with proficiently and comprehensively by José Esparza and colleagues from the WHO and Jean-Louis Excler, director of the International AIDS Vaccine Initiative in India.

The book focuses on a few critical areas that are of practical use to national AIDS control programmes, health care workers, academicians and NGOs active in the area of HIV/AIDS prevention and care. As guest editor, my goal was to encourage contributions not only from experts, but also from those who have a good understanding of programmatic issues. The assistance provided in this endeavour by Dr. Rajesh Bhatia, Mr. E. Rangarajan and Dr. Gayatri Ghadiok is gratefully acknowledged.

I hope this volume will provide a valuable insight into various issues and priority areas, and contribute towards HIV/AIDS prevention and control in the developing world in general and Asia in particular. Although by no means a complete discourse on an enormous problem that touches almost every sector of society, the book covers the most crucial aspects of the HIV/AIDS pandemic as it unfolds in Asia.

Jai P. Narain
New Delhi
India

1

AIDS IN ASIA: THE EPIDEMIC PROFILE AND LESSONS LEARNT SO FAR

Jai P. Narain

Introduction

The human immunodeficiency virus (HIV), causing acquired immunodeficiency syndrome (AIDS), is an unprecedented public health emergency, having already caused enormous ill health and mortality worldwide (Larson and Narain 2001; UNAIDS/WHO 2002). Given the scale of the epidemic, AIDS is now considered not only a health problem, but also a developmental and security threat. Although the epidemic began in the United States more than two decades ago, up to 95 per cent of new infections now occur in developing countries, which are unfortunately also the least equipped to effectively respond to the challenge. Moreover, the epidemic is affecting developed and developing countries differently. In the United States and other industrialised countries, mortality and infection rates have declined dramatically over the past few years, largely due to the availability of antiretroviral medication. AIDS in these countries is now a chronic disease and a manageable health problem. In developing countries, however, AIDS is destroying societies, nations and communities. Even now, less than 20 per cent of those at risk of HIV infection have access to basic prevention services (Jha et al. 2002). The new HIV treatments that have increased longevity of patients in industrialised countries are unfortunately beyond the reach of those in the developing world. The disease is, therefore, widening the gap between the haves and have-nots, between rich and poor nations, thereby presenting a new ethical and human rights dilemma.

Three decades into the epidemic, there is still no vaccine and no 'cure'. There is, however, considerably more information available on how the virus is spread, as well as an increased understanding about prevention strategies and what constitutes effective treatment and care. The social and economic conditions that facilitate the spread of HIV are also well understood. Despite this, risk behaviours and risk environments persist, and HIV continues to spread among individuals and across national and regional borders.

In recent times, thankfully, international consensus and commitment to respond to this global epidemic has been growing. This has resulted in increasing partnerships, greater investments and enhanced political commitments to scale up effective interventions to fight this formidable adversary (GFATM 2002; UNGASS 2001; WHO 2001). Substantial international efforts under way over the past few years hold promise for enhanced resources and efforts:

1. In July 2000 G-8 Summit leaders in Okinawa, Japan, called for a massive effort against diseases of poverty and endorsed international development targets for HIV/AIDS, tuberculosis and malaria.

2. In April 2001 at the Organisation of African Unity (OAU) Summit in Abuja, Nigeria, the UN secretary-general Kofi Annan asked for a war chest of up to US$ 10 billion per year to fight HIV/AIDS, and issued a call for the creation of a Global Fund.

3. In June 2001 the ground-breaking UN General Assembly Special Session on HIV/AIDS mobilised political and financial commitments from both the developed and developing countries. The G-8 Summit in Genoa, Italy, in July 2001 further increased the sense of urgency (GFATM 2002).

4. In January 2002 the Global Fund to Fight AIDS, TB and Malaria (GFATM) was established. This provided an unprecedented opportunity to mobilise and disburse additional resources through public–private partnerships and to enable countries to substantially scale up effective interventions to check the spread of HIV/AIDS (WHO 2001). Reversing the epidemic of HIV/AIDS is also among the Millennium Development Goals for 2015 adopted unanimously in 2000 by all members of the United Nations.

5. In September 2003 the director-general of WHO declared failure to provide antiretroviral treatment (ART) to people living with HIV/AIDS as a global health emergency and set a target of

providing ART to 3 million people in the developing countries
by 2005, '3 by 5' initiative.

Epidemic Update

At the end of 2003, WHO/UNAIDS estimated that 40 million people
were living with HIV/AIDS worldwide (UNAIDS/WHO 2002). While
37 million of these were adults, 18.4 million were women and 2.5 million
were children under the age of 15. Five million of those living with
HIV/AIDS had been newly infected during 2003, the majority under
24 years of age, while 3 million people died of HIV/AIDS-related causes.
Today, AIDS is the leading cause of death in Sub-Saharan Africa,
which has the highest number of HIV-positive individuals (26.4 million
people living with HIV/AIDS), followed by South and South-East Asia
with 6.4 million infected individuals (Figure 1.1). More than 25 million
have already died since the beginning of the epidemic, bringing the
number of infected to more than 65 million worldwide. Sub-Saharan
Africa with 70 per cent and Asia with 18 per cent of the estimated adult
HIV infections constitute nearly four-fifths of the global burden of HIV/
AIDS (Figure 1.2). During 2003 alone, nearly 1 million people in Asia
acquired HIV and 490,000 people were estimated to have died of
AIDS. More than 2 million young Asians (aged 15 to 24) were living
with HIV.

Figure 1.1
Estimated Number of People Living with HIV/AIDS: End of 2003

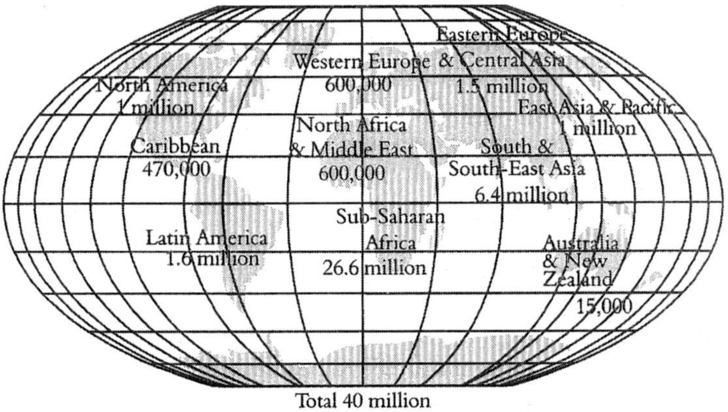

Total 40 million

Source: UNAIDS/WHO (2003).

Figure 1.2
Estimated Distribution of Adult HIV Infection and Population: 2000

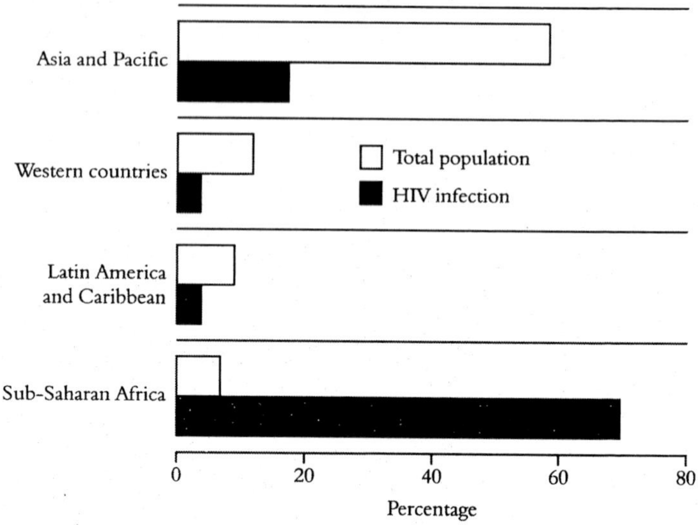

Source: WHO (2003).

While AIDS came much later to Asia, it is spreading rapidly and the epidemic is in a fairly advanced stage in many countries (Myo Thet Htoon 1994; Phoolcharoen 1998; WHO 1997). According to surveillance data, the rapid spread of HIV in Asia did not begin until the late 1980s or early 1990s when high HIV prevalence (up to 30 per cent or more) among female sex workers (FSWs) in Thailand, Cambodia and Myanmar were reported (Table 1.1). In Mumbai, India, the rate of HIV among sex workers increased dramatically, from 1 per cent in 1986 to 18 per cent in 1990, and to 51 per cent in 1996 (Larson and Narain 2001). In addition, intense and rapid spread of HIV was documented among injecting drug user (IDU) populations in Thailand, parts of north-east India (particularly in Manipur state) and the 'golden triangle' area (where the borders of China, Myanmar and Thailand meet). In Thailand, the first country to report HIV in Asia, HIV prevalence among IDUs shot up from 0 to 30 per cent between November 1987 and August 1988. In Manipur HIV infections among IDUs increased from 1 per cent in 1988 to 56 per cent in 1995. Myanmar, too, experienced similar increase among IDUs, from 17 per cent in 1989 to 59 per cent in 1990 and to 74 per cent in 1992. During the 1990s in several countries significant heterosexual transmission of HIV was noticed, primarily among sex workers and their clients, and from infected males to their regular sex partners.

Table 1.1
The HIV/AIDS Epidemic in Selected Asian Countries

Country	Adult HIV prevalence (%)	People living with HIV/AIDS (numbers)	Heterosexual	Injecting drug use
Bangladesh	<0.1	13,000	+	+
Bhutan	<0.1	<100	+	--
Democratic People's Republic of Korea	n/a	n/a	--	--
Indonesia	0.1	110,000	+	+ +
India	0.9	5,100,000	+ + +	+
Maldives	<0.1	<100	+	--
Myanmar	1.2	330,000	+ + +	+ +
Nepal	0.5	61,000	+	+ +
Thailand	1.5	570,000	+ + +	+ +
Sri Lanka	<0.1	3,500	+	--
Timor Leste	<0.1	n/a	n/a	n/a

Source: WHO.
Notes: (--) unknown or minimal HIV transmission
(+) limited HIV transmission
(+ +) moderate HIV transmission
(+ + +) major HIV transmission

Generally, the virus first affected populations with high-risk behaviour or whose work put them at risk of HIV, such as FSWs, IDUs and migrant populations such as truck drivers. These were people who are traditionally marginalised because of their social or economic status or due to lack of access to information and health services. The virus then spread to the general population through sexual contact with HIV-infected individuals, transfusion of contaminated blood or transmission from an infected mother to her offspring. Such a pattern has been noted in Thailand, India, Myanmar and Cambodia—all countries that are in an advanced stage of the HIV epidemic compared to most other countries of Asia. Both in Thailand and Myanmar the epidemic has been shown to occur in waves beginning with rapid increases in HIV infection among IDU and sex workers, followed by their partners, and then ultimately to women of childbearing age and to their children during childbirth or through breastfeeding (National AIDS Programme, Myanmar 2002; WHO 2003). The latest round of sentinel surveillance in 380 sentinel sites in India shows HIV rates higher than 1 per cent among pregnant women in six states, namely, Andhra Pradesh, Karnataka, Maharashtra, Manipur, Nagaland and Tamil Nadu.

The main modes of transmission are through heterosexual spread (80–90 per cent), injecting drug use (5–10 per cent) and mother-to-child (1–5 per cent). Transmission at the health care setting either through contaminated blood transfusion or via injecting equipment currently play a limited role.

Based on HIV prevalence rates, countries could be divided into three broad categories—those with HIV prevalence rates of more than 1 per cent among the general population, namely, Cambodia, Myanmar, Thailand and six states of India (Andhra Pradesh, Karnataka, Maharashtra, Manipur, Nagaland and Tamil Nadu); those with prevalence of less than 1 per cent in general population but with a rate of greater than 5 per cent among the population with high-risk behaviour, namely, Malaysia, Nepal, Indonesia, Vietnam, China and Pakistan; and the remaining countries with low prevalence of less than 1 per cent among high-risk populations.

While national HIV prevalence rates remain relatively low in most countries of Asia, there is no cause for complacency. The epidemic continues to spread rapidly and new infections in this region are increasing faster than anywhere else in the world. Many countries are experiencing serious localised epidemics.

In China, for example, besides localised epidemic among IDUs in nine provinces, including Beijing, HIV is spreading heterosexually in Yunnan, Guangxi and Guangdong. In 2001 a survey showed that up to 12 per cent people who donated blood in rural eastern China were infected as a result of unsafe blood donation practices (UNAIDS/WHO 2002). According to UNAIDS/WHO, 1 million people in China are currently estimated to be living with HIV, and unless effective measures are implemented, 10 million Chinese will acquire HIV by the end of this decade.

India, the second most populous country after China, has 4.58 million HIV-infected persons—the second highest in the world after South Africa. While national adult HIV prevalence is less than 1 per cent, the HIV prevalence is more than 1 per cent in six states—Andhra Pradesh, Karnataka, Maharashtra, Manipur, Nagaland and Tamil Nadu. The rates of HIV among sex workers, injecting drug users and patients with STIs remain unacceptably high in many parts of the country.

In both Indonesia and Nepal explosive epidemics have been witnessed among IDUs recently, with rates climbing up to 40 to 50 per cent over a short period of time. From virtually 0 per cent in 1998, the HIV prevalence in Indonesia increased to nearly 50 per cent in 2001 (Figure 1.3). Approximately 43,000 injecting drug users are already infected with HIV; 80 per cent of all new AIDS cases are occurring among injecting drug users.

Figure 1.3
HIV Prevalence among Injecting Drug Users at a
Drug Treatment Centre in Jakarta, Indonesia: 1997–2001

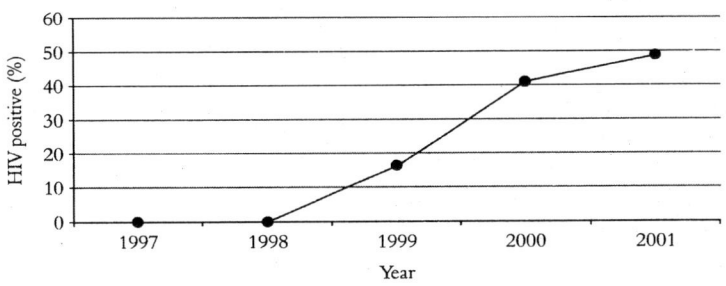

Source: UNAIDS/WHO (2002).

In Nepal HIV infection rates among IDUs in Kathmandu and other cities increased from 1.6 per cent in 1991 to 68 per cent in 2001. In at least in five countries in Asia—Malaysia, Myanmar, Nepal, Thailand and Manipur in India—up to 50 per cent of IDUs have acquired the virus.

In Asia the epidemic, therefore, remains highly dynamic and is evolving rapidly. Home to nearly half of the world's population because of its sheer size, it has the potential to significantly influence the course and overall impact of the global HIV/AIDS pandemic. The risk behaviours and vulnerability that promote, facilitate and fuel HIV transmission are present virtually in all countries and, therefore, chances of further spread are significant. The window of opportunity is rapidly closing and action is urgently needed to stem the spread of HIV in Asia. Indeed, it was Asia, in particular Thailand, which showed that HIV spread can be halted with an aggressive multi-sectoral national effort and political will. HIV is now declining in most population groups in Thailand.

Cambodia is also reporting stabilising levels of infection, as well as decreasing levels of high-risk behaviour.

Vulnerabilities, Risk Behaviours and Epidemic Potential

The region's vulnerability to HIV can be determined by various factors, including men having multiple partners and patronising sex workers, injecting drug use, relatively high prevalence of sexually-transmitted infections (STIs) and low condom use in addition to other factors including poverty, illiteracy and limited access to health and information services. Asia has in its midst 50 per cent of the world's poor, and poverty is a major contributor to the societal vulnerability. While the poor tend to die soon after developing AIDS, poverty and other social factors force women to undertake prostitution for survival and young men particularly to inject drugs, thereby enhancing their risk of acquiring HIV.

Moreover, taboos on talking about sex and sexuality, counter-productive attitudes of discrimination and stigma associated with HIV contribute to HIV/AIDS transmission. Gender inequality, condoned both culturally and socially in parts of the region, heightens the vulnerability of women and girls at many levels. The transmission of HIV to women from their husbands is on the increase. Young girls are especially vulnerable to HIV—physiologically, epidemiologically and socially. The vulnerability of women to HIV transmission has further implications for the vulnerability of children, who have a significant chance of becoming infected at birth when their mother is HIV positive.

Over 50 per cent of all new HIV infections occur among young people between 15 and 24 years—the group that has often limited access to important information and sexual health services critical to their health and well-being. Some young people are living in especially difficult situations, making them even more vulnerable to HIV infection. Those who are out of school, living on the streets, sharing needles with other drug users, engaging in commercial sex—sometimes forced into prostitution by their own parents—and those who are sexually abused are at special risk. Cultural mores are more likely to allow men to have multiple sex partners and patronise commercial sex establishments, while wives are expected to remain faithful. New trends in the epidemic are revealing that faithful, monogamous wives are now becoming infected when their husbands bring home the virus. Unprotected sexual intercourse, whether men with men or women with men, is the most common way of transmitting HIV. Across Asia commercial sex workers are largely young. Young sex workers are at particular risk of contracting HIV as their social status makes them less able to negotiate the use of condoms, and biologically they are more vulnerable to infection. One of the key factors precipitating the spread of HIV is sexually-transmitted infection. STI rates not only indicate the extent of unprotected sex. It is now known that an individual with an STI is not only more vulnerable to contracting HIV than an individual who has no other STIs, but can also spread infection to others more readily. Each year 50 million people suffer from STIs in the South-East Asia region who, unless treated early and properly, will lead to increased possibility of HIV transmission.

Needle sharing among IDUs is a high-risk activity that has fuelled the spread of HIV and AIDS in a number of Asian countries. In China, north-east India, Malaysia, Myanmar, Thailand and Vietnam, for example, the first rapid spread of HIV was among IDUs. Experience across Asia shows that the epidemic in a country or an area is often heralded by rapid spread of HIV among injecting drug users, who as a matter of camaraderie often like to share injecting equipment, fuelling rapid spread among their group members. Since drug use is illegal and covert, these high-risk populations are particularly difficult to target for interventions such as safe needle exchange and prevention education.

These factors point clearly to enormous potential for expanding the AIDS pandemic in many Asian countries. However, it is difficult to predict when this epidemic will be fuelled or how quickly this will happen. It is clear that when a threshold is established the spread occurs rapidly, as was seen among IDU in Thailand, Myanmar, north-east India and more recently in Indonesia and Nepal. And then, from IDUs, HIV can spread to their sexual partners. Studies show that the spread of HIV among sex workers and their clients is highly dependent on the consistency of condom use and the number of clients visiting sex workers per day. Countries where sex workers have a greater number of clients have witnessed higher prevalence of HIV compared to those where the number of clients per sex worker is lower.

Health, Social and Economic Impact

The future of the epidemic in Asia is contingent upon the extent and effectiveness of current and future prevention efforts. Moreover, since it takes seven to ten years for people with HIV to develop AIDS, the annual toll will continue to grow in the future, requiring further prevention efforts and increased medical and social services for the next several years. In the wake of the HIV pandemic, tuberculosis is beginning to increase in areas hit hard by HIV. There is a fear that a parallel epidemic of TB may follow HIV, as has been witnessed in Africa, where TB notifications have registered a many-fold increase during the 1990s, attributed primarily to the AIDS epidemic (Figure 1.4) (Narain et al. 1992; Yanai et al. 1996).

Figure 1.4
TB Trends in Selected African Countries: 1980–2000

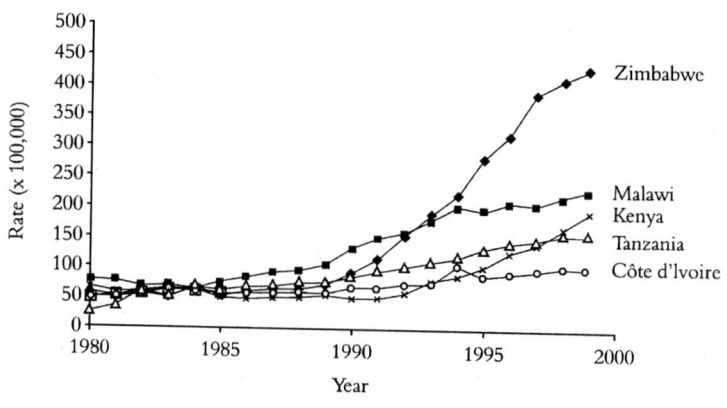

The greatest tragedy, besides the high medical and health care costs, will be the loss of thousands of lives, particularly among young adults in their most productive age and infants born to HIV-infected mothers, directly affecting child survival rates. This will have a major impact on the already fragile health and economic infrastructure in terms of direct medical and patient care costs, and indirect costs in the form of absenteeism and decreased productivity.

In some of the worst affected countries of Africa, AIDS is already eroding the development achievements of the past 10 years and undermining the capacity of health and social services. Average life expectancy has fallen by 15 years as a result of AIDS. In terms of economic impact, studies during 1990s indicated that Thailand and India may have lost up to US$ 9 and US$ 11 billion respectively due to HIV/AIDS by year 2000 (Charles et al. 1993). The economic impact is greatest because HIV primarily affects individuals in their economically productive years when they are ready to contribute to the society. Nearly 80 per cent of AIDS cases are between the age of 20 and 40 years (Figure 1.5).

Figure 1.5
Distribution of AIDS Cases by Age and Sex in the South-East Asia Region

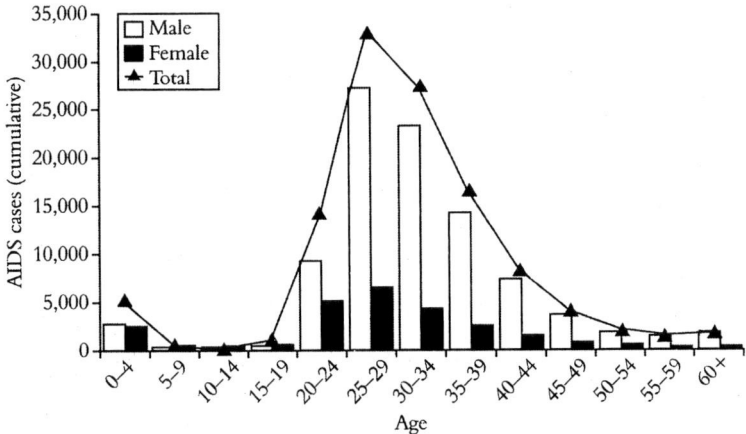

Source: WHO/SEARO (2004).

The impact of the epidemic has been documented to be most significant at the family and community level, especially in poor and marginalised groups. Poor families become poorer and lower middle-income households become poor. A study in Thailand, for example, found that once a family member developed AIDS, more than half the household reduced their food intake, 60 per cent used all of their savings for medical costs, 19 per cent sold property such as land, animals or vehicles, 15 per cent pulled their children out of school to help at home, and 11 per cent borrowed money to pay for the medical costs and help maintain household needs (Pitayanon et al. 1997).

Significant but less quantifiable are the emotional and psychological costs to the individual, family and community. The HIV/AIDS epidemic is severely affecting children. In addition to the risk of acquiring HIV infection from an infected mother, children risk losing both parents. By the end of 2002 over 13 million children globally were estimated to have lost their mother or both parents to AIDS. In Africa, for example, village after village has been destroyed and families left only with children and/or the elderly. Children under such circumstances are at increased risk of becoming malnourished and dropping out of schools. Moreover, high levels of discrimination against people living with HIV/AIDS still persist, be it in health care settings, workplaces and schools, or in neighbourhoods and communities at large.

National Responses

During the late 1980s, and throughout the 1990s, all countries established national AIDS programmes, and adopted strategies and interventions to prevent the spread of HIV and provide care for those living with HIV/AIDS. The strategies broadly included: (a) preventing HIV; and (b) providing care and support to those living with HIV/AIDS.

Prevention of sexual transmission has focused on promoting community-based interventions, particularly among populations at risk, including promotion and provision of condoms in sex work situations, strengthening of STI prevention and care, and creating an enabling environment. For example, the Thai working group on HIV/AIDS projection estimates that the highly active Thai AIDS programme has already resulted in averting more than 5 million additional HIV infections (Figure 1.6).

Figure 1.6
Number of HIV Infections Averted in Thailand
on Account of Prevention Programmes

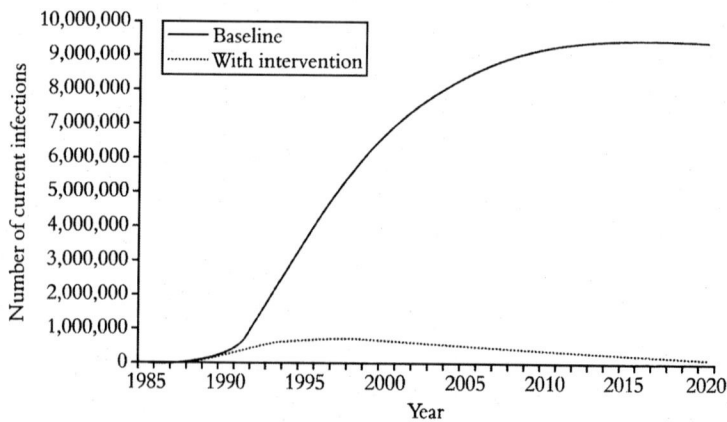

Source: The Thai Working Group on HIV/AIDS Projection, March 2001.

Interventions to prevent HIV transmission through blood and blood products include ensuring safe blood transfusion and widely implementing harm reduction approaches among IDUs. The emphasis of blood safety is on promotion of voluntary non-remunerated blood donations in place of professional blood donors, rational use of blood and screening of all donated blood for HIV.

To prevent HIV among IDUs, national AIDS programmes are promoting harm reduction approaches and providing support to innovative/effective interventions. The prevention of transmission from skin piercing practices at health care settings is ensured through consistent adherence to infection control procedures, universal precautions observed by all health care workers at all levels and in all health care settings, and dissemination and practice of infection control guidelines.

Use of antiretroviral drugs such as zidovudine or nevirapine to prevent HIV transmission from an infected mother to her child is a proven effective intervention. Pilot projects are ongoing in many countries, including India. In Thailand providing antiretroviral drugs to infected pregnant women and their newborn babies is part of national policy integrated in the existing maternal and child health services.

Provision of appropriate care and support is crucial to address the needs of those already infected. Voluntary counselling and testing (VCT)—identifying those already infected with HIV—is the entry point for care interventions. Among other components are prevention and treatment of opportunistic infections (tuberculosis in particular), nursing care and use of antiretroviral drugs. Comprehensive care along the continuum includes establishing and expanding VCT services in order to identify those infected with HIV, that is, to identify the beneficiaries of care and support services for provision of psychosocial support through counselling services. Integration of HIV/AIDS care with general health services at primary, secondary and tertiary health care levels, and involvement of community-based organisations in the provision of care at home and in the community are necessary elements.

In addition, treatment of HIV/AIDS-related diseases and provision of palliative care, through early diagnosis, prevention and treatment of common opportunistic infections, including tuberculosis, and improving access to antiretroviral therapy are now major priorities. Besides advocating for improved access to antiretroviral treatment, the rational use of such drugs must be ensured (see Narain and Gilks, in this volume).

Lessons Learnt So Far

The experience of the last two decades, globally as well as in Asia, clearly indicates that national responses should not wait for AIDS cases to soar. Instead, they should focus on responding quickly, mobilising all sectors and all echelons of the government, and recognising and collaborating with NGOs and the private sector. Involving vulnerable groups at every step of policy and programme development and implementation is crucial for programme success.

It is clear that with adequate commitment, leadership and availability of resources, HIV can be prevented. One of the success stories in the region is Thailand, where HIV is now declining in various population groups as a result of effective prevention and care programmes. Among military conscripts, for example, HIV prevalence declined from 3.6 per cent in 1993 to 2.1 per cent in 1996. Even more significantly, new cases of STIs treated in government clinics in Thailand have decreased to historical low levels accompanied by decline in HIV infection rates. High level of political commitment and adequate resources made available for a multi-sectoral response are responsible for the remarkable Thai success (Figure 1.7) (Rojanapithayakorn and Hanenberg 1996).

Figure 1.7
National AIDS Budget, Government of Thailand: 1988–2000

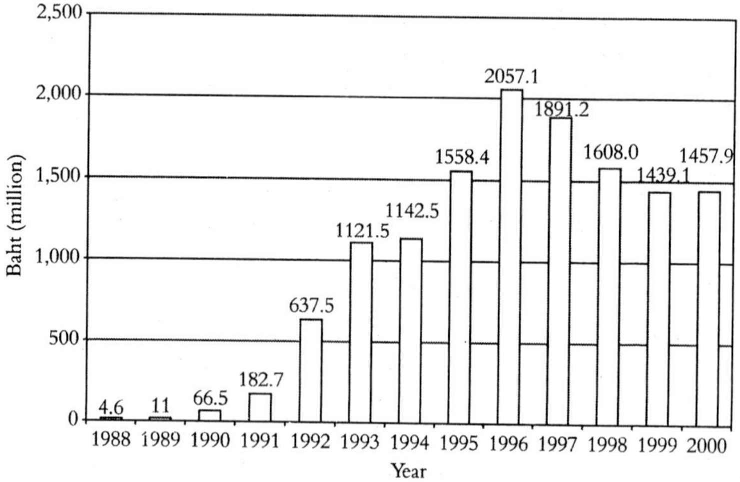

Source: Ministry of Public Health, Thailand, 2002.

In Cambodia, too, implementation of effective approaches has led to stabilising of HIV and of decreasing levels of high-risk behaviour. Condom use in sex establishments increased from less than 40 per cent in 1997 to 90 per cent in 2001. Consequently, and not unexpectedly, HIV prevalence among sex workers declined from 42 per cent in 1998 to 29 per cent in 2002, and among pregnant women from 3.2 per cent in 1996 to 2.8 per cent in 2002 (Figure 1.8).

Figure 1.8
HIV Prevalence and Consistent Condom Use among Sex Workers in Cambodia: 1997–2002

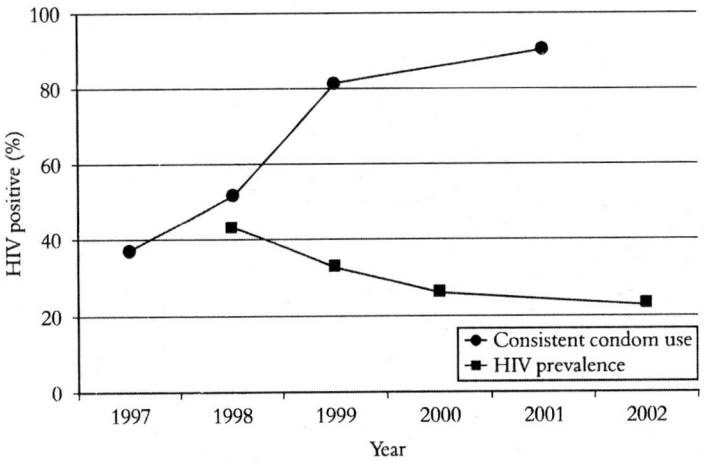

Sources: UNAIDS/WHO (2002); HSS 1998–2002; Cambodia BSS 1997–2002.

A strong public health infrastructure is essential for an effective health sector response. This includes early diagnosis and treatment of STIs using the syndromic approach, blood transfusion safety, epidemiological surveillance and research, and a continuum of HIV/AIDS care linking health institutions, the community and the home. The National Blood Safety Programme in Myanmar, launched in 1985, is a good example of a successful strategy to ensure blood safety in the entire country by strengthening the public health infrastructure. As a result, by 1998, 100 per cent safety of blood donated up to the township level was ensured (Zaw 2000).

Partnerships with communities as well as with NGOs and the private sector can be instrumental in monitoring and sustaining multi-sectoral responses and in halting the negative consequences of the epidemic.

Examples of successful, though scattered, partnerships are increasingly evident across the region (Larson and Narain 2001). In Nepal a network of local NGOs has mobilised resources to address high-risk activities along the highway. The Family Planning Association of Nepal has established clinics to offer STI treatment to truckers and the Contraceptive Retail Sales Company coordinates social marketing of condoms. New Era, a research institute, conducts baseline monitoring and evaluation surveys and Stimulus, a local advertising firm, provides media support. The value of such a network is determined by effective collaboration and coordination among various partners.

Among other lessons learned is the fact that in order to respond to the unprecedented problem of AIDS, communities must act with a true sense of participation, mobilisation and action. There are many examples of successful involvement of the community in HIV/AIDS control (Jana 1998; Tarantola et al. 1999). The Sonagachi Sex Workers Project, established in the red light area of Kolkata—in which education is delivered through peer outreach, clinical services are provided at a general and STI health clinic in the area, and condoms are distributed by peer educators—is an excellent example of community involvement.

Religious leaders in Indonesia have given a call to people not to discriminate unfairly against people with AIDS. The Department of Youth Affairs and Sports, Ministry of Human Resource Development, India, initiated a nation-wide campaign in 1991 using its voluntary student youth programme called the National Service Scheme (NSS). Presently, with 1 million student volunteers across 158 universities, 6,000 colleges and 2,000 secondary schools, NSS is well placed to reach the youth across the country with important and useful information on AIDS prevention.

The Way Forward

In spite of these examples, successes and efforts, there are still many challenges in HIV/AIDS prevention and care. There is an urgent need to significantly scale up interventions that work, both in coverage and quality, to make an impact in combating AIDS. Injecting drug use and high sex partner exchange rates are difficult subjects for governments or official agencies to deal with. Urgent and universal support for primary prevention and behaviour change interventions is necessary. Primary risk behaviour groups affected are socially marginalised and interventions aimed at behaviour change continue to remain under-funded. Overcoming denial, blame, complacency and stigma are the biggest obstacles to effective response. Finally, the health infrastructure remains poorly developed. Therefore, mounting effective prevention and care programmes in the absence of a well-developed health system is not realistic.

Some priorities that need urgent consideration are discussed in this section.

Enhancing Political Will and Commitment

Adequate political, societal and administrative commitment, and support from all sectors is crucial for HIV/AIDS prevention and control programmes. Partnerships must be mobilised, strengthened and sustained at every stage among the government, the private sector, NGOs, community groups and donor agencies. Considerable social mobilisation and advocacy is needed so that HIV/AIDS programmes continue to receive priority attention. Strategic information and the collection, analysis and rapid dissemination of data on the epidemic generated through HIV/AIDS surveillance are essential for formulating effective health sector responses and for providing an evidence base for advocacy.

Advocacy is focused on political and social commitment, winning the support of key constituencies, national and international leadership, and of donors. Although all countries have been responding positively to the HIV/AIDS epidemic, not all programmes enjoy priority status and political support, including allocation of funds. Several countries still depend on funds from donors, bilateral and international organisations such as the WHO, other UN agencies, the World Bank and NGOs. However, to make the most effective use of limited resources, programmes should: (a) focus on a few priority areas that will have maximum impact; (b) integrate HIV/AIDS with the ongoing programme; (c) develop better coordination and information sharing to avoid duplication of programmes and activities; and (d) foster collaboration with NGOs.

Forging and Sustaining Partnerships

Since the first AIDS case was reported, there has been a tremendous response from all communities and sections of society, including NGOs and various other institutions. At the country level, however, collaboration with various stakeholders and partners in fighting the epidemic is often not easy. Considerable efforts are needed by AIDS programme managers to carry out advocacy among top policy makers, other ministries, political leaders, professional organisations, donor agencies, as well as among private and business community leaders. While each partner may develop its own programmes to support national HIV/AIDS control efforts, they all must work within the framework of the national policy, strategy and according to national priorities.

Expanding the Programmes in Scale

Experience shows that in many countries prevention efforts are carried out in a few project areas. The major challenge, therefore, is to expand the coverage of the intervention programmes to benefit as many of those at risk as possible. Only then can the impact of these interventions, in terms of a decline in sexually-transmitted infections, including HIV, be seen. Moreover, although information and education is the backbone of all HIV prevention and care programmes, this alone is not enough. Education programmes must be supported with improved availability and accessibility to condoms, provision of STIs and other related health services and, most importantly, the creation of a positive social environment without discrimination and stigma to encourage appropriate behaviour change. The role of NGOs, particularly those at the community level, with full involvement of the targeted population for intervention is most crucial. The emphasis will have to shift from 'creating awareness' to 'behaviour change'.

Integrating Prevention and Care Services

Since 80 to 90 per cent of HIV transmission is related to sexual intercourse, education aimed at adoption of safer sexual behaviour by people at risk is crucial to stem the HIV/AIDS pandemic. Safer sexual behaviour includes abstinence, fidelity and use of condoms. Such behaviour can be encouraged through information and education programmes, by ensuring that condoms are easily accessible and affordable, and by empowering, providing support for, and educating women and other vulnerable groups about the risks of unsafe sex. These interventions, targeting young people, are likely to be most effective when implemented in collaboration with NGOs or by using a peer education approach integrated into existing health and development programmes.

Mobilisation of local resources is vital for the success of HIV/AIDS prevention programmes. These programmes should be a part of appropriate development plans. Local resource mobilisation could involve NGOs, the private sector, community and religious leaders, and academic communities. Sharing of effective approaches and success stories will indicate which approaches or strategies have worked in local situations and whether these could be replicated with appropriate changes, such as the 100 per cent condom use programme among sex workers. To provide comprehensive care for HIV/AIDS-infected persons and their families, a continuum of care model is being promoted. This extends across various levels of the health care system, linking facilities such as hospitals at state/provincial and district levels, health centres and village health posts, as well as families in their homes through supportive community networks. Therefore, HIV/AIDS care and treatment, integrated into all levels of the health care system, helps in the management of important HIV-associated opportunistic infections such as TB, fungal infections and diarrhoea, and to fulfil the needs of people with HIV/AIDS in terms of their medical, psychological and social needs.

Improving Access to New Drugs

Major technological breakthroughs have been reported recently in the development and use of antiretroviral (ARV) drugs in promoting and prolonging the life of those infected with HIV/AIDS and, more importantly, in preventing transmission of HIV from an infected mother to her child. A single dose of nevirapine given to a mother during labour and to the baby during the first 72 hours can reduce the risk of HIV transmission by nearly 50 per cent (Guay et al. 1999; Ying-Ru Lo and Farley 2000). Wider application of such an intervention, however, requires scaling up VCT programmes.

The availability of ART not only reduces the viral load to undetectable levels, but also reduces HIV-related morbidity, mortality, the incidence of opportunistic infections and hospitalisation by 50 to 60 per cent (Chequer et al. 2000; WHO 2002a). Unfortunately, because of the high cost of these drugs (which have declined remarkably over the past two years), ART was earlier not part of national AIDS programmes. However, this has dramatically changed since September 2003 when the

WHO declared the failure to provide ARV treatment a global emergency. Many countries have committed to providing free antiretroviral therapy, including India, Thailand, Indonesia and Nepal.

In 2003 the WHO set a target of ensuring 3 million people access to antiretroviral therapy by 2005—a 10-fold increase from the present level to be achieved in the next two to three years. To achieve this target, it is incumbent upon all countries and stakeholders in Asia not only to urgently take action to enhance access to these life-saving drugs, but also to ensure their appropriate and rational use. In this regard, strengthening the infrastructure in terms of expanding VCT services, training of health care providers on treatment practices and building laboratory capacity, particularly for CD4 enumeration and monitoring drug resistance, is a prerequisite.

WHO Support to National Programmes

The WHO Special Programme on AIDS, and later the Global Programme on AIDS (GPA), was officially established on 1 February 1987 with the responsibility for the urgent mobilisation of national and international efforts, and resources for global AIDS prevention and control. The AIDS epidemic was defined as a world health problem of extraordinary scale and extreme urgency, representing an unprecedented challenge to public health services in the world. The global AIDS strategy was endorsed unanimously by the World Health Assembly in May 1987, and presented to the World Summit of Ministers of Health in London.

Thereafter, significant funding and technical support was provided by the WHO, not only for the implementation of national AIDS control programmes, but also to community-based organisations. As an international leader coordinating international/global response to HIV, the WHO also actively encouraged the involvement of the community, respect for human rights and compassion for people living with HIV/AIDS. Involvement of people with AIDS and community organisations was part of the WHO's policy. They provided guidelines for the development of national AIDS programmes in different countries and helped in mobilising resources or by providing funds directly. The guidelines articulated the role of injecting drug use and homosexuality, and promoted the use of condoms.

In 1996 the GPA was replaced by UNAIDS, with the WHO as one of the five co-sponsors. As a founding co-sponsor of UNAIDS, the WHO now takes a lead role in the health sector response to HIV/AIDS (WHO 2002b). Specifically, the WHO's area of work includes prevention and management of sexually-transmitted diseases, blood safety, HIV/AIDS continuum of care, including ARV treatment, epidemiological surveillance and research. While focusing its attention on the public health aspects of the epidemic, the WHO continues to promote the health, social and political dimensions, and develop networks of creative partnerships throughout the world. Over the past two years the WHO has helped countries in Asia mobilise more than US$ 1 billion from the GFATM, thereby providing an opportunity to build on the successes so far (GFATM 2003).

Conclusions

HIV continues to spread in Asia, albeit unevenly in different countries. While a few countries, namely, India (in parts), Myanmar, Thailand and Cambodia, are in an advanced stage of the epidemic, HIV prevalence remains low in many others in the region. Experiences in responding to the global pandemic show that HIV can be prevented if sound, rational and effective strategies are used. These include prevention interventions promoting safer behaviour, primarily in sex and drug use, early diagnosis and management of sexually-transmitted infections, and ensuring accessibility to good quality condoms. While NGOs and community-based organisations have a critical role to play in implementing these interventions among various population groups, the government has the overall responsibility to plan, coordinate, mobilise and facilitate various HIV/AIDS prevention, care and treatment activities. Government responsibility also includes ensuring safe blood for transfusion as well as in providing care and support for those living with HIV/AIDS. Continued advocacy for enhanced political commitment and support, mobilisation of partnerships across various sectors, inter-country collaboration and sharing of country experiences, and ensuring access to new AIDS drugs and other interventions provide major opportunities in the years ahead.

REFERENCES

Charles, M., S.A. Obremskey and **Meechai Viravaidya** (1993). The economic impact of AIDS on Thailand. In D.E. Bloom and J.V. Lyons (eds.), *Economic Implications of AIDS in Asia* (pp. 7–34). New Delhi: UNDP.

Chequer, P., E.C. Sudo, M.A.A. Vittria, V.G. Veloso and **E.A. Castilho** (2000). The impact of antiretroviral therapy in Brazil. 13th International AIDS Conference, Durban, South Africa (abstract MOPE 1066).

Global Fund to Fight AIDS, TB and Malaria (GFATM) (2002). http://www.global fundatm.org.

——— (2003). Results of 2nd round, http://www.globalfundatm.org.

Guay, L.A. et al. (1999). Intrapartum and neonatal single dose nevirapine compared with zidovudine for prevention of mother-to-child transmission of HIV in Kampala, Uganda: HIVNET 012 randomized trial. *Lancet*, 354(9181), 795–802.

Jana, S. (1998). STD/HIV intervention among sex workers in West Bengal, India. *AIDS*, 12(Supplement B), S101–8.

Jha, P. et al. (2002). Improving the health of the global poor. *Science*, 295(5562), 2036–39.

Larson, H.J. and **J.P. Narain** (2001). Beyond 2000: Responding to HIV/AIDS in the new millennium. SEA/AIDS/122, WHO South-East Asia Regional Office, New Delhi.

Myo Thet Htoon (1994). HIV/AIDS in Myanmar. *AIDS*, 8(Supplement 2), S105–9.

Narain, J.P., M.C. Raviglione and **A. Kochi** (1992). HIV-associated tuberculosis in developing countries: Epidemiology and strategies for prevention, *International Journal of Tuberculosis and Lung Diseases*, 73(6).

National AIDS Programme, Myanmar (2002). *Report of HIV/AIDS surveillance*, Yangon: National AIDS Programme, Ministry of Health.

Phoolcharoen, Wiput (1998). HIV/AIDS prevention in Thailand: Success and challenges. *Science*, 280(5371), 1873–74.

Pitayanon, S., S. Kongsin and **W.S. Janjareon** (1997). The economic impact of HIV/AIDS mortality on households in Thailand. In D. Bloom and P. Godwin (eds.), *The economics of HIV and AIDS: The case of South and South-East Asia* (pp. 53–101). New Delhi: Oxford University Press.

Rojanapithayakorn, W. and **R. Hanenberg** (1996). The 100 per cent condom programme in Thailand. *AIDS*, 10(1), 1–7.

Tarantola, D. et al. (1999). Governments of Asia and the Pacific responding to the HIV/AIDS pandemic. *AIDS*, 8(Supplement 1), S186–92.

UNAIDS/WHO (2002). *AIDS Epidemic Update*, December.

——— (2003). *AIDS Epidemic Update*, December.

UNGASS (2001). United Nations General Assembly Special Session on HIV/AIDS: Declaration of Commitment on HIV/AIDS. Resolution A/RES/S-26/2, New York, 25–27 June.

WHO (1997). *AIDS: No time for complacency*. New Delhi: WHO Regional Office for South-East Asia.

——— (2001). Report of the commission on macroeconomics and health (Jeffery Sachs, ed.) Geneva: WHO.

WHO (2002a). *The use of antiretroviral therapy: A simplified approach for resource-constrained settings.* New Delhi: WHO Regional Office for South-East Asia.

——— (2002b). *Global health sector strategy for HIV/AIDS 2003–2007: Providing a framework for partnership and action.* Geneva: Department of HIV/AIDS, WHO.

——— (2003). *HIV/AIDS in Asia and the Pacific Region.* WHO Regional Office for South-East Asia, New Delhi, and Regional Office for Western Pacific, Manila.

WHO/SEARO (2004). HIV/AIDS Programme. Report, WHO/SEARO, New Delhi.

Yanai, H., W. Uthai Voravit, V. Panich, P. Sawanpanyalert, B. Chaimanee, P. Akarasewi, K. Limpakarnjanarat, P. Nieburg and T. Mastro (1996). Rapid increase in HIV-related tuberculosis, Chiang Rai, Thailand, 1900–1994. *AIDS,* 10(Supplement), S27–31.

Ying-Ru Lo and Tim Farley (2000). Trends in prevention of mother-to-child transmission. *Journal of Health Management,* 2(2), 201–18.

Zaw, Myint (2000). Epidemiologic programming to present transfusion-related HIV infection. *Journal of Health Management,* 2(2), 257–62.

2

THE ECONOMIC AND SECURITY DIMENSIONS OF HIV/AIDS IN ASIA

Jette Nielsen and Bjorn Melgaard

An estimated 7.2 million people are living with HIV/AIDS in Asia and the Pacific with almost 1 million new infections estimated to have occurred in 2002 (UNAIDS 2003). With national prevalence rates above 1 per cent, Cambodia, Myanmar and Thailand are the worst affected countries in the region. Cambodia has the highest national prevalence with an estimated 2.6 per cent of the adult population (Kingdom of Cambodia 2003). Other countries are experiencing serious, localised epidemics among vulnerable populations. In India an estimated 4.58 million people were living with HIV/AIDS in 2003—the second highest national figure in the world after South Africa. In China official estimates put the number of people living with HIV/AIDS at 1 million in mid-2002. Without effective responses in the country, as many as 10 million Chinese could have acquired HIV by the end of this decade (UNAIDS 2002a).

In over two decades of dealing with HIV/AIDS, the international community has come to realise that there are more aspects to the epidemic than health. In the worst affected countries of the world, HIV/AIDS has influenced all sectors of society by making economies stumble and undermining human security (International Crisis Group 2001; UNAIDS 2003).

The economic and security dimensions of HIV/AIDS in Asian countries are not fully understood, but as HIV/AIDS continues to spread in Asia, it is important to understand its potential impact on various sectors beyond health. This is obviously important for countries in Asia, but the international community should pay attention as well. Asia hosts more than half the world's population, it has a substantial and increasing share of the global economy, and is home to large national defence forces, including three of the world's seven declared nuclear states. If HIV incidence rates continue to increase in Asia, the epidemic has the potential to hamper the economic prospects of billions as well as affect political and military stability (Eberstadt 2002; UNAIDS 2003).

HIV/AIDS and the Economy: A Real but Elusive Connection

Through its impact on the labour force, households and enterprises, HIV/AIDS can act as a brake on economic growth and development. A number of studies conclude that the epidemic has a negative effect on GDP growth in high-prevalence countries. Calculations from Sub-Saharan Africa suggest that the annual loss of GDP as a result of AIDS ranges between 0.3 and 1.5 per cent (Bell et al. 2003). It is, however, often pointed out that more complete data is required to achieve greater precision in the modelling of macroeconomic impact of HIV/AIDS (Bloom et al. 2001a; Cornia 2002; UNAIDS 2002a; Whiteside 2002).

In Asia national economies seem unaffected by HIV/AIDS. In the immediate and mid-term perspective, traditional indicators such as growth in GDP, life expectancy and infant mortality are unlikely to change significantly due to the relatively low national HIV prevalence rates. The impact of the disease is more likely to be seen on households, the private business sector as well as on additional costs to the health sector.

Households: Impact and Coping Strategies

Studies show that the socio-economic impact of an HIV/AIDS-related death on a rural household is often greater than the costs of disease and death from other causes (Bloom et al. 2001b; Pitayanon et al. 1997). The cost of treatment and care over several years when HIV/AIDS is present in a household drains the family of savings and assets to a larger degree than in the case of accidental deaths or deaths from diseases with a shorter time span. Eventually, the household will dissolve, as parents die and orphaned children are sent to relatives for care and upbringing (UNAIDS 2002a).

Research from China, India and Thailand concur that the cost of treatment of an HIV-infected family member has a severe impact on the rural household economy. A study from India shows that families affected by HIV/AIDS spent an average of 49 per cent of the household income on medical treatment. In low-income families this percentage increased to as much as 82 per cent (Duraisamy 2003). A study in Yunnan province of China found that in rural areas an average AIDS patient spent around RMB 800 (approximately US$ 100) on medical treatment, which is slightly more than half of an average annual per capita income of RMB 1,478 (approximately US$ 185) (China HIV/AIDS Socio-economic Impact Study Team 2002). Another study in rural Thailand shows that some HIV/AIDS affected households spent up to US$ 974 on treatment ranging from hospital care to traditional healers out of an annual income of approximately US$ 2,000 in 1997 (Alban 2002; ESCAP 2003; Pitayanon et al. 1997). AIDS is thus associated with large out-of-pocket expenditures, often of catastrophic magnitude.

In addition to the increased medical expenditures and possible lost earnings of the person living with AIDS, households also lose income as other family members give up work opportunities outside to stay at home and take care of the sick relative.

To cope with the consequences of HIV/AIDS, households pursue various strategies. In Yunnan some families started to sell their land illegally or lease it at a reduced rent in order to sustain themselves (China HIV/AIDS Socio-economic Impact Study Team 2002). In rural Thailand 60 per cent of HIV/AIDS-affected households had their savings drained by medical care costs; 19 per cent had to sell their assets ranging from land, vehicles, jewellery to live stock, and 11 per cent turned to borrowing money for increased medical expenditure as well as maintaining household consumption (Pitayanon et al. 1997).

A study in Maharashtra state in India suggests that households affected by an HIV/AIDS-related death had been forced to sell their means of production to cover for the economic burden of high treatment and other costs of HIV/AIDS. Compared to households not affected by HIV/AIDS, fewer of the HIV/AIDS death households owned means of production, land and animals (Verma et al. 2002). It is possible that the lack of assets in HIV-affected households mainly is an indication of the level of poverty, which could have been present before HIV/AIDS became part of the equation. It is also likely that HIV/AIDS is a factor that fuels the process whereby poor families lose, for instance, means of production or land.

One of the more unfortunate responses to a prime-age adult death in poorer households is that of removing the children, especially girls, from schools. The demise of a family breadwinner is likely to cause a reallocation of household tasks and girls' income-generating potential will be required to make ends meet. In addition, school uniforms and tuition fees can become unaffordable. In Thailand 15 per cent of households affected by HIV/AIDS withdrew their school-age children from their education (Pitayanon et al. 1997; UNAIDS 2002a; Whiteside 2002). Figure 2.1 summarises the effects of an HIV/AIDS-related death within a family from the illness and death of the breadwinner to the dissolution of household. In a larger perspective, the reduced household income and shift in expenditures from consumption goods to medical care could have a negative impact on the private sector and could strain services in the health sector.

Figure 2.1
Impact of HIV/AIDS on Rural Households in Asia

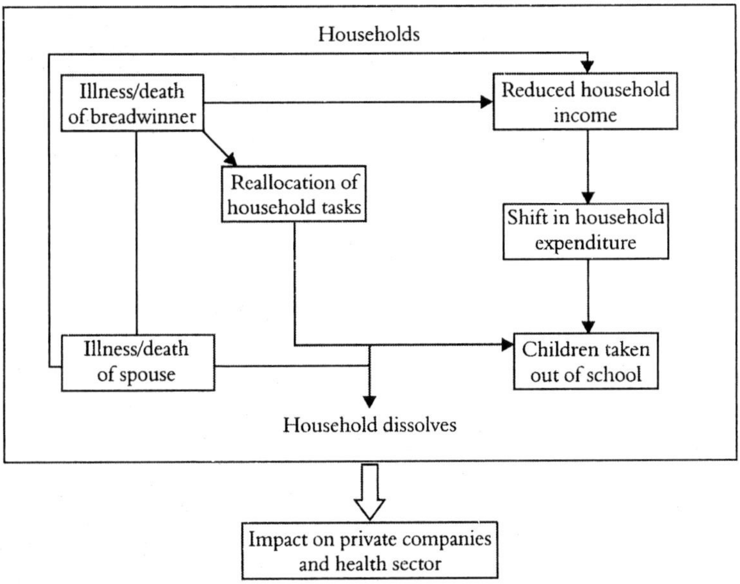

Source: Adapted from Centre for International Economics (2002).

Household studies have been criticised for only focusing on the impact of HIV/AIDS in the worst affected rural areas. The studies only provide a snapshot of the situation in a particular household setting as opposed to a broader overview of the impact of HIV in different types of households (Bloom et al. 2001b). At the same time, it has been pointed out that household studies tend to underestimate the impact because they fail to capture the most seriously affected households, which had disintegrated before the study commenced (Whiteside 2002). Still, rural household studies bring important insight into the HIV impact and coping strategies of surveyed families. Although it is difficult to determine the cause-and-effect relation between poverty and AIDS, the studies do seem to suggest a close relationship between a household affected by HIV/AIDS and its subsequent impoverishment (ibid.).

Private Business Sector: HIV/AIDS and Workplace Conflict

As the vast majority of people living with HIV/AIDS are in the prime of their working lives, between the ages of 15 and 49, the epidemic can have an impact on labour and set back economic activity (Asian Business Coalition on HIV/AIDS 2002; UNAIDS 2002a).

From countries with high HIV/AIDS prevalence rates it is known that AIDS weakens economic activity by squeezing productivity, adding costs, diverting productive resources and depleting skills. The epidemic hits productivity mainly through increased absenteeism, organisational disruption, and the loss of skills and organisational memory. In addition, as the impact on households grows more severe, market demand for products and services can shrink (Asian Business Coalition on HIV/ AIDS 2002; Global Business Council on HIV/AIDS 2001, 2002; ILO 2001; UNAIDS et al. 2000).

Companies in Asia are beginning to feel the impact of the epidemic. A survey of a small company in Thailand estimated that AIDS was resulting in a loss of US$ 80,000 annually (UNAIDS 1998). This estimate may, however, be a little high for a company in Thailand since it equals calculated costs of HIV/AIDS to larger companies in some of the worst affected countries in Africa (Alban 2002). Still, in India, Tata Tea Limited decided to implement an HIV/AIDS workplace programme after experiencing an increase in HIV/AIDS-related deaths, and a baseline study indicated that the number of infected employees was likely to increase further (Global Health Initiative 2002; ILO 2002).

However, for most companies in Asia the impact of the epidemic is not yet a bottom-line issue and enterprises tend to dismiss the epidemic as a threat to their business. Due to the long latency period between infection and the onset of a patient's symptoms, a company is not likely to see the cost of HIV/AIDS in terms of increased medical care and absenteeism until five to ten years after an employee is infected (Rosen et al. 2003). Still, lack of awareness and understanding of HIV/AIDS can drive stigma and discrimination, and ultimately result in critical workplace conflict and disruption at managerial levels. These factors can have a negative impact on the productivity of a company. In Thailand production line stoppages have occurred due to employees' fear of HIV transmission from co-workers (Asian Business Coalition on HIV/AIDS 2002).

Burden on the Health Sector

In all affected countries the HIV/AIDS epidemic is bringing additional pressure to bear on the health sector depending on the number of people who seek services, the nature of the demands for health care and the capacity to deliver that care. In the early stages of the epidemic HIV-infected persons tend to use primary health care and outpatient services to treat opportunistic infections. As HIV infection progresses to AIDS, there will be an increase in total hospitalisations related to HIV/AIDS (UNAIDS 2002a).

Projections on mortality from infectious diseases in India show that by the year 2033 HIV/AIDS could cause 22 per cent of all deaths and 40 per cent of deaths from infectious diseases. By comparison, data from 1998 showed that only 2 per cent of all deaths were caused by HIV/AIDS and 6 per cent of deaths from infectious diseases were related to HIV/AIDS (Over et al. 2003). Other estimates show that countries in the region with HIV prevalence rates above 1 per cent could expect annual AIDS deaths to increase the total annual deaths in the 15 to 49 age group by up to 40 per cent during this decade (WHO 2001).

Increased infections and HIV/AIDS-related deaths could strain public health resources. In hospitals more beds would be occupied by AIDS patients. In Chiang Mai, northern Thailand, an estimated half of the beds have been occupied by people living with HIV/AIDS in recent years (ESCAP 2003). In addition to the increased bed occupancy by AIDS patients, the health system would need to respond to demands for universal blood screening, improved services for patients with other STIs as well as treatment of opportunistic infections such as tuberculosis (Alban 2002).

Providing medical care for people living with HIV/AIDS could add substantially to the expenses of the public health sector. The cost of providing ART in India has been calculated in a recent World Bank study. Assuming that the government covers 100 per cent of ART in the public sector as well as testing and monitoring facilities in the private sector, the cost per year could be between US$ 1.7 billion to US$ 7 billion depending on the choice of treatment options. India currently spends around US$ 300 million per year on central health. The combined central health and social welfare expenditures amounts to approximately US$ 1,200 million per year. As such, the least expensive ART treatment option for the Indian government would consume 59 per cent of the current health budget and the most expensive option would cost 62 per cent of the combined health and social welfare budget (Over et al. 2003).

An accurate estimate of the impact on health expenditures would need to factor in that HIV-affected rural households possibly had limited access to public health care service already before they became infected, and may not seek health care until the last stage of AIDS. This means that the burden of disease on the health sector may not be exactly proportional to an increase in HIV infections.

In summary, the economic impact of HIV/AIDS is significant for affected rural households because the epidemic drains savings for medical expenditure and reduces income opportunities. The impact on the private business sector and the health sector is also visible, but less substantial. The connection between HIV/AIDS and the economy is elusive, but the potential negative impact of the epidemic is indisputable. By undermining the health and economic future of individuals, the HIV/AIDS epidemic becomes a potential threat to human security in general.

A Threat to Human Security

The concept of human security has evolved from the traditional concept of national security. It recognises that, in an interdependent world, the greatest threat to security does not come from the military might of other states, but from diseases, hunger, environmental contamination and crime, affecting individuals and communities. It is, therefore, the individual and not the state that is in focus for human security (UNDP 1994). Since its introduction, the human security terminology has become widely accepted.

The United Nations Security Council debated on HIV/AIDS and its implications for the maintenance of international peace and stability in the year 2000. This was significant as it represented the first time the

Security Council discussed a health issue as well as the concept of human security. The initial debate has been followed by two Security Council Resolutions, which invite UN member states to provide HIV/AIDS awareness training for military and civilian police in preparation for deployment (UN Security Council Resolution 1308/2000 and 1325/ 2000).

The Human Security Network of Ministries of Foreign Affairs from 13 countries across the world have also acknowledged the link between AIDS and human security. The Network convened an inter-sessional meeting on HIV/AIDS and human security in the Greater Mekong sub-region in January 2002. At the following ministerial-level session of the Network the importance of the implementation of the Declaration on Commitment on HIV/AIDS, which was the outcome of the United Nations General Assembly Special Session on HIV/AIDS held in June 2001, was stressed (Human Security Network 2002a, 2002b).

The threats to human security have been divided into seven categories: economic security, food security, health security, environmental security, personal security, community security and political security. With the possible exception of environmental security, all these aspects of security could be affected by HIV/AIDS (UNAIDS 2001; UNDP 1994).

The epidemic obviously has an impact on people's health security as it reduces the ability of the human immune system to cope with diseases. At the same time the burden of the epidemic on the health sector means that health care services could become strained. In addition, the effects of HIV/AIDS on the microeconomy, where affected rural households give up assets and slide into poverty, means that availability of and economic access to basic food decreases. As a result, food security becomes an issue for the people concerned (UNAIDS 2002a; UNDP 1994). HIV-infected people in both urban and rural areas risk losing their jobs and employment opportunities. Their physical condition does not prevent them from carrying out their tasks, but the stigma and discrimination that is often directed towards HIV-positive people could limit their access to the job market (Asia Pacific Network of People Living with HIV/AIDS 2003). This affects the economic security of individuals, as they are no longer assured a basic income. Likewise, children of HIV-affected households who are taken out of school will not receive proper education, which could have a negative impact on their employability and income as adults. The stigma and discrimination that is connected with HIV/AIDS also has implications for the personal security of people living with and affected by HIV/AIDS. In the worst cases people living with HIV/AIDS have been targets of physical violence and even murder (UNAIDS 2001).

Table 2.1 provides an overview of the estimated impact of HIV/AIDS on human security in Asia. It is estimated that HIV/AIDS has the most impact on health, economic, food and personal security. The impact is minimal on community and political security. The table indicates that the impact of HIV/AIDS at the national level in Asian countries is still modest. If the assessment were applied to specific sections of population, such as rural households, the pattern would change.

Table 2.1
The Impact of HIV/AIDS on Human Security in Asia

Human security categories	Scale of impact of HIV/AIDS
Economic	+ +
Food	+ +
Health	+ + +
Environment	–
Personal	+ +
Community	+
Political	+

The distinction between the seven categories of threats to human security is useful, but in reality the different threats are likely to overlap and affect each other in a complex and multi-causal interaction. The human security approach is useful to help conceptualise the impact of HIV/AIDS on the foundation for human development. As the epidemic affects human security, it also limits people's ability to freely and safely exercise fundamental choices in life. Without human security it is unlikely that human development will progress (UNDP 1994, 2003).

HIV/AIDS: A Matter of National Security in Asia

It has been argued that HIV/AIDS has an impact on national security in the more traditional sense of security as protection of territory from external aggression. The relationship between the epidemic and national security is mostly indirect and the synergy between the two is not easily captured. AIDS does not cause war itself. In the worst affected parts of the world it is claimed that HIV/AIDS stands to increase poverty and undermine the credibility and operational effectiveness of the state.

These dynamics may exacerbate or even provoke social volatility and political instability. Combined with a national military that is weakened by HIV/AIDS, a country may not be able to prevent emerging internal conflict or protect itself from external aggressors (International Crisis Group 2001; UNAIDS 2002a).

HIV/AIDS and Uniformed Services

Countries in Sub-Saharan Africa report HIV/AIDS prevalence averages of 20 to 40 per cent within their armed forces, and prevalence rates among militaries are estimated to be as much as five times higher than that of the civilian population (UNAIDS 2002a). In national defence forces across Asia, HIV prevalence rates are much lower and there is no evidence to suggest that HIV/AIDS is about to destabilise countries in the region in the foreseeable future. Still, it remains a fact that uniformed services, such as police, military and peacekeepers, are groups highly vulnerable to HIV/AIDS.

Several aspects of the military environment put its uniformed services at risk, including the fact that most soldiers are in the age group where there is greatest risk of HIV infection (15 to 49 years), as well as the risk-taking tradition that characterises the military. One of the most important factors that increases the risk of infection is the practice of posting personnel away from their own communities and families. Not only does this free soldiers from the social control they might be subject to in their own communities, it also removes them from their spouses or regular sexual partners. The resulting lonliness, stress and sexual tension tend to increase risk taking (UNAIDS 2002b). Behavioural surveys among uniformed services conducted in a few countries in Asia suggest that military and police personnel engage in high-risk sexual behaviour (Kingdom of Cambodia 2002; Lao PDR 2002; Ting et al. 1996).

In Cambodia HIV prevalence among surveyed uniformed personnel is slightly higher than the national average but decreasing. The HIV prevalence rate among the military was recorded as 7.1 per cent in 1997 compared to a prevalence rate of 2.8 per cent of civilian males aged between 15 and 49 (Kingdom of Cambodia 2002). After 1997 the military was dropped from the National HIV Sentinel Surveillance because of the similarity with the police in risk behaviour. Data from the 2002 HIV Sentinel Surveillance recorded an HIV infection rate among the police of 3.9 per cent compared to the national prevalence rate of

2.6 per cent. There is some evidence of decreasing risk behaviour among uniformed services. Military personnel claiming they always use condoms during commercial sex rose from 42.9 per cent in 1997 to 86.7 per cent in 2001 (Kingdom of Cambodia 2002, 2003).

The Armed Forces Research Institute of Medical Sciences of the Royal Thai Army reports that HIV prevalence amongst army conscripts decreased from a peak of 3.6 per cent in 1993 to 0.7 per cent in 2001, which is lower that the estimated 1.8 per cent national prevalence rate by the end of 2001 (Avert 2002; Sangkharomya 2003; UNAIDS 2002b). These data may say more about successful prevention efforts for young men before they enter the armed forces and less about risk behaviours and prevalence rates during the time of military service. However, it seems reasonable to assume that young recruits will not forget prevention messages as they commence military service. It is also worth mentioning that the Royal Thai Army in the late 1980s already acknowledged that HIV/AIDS constituted a potential threat to national security. The army successfully framed HIV/AIDS as a so-called high politics issue and ensured an allocation in the national budget for awareness programmes within the army (Holloran 2002; Sangkharomya 2003).

Experiences from Cambodia and Thailand highlight that uniformed services can change their behaviours and that they can contribute to national responses to HIV/AIDS. It is worth underlining that very little is known about risk behaviour within national military forces in other countries of the region. Most countries conduct mandatory HIV/AIDS testing both during recruitment and regularly during military service. In most cases HIV-positive recruits are rejected and HIV-positive personnel discharged from service. Reports of new HIV incidents within uniformed services will, consequently, be low and can appear even lower than the national average (Healthlink Worldwide 2002). For instance, the most recent figures on HIV prevalence within the Indian army show that only 1,400 soldiers were living with HIV in 1999 (UNDP 2003). Despite the fact that the Indian army conduct HIV/AIDS awareness programmes for its personnel, this figure seems remarkably low in a 1.1 million strong army in a country with almost 4 million infected people. In countries where information on risk behaviour and HIV prevalence is made public, it is not always possible to obtain information on the methodology used. This means that the quality of published data is often uncertain and firm conclusions are difficult to draw.

The potential impact of HIV on the military may be hard to distinguish from the impact on the nation as a whole, including other state institutions. Some argue that widespread HIV infection in the armed forces of one or more countries may lead to destabilisation and conflict. Others claim that recent wars and conflicts in, for instance, Afghanistan, Columbia and Sierra Leone have been enabled by the weakness of all national institutions rather than the military alone (Healthlink Worldwide 2002).

HIV Vulnerability of International Peacekeepers

Personnel sent on peacekeeping missions often have more financial resources than local people, which give them better means to purchase sex. As a result, local sex industries grow in response to demand from military bases and units. A study of Dutch soldiers on a five-month peacekeeping mission in Cambodia found that 45 per cent had sexual contact with prostitutes or other members of the local population during their deployment (International Crisis Group 2001; UNAIDS 2002a).

Currently, Bangladesh, India and Pakistan along with Nigeria are the top four countries contributing troops to UN peacekeeping operations. The three South Asian countries combined have close to 9,000 soldiers on missions globally (UN Department of Peacekeeping Operations 2003). One-third of police officers and soldiers under UN command are stationed in Africa (International Crisis Group 2001). Some of them may not receive pre-deployment training on sexual health in missions, and peacekeepers from Asia may arrive in Africa with a very limited understanding of the HIV/AIDS situation on that continent. International peacekeepers are, therefore, often particularly at risk of HIV during missions. After they return home they may unknowingly transmit HIV/AIDS from a high-prevalence location to a low-prevalence population (ibid.).

At the same time it should be stressed that the extent to which peacekeepers spread HIV is uncertain. In the case of Cambodia some attribute the emergence of a commercial sex industry and the introduction of HIV to the presence of international peacekeepers during the 1990s. Others argue that poverty and the rapid social change that followed the collapse of the Khmer Rouge are more significant factors (Healthlink Worldwide 2002).

Based on the limited and incomplete information that is currently available, HIV/AIDS does not seem to pose an immediate threat to national security and regional stability in Asia. But the vulnerability of the uniformed services, especially personnel posted out, must be

addressed by national defence forces within their ranks and among those
they have a mandate to protect. Appropriate prevention programmes
are also important because there are situations where armed forces have
been known to abuse their power. One of the most common ways in
which this occurs is through sexual abuse, particularly rape, during times
of war and conflict (Healthlink Worldwide 2002).

Conclusion

The economic and security dimensions of HIV/AIDS are complex, but
should not be dismissed, although the lack of concrete data makes it
complicated to draw firm conclusions. The HIV/AIDS epidemic in Asia
has a substantial impact on rural household economy. The disease has a
limited impact on the private business sector and is only starting to
show on the health sector in the worst affected countries. With its potentially negative impact on household income, food and personal security,
the epidemic could become a threat to human security and has the
potential to undermine human development. Uniformed services continue to be vulnerable to HIV/AIDS and, despite low prevalence rates
among military and police, uniformed services, especially personnel
posted out, must be targeted in HIV/AIDS awareness programmes.

To prevent the epidemic from spreading and becoming a greater threat
to economic and national security in Asia, government leaders in the
region need to demonstrate high levels of personal commitment and
political will in guiding national and regional responses to HIV/AIDS.
And the international donor community needs to be aware that the
window of opportunity for bringing the epidemic under control is narrowing rapidly in Asia.

REFERENCES

Alban, Anita (2002). The socio-economic impact of HIV/AIDS: DANIDA's HIV/AIDS
programme of action. Unpublished presentation, Ease International, Copenhagen.
Asia Pacific Network of People Living with HIV/AIDS (2003). Final report of the
APN+ human rights initiative (Draft 10 only). Documentation of AIDS-related
discrimination in Asia, Bangkok.

Asian Business Coalition on HIV/AIDS (2002). *Business taking action to manage HIV/ AIDS: A selection of business practices responding to HIV/AIDS in- and outside the Asian workplace.* Bangkok: Asian Business Coalition on AIDS.

Avert (2002). South East Asian HIV/AIDS Statistics, http://www.avert.org/aidssoutheastasia.htm.

Bell, Clive, Shantayanan Devarajan and **Hans Gersbach** (2003). *The long-run economic cost of AIDS: Theory and an application to South Africa,* http://www.worldbank.org/ hiv_aids/docs/BEDEGE_BP_total2.pdf.

Bloom, David E., **Ajay Mahal, Jaypee Sevilla** and **River Path Associates** (2001a). AIDS & economics. Paper prepared for Working Group 1 of the WHO Commission on Macroeconomics and Health, http://www.iaen.org/files.cgi/7055_bloom_ economics.pdf.

Bloom, David E., **River Path Associates** and **Jaypee Sevilla** (2001b). Health, wealth, AIDS and poverty: The case of Cambodia, http://www.iaen.org/files.cgi/7054_ bloom_cambodia.pdf.

Centre for International Economics (2002). Potential economic impact of an HIV/ AIDS epidemic in Papua New Guinea. Report prepared for AusAID, Canberra, February.

China HIV/AIDS Socio-economic Impact Study Team (2002). Limiting the future impact of HIV/AIDS on children in Yunnan (China). In Giovanni Andrea Cornia (ed.), *AIDS, public policy and child well-being.* Nairobi: UNICEF Eastern and Southern Africa Regional Office.

Cornia, Giovanni Andrea (2002). *The HIV/AIDS impact on the rural and urban economy.* In Giovanni Andrea Cornia (ed.), *AIDS, public policy and child well-being.* Nairobi: UNICEF Eastern and Southern Africa Regional Office.

Duraisamy, Palanigounder (2003). Economic impact of HIV/AIDS on patients and households in south India. Presentation, 11th IAEN Face-to-Face Conference, http:/ /www.iaen.org/papers.

Eberstadt, Nicholas (2002). The future of AIDS. *Foreign Affairs,* 82(6).

Economic and Social Commission for Asia and the Pacific (ESCAP) (2003). *Economic and social progress in jeopardy: HIV/AIDS in the Asian and Pacific region— Integrating economic and social concerns, especially HIV/AIDS, in meeting the needs of the region.* New York: ESCAP, UN.

Global Business Council on HIV/AIDS (2001). *Business action on AIDS: A blueprint.* London: Global Business Council on HIV/AIDS.

——— (2002). *Employees & HIV/AIDS: Action for business leaders.* New York: Global Business Council on HIV/AIDS.

Global Health Initiative (2002). *Private sector intervention case example: Prevention through education and community outreach.* Geneva: World Economic Forum.

Healthlink Worldwide (2002). *Combat AIDS.* London: Russell Press.

Holloran, Richard (2002). Fighting AIDS in Asia: In Thailand, the armed forces help beat back an epidemic. *Baltimore Sun,* 13 October 2002, http://www.thebody.com/ cdc/news_updates_archive/oct25_02/aids_epidemic.html.

Human Security Network (2002a). Report of the status of the Human Security Network's main action areas: Annex no. 2. Chairman's summary, Fourth Ministerial Meeting, 2–3 July, Santiago, Chile, http://www.humansecuritynetwork.org/docs/ santiago_annex2-e.php.

——— (2002b). Excerpts from the intersessional meeting on human security and HIV/ AIDS. Chairman's summary, Intersessional Meeting of the Human Security

Network on Human Security and HIV/AIDS, 21–22 January, Bangkok, http://www. humansecuritynetwork.org/docs/aids-e.php.

ILO (2001). *An ILO code of practice on HIV/AIDS and the world of work.* Geneva: ILO.

——— (2002). *Enterprises & HIV/AIDS in India.* New Delhi: ILO.

International Crisis Group (2001). *HIV as a security issue.* Washington and Brussels: International Crisis Group.

Kingdom of Cambodia (2002). *Ministry of National Defense: HIV/AIDS strategic plan 2002–2006.* Pnom Penh: Kingdom of Cambodia.

——— (2003). *National HIV sentinel surveillance, 2002.* Pnom Penh: National Centre for HIV/AIDS, Dermatology and STDs (NCHADS).

Lao PDR (2002). Behavioral surveillance survey 2000–2001. Summary report, Lao PDR, National Committee for the Control of AIDS Bureau, Ministry of Health.

Over, Mead, Peter Heywood, Sudhakar Kurapati, Julian Gold, Indrani Gupta, Abhaya Indrayan, Subhash Hira, Elliot Marseille, Nico Nagelkerke and Arni S.R. Srinivasa Rao (2003). Integrating HIV prevention and antiretroviral therapy in India: Cost and consequences of policy options. Presentation, International AIDS Economics Network, 25 April, Virginia, http://www.iaen.org/files.cgi/10191_Mead-Over--IndiaART11_short.pdf.

Pitayanon, Sumalee, Sukontha Kongsin and Wattana S. Janjaroen (1997). The economic impact of HIV/AIDS mortality on households in Thailand. In David Bloom and Peter Godwin (eds.), *The economics of HIV and AIDS: The case of South and South-East Asia* (pp. 53–101). New Delhi: Oxford University Press.

Rosen, Sydney, Jonathon Simon, Jeffrey R. Vincent, William MacLeod, Matthew Fox and Donald M. Thea (2003). AIDS is your business. *Harvard Business Review*, 81(2), 30–37.

Sangkharomya, Suebpong M.G. (2003). HIV/AIDS in Thailand: An army doctor's perspective. Presentation, Armed Forces Research Institute of Medical Science, Royal Thai Army, Bangkok.

Ting, Douglas L., Grace B. Abad-Viola and Concepcion R. Roces (1996). Survey on HIV-related risk behaviours among regular personnel of the armed forces of the Philippines. Department of Health, Manila.

UNAIDS (1998). *HIV/AIDS and the workplace: Forging innovative business responses.* Geneva: UNAIDS.

——— (2001). AIDS and human security. Speech by Peter Piot, UNAIDS Executive Director, United Nations University, Tokyo, 2 October.

——— (2002a). *Report on the global HIV/AIDS epidemic 2002.* Geneva: UNAIDS.

——— (2002b). *HIV/AIDS and uniformed services: Fact sheet No. 3.* Geneva: UNAIDS.

——— (2003). *AIDS epidemic update.* December.

UNAIDS, Global Business Council on HIV/AIDS and Prince of Wales Business Leaders' Forum (2000). The business response to HIV/AIDS: Impact and lessons learned. Geneva.

UNDP (1994). *Human development report 1994.* New York: Oxford University Press, http://www.undp.org/hdro/hdrs/1994/english/94.htm.

——— (2003). *Regional human development report: HIV/AIDS and development in South-East Asia 2003.* New Delhi: UNDP.

UN Department of Peacekeeping Operations (2003). Contributors to United Nations' peacekeeping operations: Monthly summary of contributions, July 2003, http://www.un.org/Depts/dpko/dpko/contributors/July2003Countrysummary.pdf.

Verma, Ravi K., S. Salil, Veera Mendonca, S.K. Singh, R. Prasad and R.B Upadhyaya (2002). HIV/AIDS and children in the Sangli district of Maharashtra (India). In Giovanni Andrea Cornia (ed.), *AIDS, public policy and child well-being*. Nairobi: UNICEF Eastern and Southern Africa Regional Office.

Whiteside, Alan (2002). The economics of HIV/AIDS. Plenary presentation at the International AIDS Economics of AIDS in Developing Countries Symposium, Barcelona, 6 July, http://www.iaen.org/files.cgi/7341_whiteside.pdf.

WHO (2001). HIV/AIDS in Asia and the Pacific region. WHO Regional Offices for the Western Pacific and for South-East Asia. WHO Library Cataloguing in Publication Data, http://www.who.int/hiv/strategic/en/wpraids2001.pdf.

3

THE PANDEMIC OF HIV INFECTION:
LESSONS FROM AFRICA

Ahmed S. Latif

The joint United Nations Programme on AIDS and the World Health Organisation (WHO) estimates that close to 40 million people have become infected with HIV infection throughout the world (Table 3.1). The majority of people with HIV infection and AIDS live in Sub-Saharan African, and South and South-East Asian countries. With estimates of adult HIV prevalence of 8.8 per cent in Sub-Saharan Africa, the region is experiencing the worst HIV epidemic in the world. In 1998 HIV prevalence rates among antenatal clinic attenders in Botswana, Zimbabwe, Swaziland and South Africa were 38.8 per cent, 35 per cent, 31.6 per cent and 22.8 per cent respectively. Prevalence rates of HIV

Table 3.1
Global Estimates of HIV Infection and AIDS

Region	Adults and children living with HIV infections
Sub-Saharan Africa	26,600,000
North Africa and Middle East	600,000
North America	1,000,000
South America and Caribbean	2,070,000
Western Europe	600,000
Eastern Europe and Central Asia	1,500,000
South and South-East Asia	6,400,000
East Asia and Pacific	1,000,000
Australia and New Zealand	15,000
Total (approx.)	**40,000,000**

Source: UNAIDS (2002).

infection in countries in South and South-East Asia are not as high as those found in Southern Africa. However, the epidemic continues to grow in most parts of this region as well. The case scenario of the effects of the epidemic in Africa may well be replicated in other parts of the world if efforts are not made to curtail the spread of infection. The epidemic is growing fast in many parts of the South-East Asian region, and with the recent slump in the economies of many countries in the region, effects similar to those seen in parts of Sub-Saharan Africa may well occur. In Sub-Saharan Africa the epidemic spread early and reached pandemic proportions before the aetiology and methods of controlling it became known. Asia has the benefit of this knowledge and it is imperative that interventions known to positively influence prevention and control of HIV infection be implemented as a matter of urgency.

The Impact

The effect of the epidemic is seen on all sectors of society. The epidemic has had an adverse effect on life expectancy in Sub-Saharan Africa (Figure 3.1). Gains made in life expectancy in the years before 1980 have been lost and it is estimated that life expectancies in countries affected badly by HIV infection and AIDS may be less than 40 years (UN Population Division 2001).

Figure 3.1
Projected Changes in Life Expectancy in
Selected Southern African Countries: 1955–2000

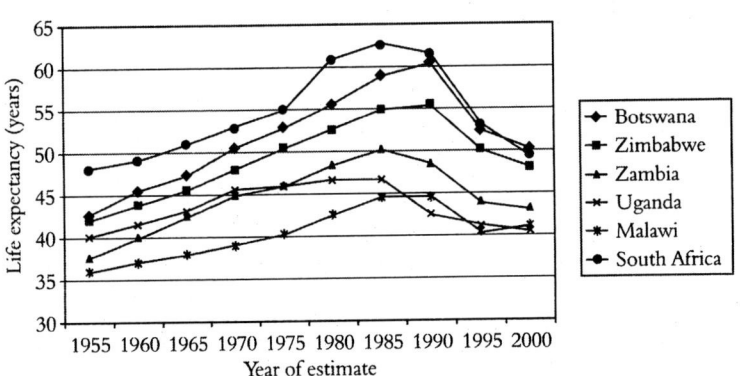

Source: UN Population Division (2001).

The epidemic has effects on the agriculture, education, health, labour and transport sectors. Development has ceased in many countries where struggling economies are no longer able to repay loans taken to strengthen the health and agriculture sectors.

The epidemic is growing fastest in South Africa (Figure 3.2) where it is estimated that over 1,500 new infections occur daily (UNAIDS 2002).

Figure 3.2
Changing Prevalence of
HIV Infection in South Africa: 1990–98

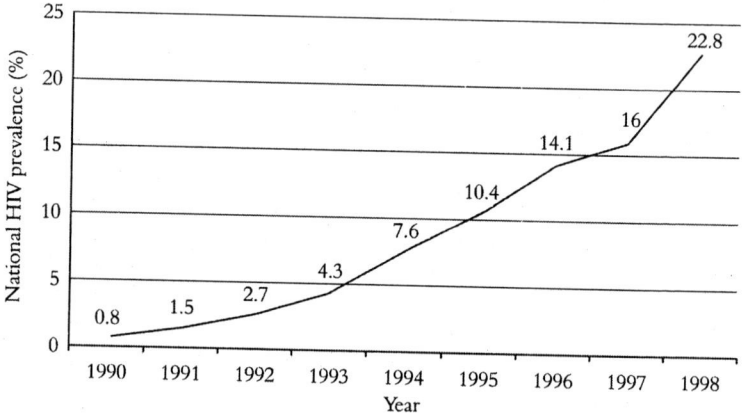

Source: UNAIDS (2002).

With high HIV prevalence, the rates of tuberculosis have increased tremendously in Southern Africa. Of the 15.3 million people in the world estimated to be infected with HIV and *Mycobacterium tuberculosis* at the end of 1997, 11.7 million (75 per cent) live in Sub-Saharan Africa. HIV infection is the single strongest risk factor for progression of TB from latent infection to active disease. As a result, TB has been increasing in nine African countries, attributed primarily to HIV/AIDS. TB is one of the commonest opportunistic infections encountered in immuno-suppressed persons with HIV infection in developing countries (Corbett et al. 2002). TB is eminently curable, and because of this it is necessary that facilities for its accurate diagnosis and treatment be available in all countries with high HIV prevalence rates.

Risk Factors Contributing to HIV Transmission in Africa

Poverty-related Factors

Separation of Marital Partners

For economic reasons marital partnerships may be split, usually with the husband seeking paid employment in urban areas and cities in places far away from home, while the wife remains at home looking after the children and tending the fields and the livestock. Often the husband is away from the wife for periods of over three months at a time. This prolonged separation may lead a partner to develop a non-permanent relationship with a non-regular partner who may well have other partners. In relationships such as these the use of condoms is not considered necessary.

This situation has been in place for many decades now and it is essentially the result of the search for economic survival. However, not many AIDS control programmes in the sub-region have addressed these issues.

Sex for Commercial Gain

Female commercial sex workers engage in sex for money for economic survival. Multiple sexual partners and unprotected sexual intercourse have given rise to high HIV prevalence rates with up to 80 per cent of female sex workers being HIV seropositive (Buve et al. 2001; Weiss et al. 2001). Most countries in the sub-region have embarked on educating women on the use of the female condom and making these widely available.

Prevalence of Other Sexually-transmitted Infections

Prevalence of STIs in Sub-Saharan Africa is high, which facilitates the transmission and acquisition of HIV (Laga et al. 1993; Latif et al. 1989; Mbizvo et al. 1997; Weiss et al. 2001). As STIs are only transmitted from person to person, it is necessary to treat all persons who may be infected, whether they have the symptoms or not. All countries in the sub-region have realised the importance of partner referral and treatment, and have implemented activities to address this issue. The setting up of formal contact tracing facilities, where health personnel go out to seek contacts of persons with STIs, has been found difficult to implement in view of resource constraints.

Unsafe Sexual Behaviour

Multiple Concurrent Partnerships   Education programmes addressing these issues are incorporated within the national prevention strategies of all countries in the sub-region. However, the knowledge of prevention methods seems not to affect behaviour change. Targeted intervention programmes addressing specific groups of the population such as peer-led education programmes for factory workers, sex workers, and youth in and out of school have yielded encouraging results.

The Reluctance of Men to Use Condoms   All HIV/AIDS control programmes in the sub-region have a strong focus on condom promotion and distribution as part of the primary prevention strategy (Bassett et al. 1992). Despite the widespread promotion of condoms, there is a general reluctance of men in the sub-region to use condoms both in regular and in casual or non-regular partnerships. Sex workers indicate that men are reluctant to use condoms and if the sex worker insists on it, then she will lose trade and therefore income. Programmes targeting sex workers aim for 100 per cent condom use. However, this target has not been reached in any of the countries. Studies among sex workers have shown that the use of condoms by men during sexual relationships has increased over the last few years in Zimbabwe, Zambia, Malawi, Botswana and Mozambique.

Since the female condom has become available, women now have the ability to protect themselves. Most countries in the sub-region have made these available for a small, subsidised charge. Only in Botswana and Namibia are female condoms distributed free at health facilities.

Customs, Beliefs and Practices

Sexual Partnerships across Age Groups

Men in general tend to develop sexual partnerships with women and girls much younger than themselves. There appears to be a belief that younger women and girls have less likelihood of being infected. Younger women tend to accept such relationships in part because of the monetary rewards that may result. However, it is known that the physiological make-up of a young girl makes her more likely to become infected with HIV should she have her first sexual experience with an infected man.

Use of Intra-vaginal Desiccants

In a number of countries in the sub-region sexually active women tend to use chemical and herbal substances intra-vaginally in order to 'keep themselves dry' (Latif et al. 1999). Men encourage this practice as they believe that being dry indicates the absence of STIs. This practice, however, alters the normal microbiological flora of the vagina that has some protective role against STIs (Gray et al. 1997). However, national AIDS programmes in the sub-region are yet to address this issue.

Use of Alcohol and Drugs

The use of alcohol is a major problem in Africa. Many working men in the sub-region drink alcohol in public places where it is easy to set up relationships with sex workers. Studies in Zimbabwe have shown that drinking in public places is an independent risk associate for HIV acquisition. Figure 3.3 shows the prevalence of HIV infection amongst consumers and non-consumers of alcohol in the mining town of Carletonville in South Africa.

Figure 3.3
HIV Prevalence among Consumers and
Non-consumers of Alcohol in Carletonville, South Africa: 1998

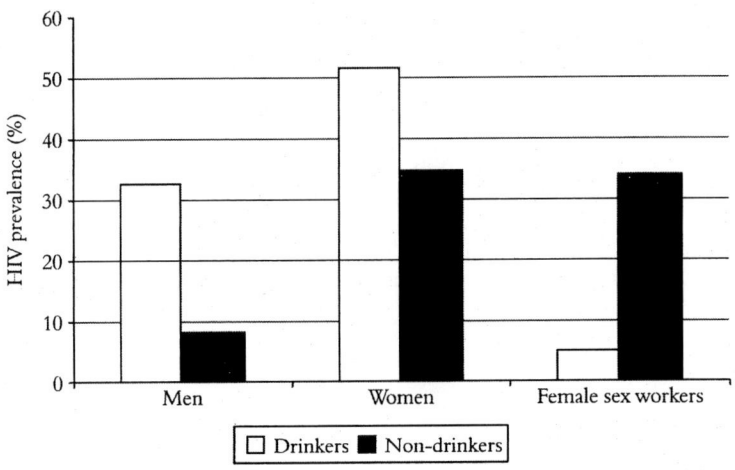

Source: UNAIDS.

The Non-circumcision of Men

Male circumcision is incriminated in some studies to play a protective role against STIs (Moses et al. 1990, 1998). However, only a small number of men undergo circumcision. There are various biological reasons for the intact foreskin being a risk factor for acquisition of HIV. One reason is that the inner mucous surface of the foreskin acts as a receptacle for bacteria and viruses. In addition, the foreskin is prone to trauma during sex and it is known that microscopic tears may appear on the foreskin, opening a portal for the entry of STI agents and HIV. There are no controlled studies assessing the role of circumcision in HIV acquisition and transmission.

Successful Interventions

Despite there being no cure for HIV/AIDS, there is sufficient evidence in Africa and elsewhere to suggest that certain interventions are successful in preventing the infection and in alleviating the suffering that is associated with the illness. These interventions are discussed in this section.

Primary Prevention Activities

Modified sexual behaviour may prevent infection in the first place. Primary prevention can also be achieved through engaging only in safer sexual activities, activities that may result in persons changing their sexual behaviour and ensuring safe sex. This can be achieved through educating communities on:

- dangers of HIV/AIDS/STIs;
- ways of preventing infection by changing one's behaviour;
- ways of preventing infection by engaging only in safer sexual activity; and
- promoting and providing condoms.

Primary prevention activities in many parts of Africa have resulted in changed sexual behaviour. With the incorporation of sex education in schools, the knowledge of adolescents on HIV/AIDS and STIs has increased tremendously. Demographic and health surveys performed between 1994 and 1998 in a number of Sub-Saharan African countries have shown that over 90 per cent of men and women aged between

15 and 19 years had heard of AIDS and over 60 per cent knew of one or more ways of preventing the sexual transmission of HIV (Table 3.2).

Table 3.2
Awareness of HIV/AIDS among Adolescents in
Selected Sub-Saharan African Countries

Country	Adolescents who have heard of AIDS (%)		Adolescents who know of one or more ways to prevent HIV (%)	
	Men	Women	Men	Women
Cote d'Ivoire	96	95	77	49
Ghana	97	97	56	50
Kenya	99	99	81	72
Madagascar	–	63	–	22
Mali	90	80	67	49
Mozambique	90	81	28	15
Senegal	–	90	–	53
Tanzania	97	96	59	43
Uganda	100	99	79	64
Zambia	99	99	81	63
Zimbabwe	99	98	77	64

Source: Population Reference Bureau (2000).

Targeted interventions aimed at groups at greater risk for infection have also demonstrated success in reducing the acquisition of HIV infection. In one study carried out in Harare, Zimbabwe (Mbizvo et al. 1997), a significant reduction in HIV incidence was achieved through a well-developed and well-implemented workplace-based peer-led education initiative. In the study carried out in 40 factories, condom use was promoted and condoms were distributed, appropriate health education was provided, appropriate STI care-seeking behaviour was promoted and easy access to free STI care was provided. In half the factories, selected randomly, this workplace-based peer-led education intervention was set up. At the end of the study, which lasted three years, the incidence of HIV infection among workers in the intervention sites was significantly lower than among workers in the control sites.

Secondary Prevention Activities

In all countries in the Southern African region STI care is available in all primary health care and reproductive health care facilities in the private and public sectors and STI care is provided through the syndromic case management approach. Most countries in the region have developed national guidelines for the management of STIs, and these form part of the essential drugs programme.

This requires training of care providers. Most Southern African countries have incorporated training activities within the National HIV/ AIDS/STI Strategic Plan. Training programmes have been undertaken to train not only doctors, but other health workers in the provision of high-quality STI care. Guidelines for the management of STIs have been developed and are widely used in the region. A number of countries have instituted programmes for the reporting of STI episodes from primary care clinics. Reporting systems usually are based on the syndromic diagnosis of STIs, and data collection is based on the use of tally sheets on a daily basis. In this way universal reporting of episodes of STI syndromes has been implemented.

The effect of STI control on HIV incidence is difficult to assess. Three trials have been conducted in East Africa in order to address this question:

1. In Mwanza, Tanzania, a study demonstrated that improved STI treatment services reduced HIV incidence in the general population by about 40 per cent (Grosskurth et al. 1995). The incidence of new cases of active syphilis also fell sharply (Mayaud 1997). The syndromic management approach was used in treating symptomatic persons with STIs in the study.

2. In Rakai, Uganda, the effect of mass treatment of the population for common bacterial STIs was measured along with rates of HIV infection. Disappointingly, although reductions were seen in some STIs, there was no significant effect on HIV incidence (Wawer et al. 1999).

3. A third trial was carried out in Masaka, Uganda. In this study the effect of a community-based behavioural intervention with or without the provision of improved STI care through the syndromic management approach was assessed. Despite reductions in STIs and changes in reported behaviour, neither the behavioural nor the STD treatment intervention had a significant effect on HIV-1 incidence.

These findings have important implications for HIV and STI control programmes. The importance of early effective treatment of STIs has a beneficial effect on HIV control.

Voluntary Counselling and Testing for HIV

Knowing one's HIV status has been shown to prevent acquisition and transmission of HIV. Persons who are at risk for HIV should be able to be tested for infection. Such persons should receive appropriate pre-test counselling and should be given post-test counselling as well when the results of the test are available. HIV-negative persons should receive intensive counselling in order for them to remain negative. In this situation an assessment of risk status and reasons for risk-taking behaviour should be made, and the client should be offered appropriate advice to reduce risk and to cope with behaviour change. Persons who are HIV positive should also receive appropriate counselling to cope with the infection and to live a positive lifestyle.

A number of countries in Africa have set up centres where persons may be tested for HIV infection after receiving appropriate counselling (Box 3.1).

Box 3.1
Voluntary Counselling and Testing (VCT) for HIV Infection

- Knowing one's HIV status assists in modifying one's sexual behaviour.
- Provision of services for voluntary HIV testing with pre- and post-test counselling is an intervention being widely accepted throughout the sub-region as a means for the prevention of acquisition and transmission of HIV.
- National AIDS control programmes in the sub-region have plans for implementing VCT.
- VCT centres are found in Zimbabwe, Zambia, Botswana, Malawi, Namibia and South Africa.

Prevention of Mother-to-Child Transmission of HIV

There is sufficient evidence that antiretroviral agents given to a pregnant woman at the appropriate time during pregnancy and/or labour reduce mother-to-child transmission of HIV. Studies carried out in Thailand and in Uganda have shown that zidovudine given during the last month of pregnancy to pregnant women and nevirapine given in a single dose during labour together with a single dose to the neonate significantly reduce mother-to-child transmission of HIV. However, it should be noted that HIV-infected women can infect their infants through breast-feeding. They should ideally be counselled about this risk so that they are able to make an informed choice regarding abstaining from breast-feeding, and be educated on safe and hygienic ways of formula-feeding their babies. A number of countries in Sub-Saharan Africa have incorporated strategies for the prevention of mother-to-child transmission of HIV using antiretroviral agents.

Mitigating the Effects of HIV/AIDS

Though no cure is available for HIV infection, much can be done to mitigate its effects on individuals and communities. Persons with HIV infection and their families need a great deal of support.

Protecting the Rights of People Living with HIV Infection and AIDS

Unfortunately, the stigma of being HIV positive still remains. Most countries in the region have developed and adopted policies on HIV infection and AIDS. Such national policies and guiding principles form the basis of the national response to the epidemic. In most countries policies backed by legal instruments have been implemented to protect the rights of the HIV-infected individual. Mandatory testing of persons for any reason is discouraged and persons known to be HIV infected are not denied jobs and staff development opportunities. The development of a national policy on HIV/AIDS is an important and a necessary strategy for mitigating the effects of the infection.

Persons with HIV infection need support at the national level, the community level as well as at the family level. Education of family members and the community is an essential requirement for the provision of care and support for infected persons.

There is need for strong advocacy on the needs and rights of the HIV-infected person and support should come from the highest authority in the land. In this way a number of adverse effects of HIV infection on individuals, families, communities and society may be mitigated.

Provision of Counselling Services

In view of the incurable nature of the infection, HIV-infected individuals need counselling to enable and assist them to cope with a potentially life-threatening and infectious condition. Counselling begins before an individual is tested for HIV and continues after the result of the test becomes available, regardless of whether the test is positive. Persons who have been tested for HIV infection and are found to be negative should be counselled about the window period and also on how they should modify their behaviour and activities in order to remain negative. Those found to be HIV positive should be counselled regarding living a positive lifestyle and not becoming infected with STIs of any nature in future. Most Sub-Saharan African countries have established services for HIV pre-test and post-test counselling. In view of the large number of persons requiring these services, countries have trained doctors, nurses, and other health and paramedical workers to provide this important need. In addition, persons with HIV infection require repeated counselling regarding living a healthy and positive lifestyle. Periodically they will need counselling to overcome crises and to cope with the illness as it develops. Hence, the need for training of personnel is very high.

Provision of Care

Apart from social and psychological support, persons with HIV infection periodically require care for HIV-related and non-HIV-related illnesses. Like anyone else, an HIV-infected person may develop illnesses that require standard treatment or specialist attention for surgical, dental, or obstetric and gynaecologic conditions. HIV status should not preclude any person from receiving standard care. No HIV-positive patient should be denied care when it is required. There is a need for all doctors and health workers to be aware of universal precautions for the prevention of transmission of infection and there is need for health institutions to have a policy on implementing and practising universal precautions.

Persons with HIV infection tend to develop illnesses that may not be life-threatening and will respond to appropriate treatment. Such treatment should be readily available and health workers should be trained to manage such illnesses.

Most Southern African countries have developed community-based care programmes for terminally-ill patients. Home-based care is provided by members of the community and is supervised by health professionals based at district hospitals and health centres. The need for this type of care became apparent when it was realised that large numbers of persons had become infected and would become ill. Guidelines for the provision of community home-based care have been developed, and members of the community and members of the patient's family are trained in providing care.

Preventing Opportunistic Infections

Certain opportunistic infections that HIV-infected immunosuppressed individuals suffer from may be prevented by using antibiotics on a long-term basis as chemoprophylaxis. Tuberculosis is the commonest opportunistic infection seen among HIV-infected individuals throughout the developing world. It usually occurs as the patient becomes immunosuppressed. By giving patients anti-TB drugs such as rifampicin and isoniazid INH, its occurrence may be prevented.

In addition, some of the other opportunistic infections such *Pneumocystis carinii* pneumonia, toxoplasmosis, some bacterial pneumonias and salmonelloses may be prevented by cotrimoxazole as long-term chemoprophylaxis. The use of cotrimoxazole has been shown to be effective in preventing many of these infections if given in appropriate doses over a long term.

Provision of Antiretroviral Therapy

Antiretroviral therapy given appropriately and in a timely fashion prolongs life and delays the onset of AIDS in persons with HIV infection. Studies addressing the question of feasibility of use of antiretroviral agents in resource-constrained settings show that treatment has doubled in Africa. With the reduction of prices and availability of funding from many sources including the GFATM, the treatment scale-up has become a reality now.

Lessons for Asia

National-level Commitment, Leadership and Support

An essential component of HIV/STI control anywhere in the world is the support and commitment of leaders and policy makers. In Africa the problem of HIV/AIDS has received the recognition of most leaders, and many countries have declared the pandemic a national disaster. Direction and support at the highest level, and political leadership and commitment are necessary as the epidemic is not simply a medical problem, but affects all sectors of society. Multi-sectoral participation and involvement of the community are needed for successful implementation of interventions that work.

Uganda was one of the first countries in Africa to realise the need for action from the highest level. The Uganda National AIDS Commission was formed, with its head of being equivalent to a cabinet minister reporting directly to the country's president. The spread of the epidemic in Uganda has slowed considerably. There are a number of reasons for this:

1. The national government gave its full support to prevention and control efforts, and formed the National AIDS Commission to develop policy and direct interventions.
2. There has been a change in the sexual behaviour of the younger section of the population, probably as a result of improved knowledge and awareness of the dangers of unsafe sexual behaviour and practices, easy access to condoms and improved services for the treatment of the treatable STIs.
3. Many people may have been motivated to change their behaviour after seeing large numbers of people die from the illness.
4. Uganda was the first country in Africa where persons infected and affected by HIV/AIDS came out into the open and made public statements. Members of the general public were now able to relate to persons affected by HIV/AIDS. Role models joined in the struggle against the transmission of HIV infection, and singers, movie stars and sportspersons all supported the cause and gave their time to spread prevention messages.

The Devastating Impact of the HIV Epidemic

Data on the health, social and economic impact of HIV in most African countries reveals that the epidemic has a tendency to devastate families and communities, and undermine the economic development of nations. From impact at the individual to national level, the consequences are indeed beyond imagination. Villages and communities have been decimated, and hard-won health and economic development gains wiped out by the HIV/AIDS epidemic in country after country in Africa, particularly those in the Sub-Saharan region.

Primary Prevention of HIV Infection

Primary prevention activities directed towards behaviour change work. It is evident from a number of African countries that incorporating education on sexuality within the school curriculum helps adolescents make informed choices later in life. Studies carried out in Ghana, Cote d'Ivoire and Senegal have shown that sexual debut may be delayed through education and counselling of in-school youth on the importance of maintaining sexual health and the dangers of STIs and HIV infection. Through such interventions knowledge, awareness, practices and attitudes can be changed in young people. Targeted interventions among groups of the population considered to be at higher risk of infection also work. It has been shown in Zimbabwe, Tanzania and Malawi that among sex workers condom use can be improved through peer-led education interventions. Studies carried out among male factory workers and long-distance drivers in Zimbabwe have shown that the incidence of HIV infection may be reduced through workplace-based peer-led prevention initiatives.

Provision of STI Care

The rapid and effective treatment of treatable STIs is shown to be an effective method in reducing the transmission of HIV infection. In a controlled study performed in Mwanza, Tanzania, it was shown that by providing high-quality STI care through the syndromic management approach the incidence of HIV infection was significantly reduced.

In Zimbabwe the number of episodes of STIs reported annually reduced tremendously over a period of 10 years (Figure 3.4). One reason for this is that STI services are fully integrated within primary and reproductive health care facilities in the public and private sectors. The STI syndromic management approach has been in practice in Zimbabwe for nearly 20 years now.

Most countries in Africa now provide STI care through this approach at all primary and reproductive health care facilities. Decentralisation and integration of STI services has required a functioning network of primary and reproductive health facilities, personnel trained in the provision of STI care, standardised STI management guidelines and essential STI drugs. Most HIV/AIDS/STI control programmes in Sub-Saharan Africa have included training of health workers in the management of STIs as a major control strategy.

The Prevention of Mother-to-Child Transmission of HIV

Studies carried out in South-East Asia and Sub-Saharan Africa have shown that by using single-dose and multiple-dose regimens of anti-retroviral agents, it is possible to significantly reduce mother-to-child transmission of HIV. In order to implement this, it is obviously necessary

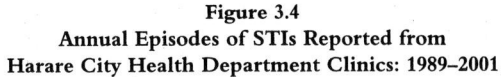

Figure 3.4
Annual Episodes of STIs Reported from
Harare City Health Department Clinics: 1989–2001

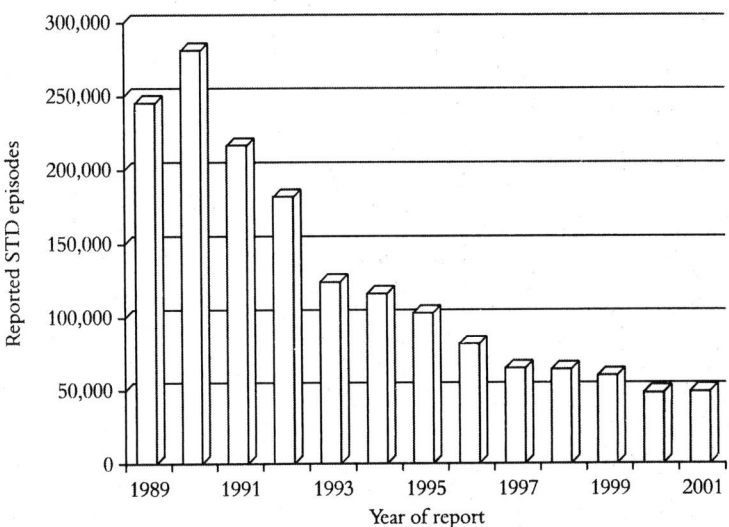

to identify those pregnant women who may be infected. This requires large-scale screening programmes together with pre-test counselling. Once HIV-infected pregnant women are identified, it is necessary to counsel them about the risks of transmission of the infection to their babies and also about their own HIV infection. In addition, it is known that HIV-positive women who continue to breastfeed their infants pose a significant risk of infection to their infants. Ideally, HIV-positive mothers should be counselled regarding this risk and should be offered alternatives to breastfeeding.

Voluntary Counselling and Testing for HIV

Knowing one's HIV status may help modify sexual behaviour. Provided that people who are to be tested are counselled adequately before and after the test, this intervention has been found to be effective in changing sexual behaviour. Most countries in Africa have established VCT centres where persons may go to be tested for HIV after being counselled. For this intervention to be acceptable, it is necessary that persons seeking testing be assured of confidentiality and are advised appropriately.

Mitigating the Effects of HIV Infection

Persons who are infected with HIV can remain productive members of society for a long time. HIV-infected individuals and their dependants need psychological support in order to cope with an illness that is not only incurable but results in serious social problems. Trained counsellors may be able to provide the support that is commonly needed by people who have recently found out that they are HIV infected. As HIV disease progresses, patients will require additional psychological support, especially in times of crises. Studies have shown that simple reassurance and explanation may be sufficient to alleviate the stress that many patients with HIV infection go through periodically.

As patients become ill, they will require care and treatment for HIV-related illness. Patients with minor illnesses and minor opportunistic infections respond well to standard treatment recommendations. Zimbabwe, Zambia and Botswana have developed standardised guidelines for the treatment of HIV-related illnesses and in Zimbabwe the guidelines form part of the Essential Drugs Programme.

As the epidemic matures and more people become infected, it has been realised in most Southern African countries that existing health facilities do not have the bed capacity to admit and manage in hospital all those who require long-term and terminal care. As a result, community home-based care programmes have been developed and implemented. Chronically-ill patients with HIV infection are usually managed at home with family and community members assisting in care provision. Such programmes in Southern Africa have shown to have a beneficial effect for the patient and his/her family. Training of family members, community members and health workers is necessary for the successful implementation of the service.

The epidemic of HIV infection continues to enlarge in Africa, and most countries have noted massive increases in mortality rates, especially in persons aged between 29 and 49 years. Most Southern African countries are now seriously considering the use of ART. These drugs are extremely costly, as is monitoring patients receiving ART. However, they are now becoming available on a generic basis. Currently a multi-centre study is under way in Uganda and Zimbabwe, examining the possibility of effective use of antiretroviral agents to treat persons with HIV infection using clinical monitoring indicators.

Conclusion

The HIV/AIDS epidemic has affected every country in the world. The majority of persons living with HIV infection and AIDS are found in the developing world where resources are poor, and access to care and new treatments is limited. Despite the high prevalence rates, care for persons with HIV infection living in these countries is not given high priority as a result of the high burden of disease due to other illnesses. In areas where the epidemic is most severe the provision of care is further compromised by the rapidly weakening economies and the costs of effective medications. Sub-Saharan Africa has been badly hit by the pandemic and various lesson can be learnt from local experiences by the international community, especially people living in South-East Asia.

R EFERENCES

Bassett, M.T., A.S. Latif, D.A. Katzenstein and J.C. Emmanuel (1992). Sexual behavior and risk factors for HIV infection in a group of male factory workers who donated blood in Harare, Zimbabwe. *Journal of Acquired Immune Deficiency Syndromes*, 5(6), 556–59.

Buve, A. et al. (2001). The multicentre study on factors determining the differential spread of HIV in four African cities: Summary and conclusions. *AIDS*, 15(Supplement 4), S127–31.

Corbett, Elizabeth L., Richard W. Steketee, Feiko O. ter Kuile, Ahmed S. Latif, Anatoli Kamali and Richard J. Hayes (2002). HIV-1/AIDS and the control of other infectious diseases in Africa. *Lancet*, 359(9324), 2177–87.

Gray, R.H., M.J. Wawer, N. Sewankambo and D. Serwadda (1997). HIV-1 infection associated with abnormal vaginal flora morphology and bacterial vaginosis. *Lancet*, 350(9093), 1780.

Grosskurth, H. et al. (1995). Impact of improved treatment of sexually transmitted diseases on HIV infection in rural Tanzania: Randomised controlled trial. *Lancet*, 346(8974), 530–36.

Laga, M. et al. (1993). Non-ulcerative sexually transmitted diseases as risk factors for HIV-1 transmission in women: Results from a cohort study. *AIDS*, 7(1), 95–102.

Latif, A.S., D.A. Katzenstein, M.T. Bassett, S. Houston, J.C. Emmanuel and E. Marowa (1989). Genital ulcers and transmission of HIV among couples in Zimbabwe. *AIDS*, 3(8), 519–23.

Latif, A.S., P.R. Mason, E. Marowa, L. Gwanzura, A. Chingono and O.L. Mbengeranwa (1999). Risk factors for gonococcal and chlamydial cervical infection in pregnant and non-pregnant women in Zimbabwe. *Central African Journal of Medicine*, 45(10), 252–58.

Mayaud, P. et al. (1997). Improved treatment services significantly reduce the prevalence of sexually transmitted diseases in rural Tanzania: Results of a randomized controlled trial. *AIDS*, 11(5), 1873–80.

Mbizvo, M.T., A.S. Latif, R. Machekano, W. MacFarland, M.T. Bassett, S. Ray and D. Katzenstein (1997). HIV seroconversion among factory workers in Harare: Who is getting newly infected? *Central African Journal of Medicine*, 43(5), 135–39.

Moses, S. et al. (1990). Geographic patterns of male circumcision practices in Africa: An association with HIV seroprevalence. *International Journal of Epidemiology*, 19, 693–97.

Moses, S., R.C. Bailey and **A.R. Ronald** (1998). Male circumcision: Assessment of health benefits and risks. *Sexually Transmitted Infections*, 74(5), 368–73.

Population Reference Bureau (2000). *Youth in Sub-Saharan Africa: A chartbook on sexual experience and reproductive health*. Washington, DC: Population Reference Bureau.

UNAIDS (2002). *Report on the global HIV/AIDS epidemic*. Geneva: UNAIDS.

UN Population Division (2001). *World population prospects: The 2000 revision*. New York: UN Population Division.

Wawer, M.J. et al. (1999). Control of sexually transmitted diseases for AIDS prevention in Uganda: A randomized community trial. *Lancet*, 353(9152), 525–35.

Weiss, H.A. et al. (2001). The epidemiology of HSV-2 infection and its association with HIV infection in four urban African populations. *AIDS*, 15(Supplement 4), S97–108.

THE 100 PER CENT CONDOM USE PROGRAMME: A SUCCESS STORY

4

Wiwat Rojanapithayakorn

By the end of 2003, 40 million people worldwide were living with HIV/ AIDS. Of these, more than 6 million were in Asia and the Pacific region (UNAIDS/WHO 2003). The main mode of HIV transmission in the Asia Pacific is sexual. Extensive heterosexual transmission mediated through large-scale sex industries has been observed in Thailand, Cambodia, India, Myanmar and many other countries in the region. Transmission from sex workers to customers has resulted in expansion of infection to the general population. HIV spread from infected male clients to sex workers, from infected sex workers to their clients, and subsequently from infected clients to their wives and also from infected wives to newborns.

Interventions for the prevention of sexual transmission of HIV include information, education and communication (IEC), prevention and care of sexually-transmitted infections and condom promotion. Condom promotion has been considered a major strategy to prevent sexual transmission of HIV. However, most such campaigns have not been effective in achieving a high enough level of condom use to stop transmission.

One of the most successful condom promotion campaigns in the Asia region is the 100 per cent condom use programme successfully implemented in Thailand (Rojanapithayakorn and Hanenberg 1996). This is now being expanded to Cambodia, Myanmar, China, Vietnam and a few other countries in the region. The programme has been found to be a very effective strategy in the target populations in a short time period.

The 100 Per Cent Condom Use Programme in Thailand

The 100 per cent condom use programme in Thailand originated from an evaluation of STI control strategies during the 1980s, which showed that these strategies were not enough to curb the high STI incidence. These included the promotion of health-seeking behaviour, provision of STI services and routine STI check-up of sex workers. It was perceived that the provision of STI services alone might not be effective enough to prevent spread of infections. A better way was to promote safe sex and promote condom use among sex workers and their clients.

However, people working in STI/HIV/AIDS prevention and control realised that it was not easy to promote condom use in sex work. Many programmes to train sex workers on negotiating skills on condom use were found ineffective because sex workers had no power to say 'no' to clients who insisted on not using a condom. When sex workers insisted on condom use, the customer would resist. Some of them even increased the price of condom-free sex, and most of the time sex workers had to comply with clients' demands. On many occasions the owners of sex establishments forced their workers to comply with whatever their customers wanted, including the provision of condom-free sex.

The 100 per cent condom use programme was developed with an attempt to empower sex workers. The main idea behind the programme was to 'monopolise' sex work in such a way that all sex services required condom use. All sex establishments were requested to adhere to the same rule of 'no condom, no sex' so that customers would have no choice except to use condoms. Implementation of the strategy required participation of the owners of sex establishments (as sex work in Thailand has been mainly of the establishment type, both direct and indirect forms). They could instruct sex workers in their place to provide condom-only services. Since the owners of sex establishments always listen to the local authorities, there was a need to convince and get approval from local authorities, particularly the police, so that they understood the strategy and could work more closely with the establishment owners.

In August 1989 the project was started in the Ratchaburi province of Thailand. The province was selected because of the good understanding of the government authorities, especially the provincial governor, on the HIV/AIDS problem and their willingness to implement the 100 per cent condom use approach. There was a very fruitful collaboration from various sectors within the province. After a few months of implementation, it was found that the project was extremely successful. STI prevalence in sex workers dropped remarkably; in fact, it became rare among sex workers in the province.

After the successful implementation in Ratchaburi, the programme was gradually expanded to cover 13 provinces by mid-1991. The approach was found to be as successful in all participating provinces. In Samut Sakhon province (adjacent to Bangkok) the prevalence of STI in sex workers dropped from 13.5 per cent to 0 after the implementation (Figure 4.1). Similarly in Pitsanuloke, a northern province in Thailand, prevalence of STI in sex workers decreased from 30 per cent to 1 per cent (Figure 4.2). In August 1991 the 100 per cent condom use policy and its successful findings were presented to the National AIDS Committee chaired by the prime minister, and it was agreed to implement it in all provinces.

Figure 4.1
Prevalence of STI in Sex Workers in Samut Sakhon Province, Thailand, after Implementation of the 100 Per Cent Condom Use Programme

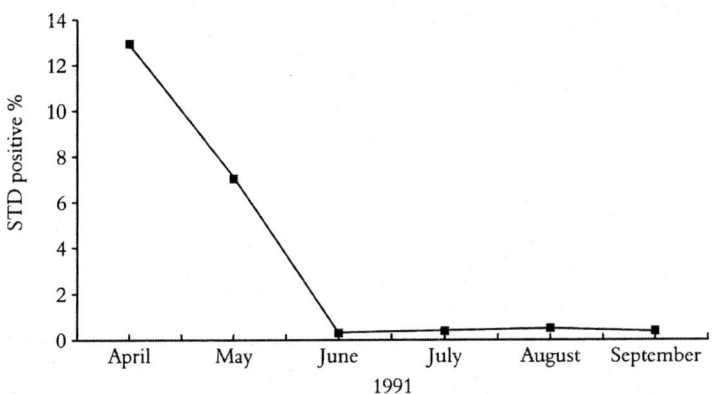

Source: Samut Sakhon Health Office.

How Does the Programme Work?

The principle of this programme is to gain cooperation from owners of all sex establishments to instruct or require their sex workers to use condoms in all sexual encounters. If their customers refuse to use a

Figure 4.2
Increase in Condom Use and Decrease in STDs among Sex Workers
During the 100 Per Cent Condom Use Intervention in Pitsanuloke, Thailand

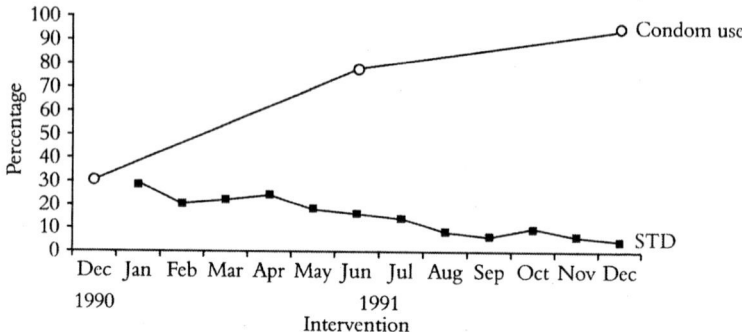

Source: Ministry of Public Health, Thailand.

condom, they are urged to withhold service and refund those customers' money. It is important that this measure must cover all sex establishments so that customers will not be able to purchase sex services without using condoms anywhere. Through this measure HIV transmission has been greatly reduced.

Steps to implement the 100 per cent condom use programme include holding of joint meetings between government officials and owners of all sex establishments to declare the initiation of this programme. Owners of sex establishments will be encouraged to prevent the disease by instructing or ordering their workers to use condoms in all sexual encounters and to withhold sex service to customers refusing condom use. They are informed to be aware of the methods of investigation into condom use that would be employed as part of the programme's monitoring process. Sanctions administered to those establishments found to be uncooperative include temporary and indefinite closure of their establishments by the police.

In the programme, condom use is monitored by a list of indicators, including:

- interviewing male STI patients on the source of infection;
- decoys posing as clients;
- regular screening of sex workers for STI; and
- condom supply or sales in entertainment establishments.

Although many sex workers in Thailand regularly attend STI clinic for health checks, the results of the examinations are used as evaluation indicators. In general, STI in sex workers can be the result of one of the following possibilities: (*a*) she did not use a condom and thus got the STI from her client; (*b*) she used condoms all the time, but one broke and she got the STI from such incident; or (*c*) she used condoms all the times with her customers, but not with her husband or boyfriend, and she got the STI from him. The Thai 100 per cent condom use programme mainly utilises information on condom use from male clients of STI clinics. Such information has been routinely collected in all STI clinics throughout the country since the beginning of the programme.

The Ministry of Public Health (MOPH) and some related organisations have supplied condoms to users at no cost since the introduction of this device in the national family planning programme 30 years before the AIDS epidemic. There are currently two main suppliers of condoms in the country: the MOPH supplying free condoms through its disease prevention and family planning infrastructure, and the private sector (chemists and various convenience stores) selling condoms to users through the market mechanism. The availability and accessibility of condoms have facilitated the implementation of the 100 per cent condom use programme.

The programme in its current form in Thailand is quite sustainable because it has been well integrated into existing health structures with a division of responsibility to avoid overburdening any one unit. This has also reduced the need for extensive special budgeting for the local health authorities beyond the provision of free condoms.

The programme has got quite a lot of attention in the last few years (Boonchalaksi et al. 1998; Chamratrithirong et al. 1998; WHO Western Pacific Regional Office 2000). One can see how popular the topic is by simply searching the Web using '100 per cent condom' as a search phrase. Over 1,000 leads can be observed by just a single search through a popular Internet search engine. Many of them provide information and discussion on the implementation and the success of the 100 per cent condom use programme in Thailand.

Effectiveness of the Programme

There has been a marked increase in condom use in sex establishments to a level as high as 95 per cent since December 1993 (Figure 4.3). The

Figure 4.3
Percentage of Condom Use among
Direct Sex Workers in Thailand: 1989–2001

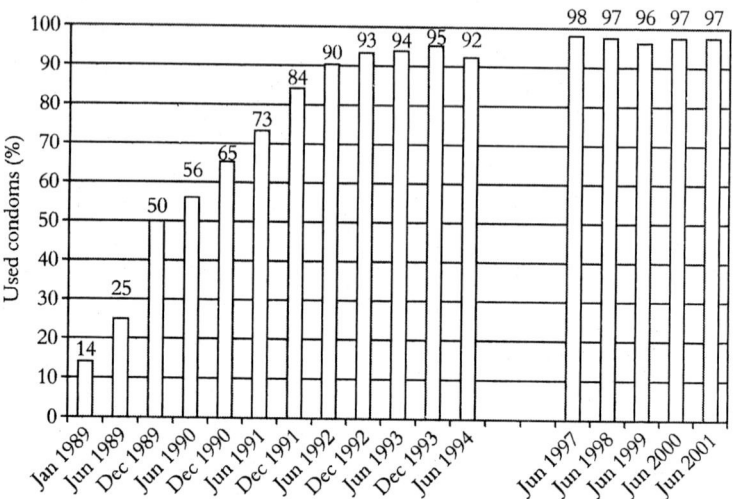

Source: Department of Communicable Disease Control (CDC), Ministry of Public Health, Thailand.

national incidence of STIs has decreased from 400,000 cases per year (6.5 per 1,000 population) in 1989 to fewer than 15,000 cases (0.25 per 1,000) in the year 2000, a reduction of over 95 per cent (Figure 4.4). On an average, the programme has prevented approximately over 260,000 STI cases per year in the government STI service system, plus three to four times more in patients attending private clinics and chemists.

Evidences of declining HIV prevalence are observed among various risk groups, including sex workers, male STI clients, blood donors and pregnant women. For example, the mean HIV prevalence rate among military conscripts has dropped from a peak of 4 per cent in 1993 to 1 per cent in 2000 (Figure 4.5). The decline in HIV prevalence has not been observed in the group with injecting drug use.

An independent research group came to Thailand in the mid-1990s to study the impact of the programme, and they concluded in their presentation at the International Conference on HIV/AIDS in Vancouver in 1996: 'The 100 per cent condom programme adopted by the Thai government may have already prevented more than 2 million HIV infections in Thailand.'

Figure 4.4
Number of STD Cases in Thailand: 1970–2001

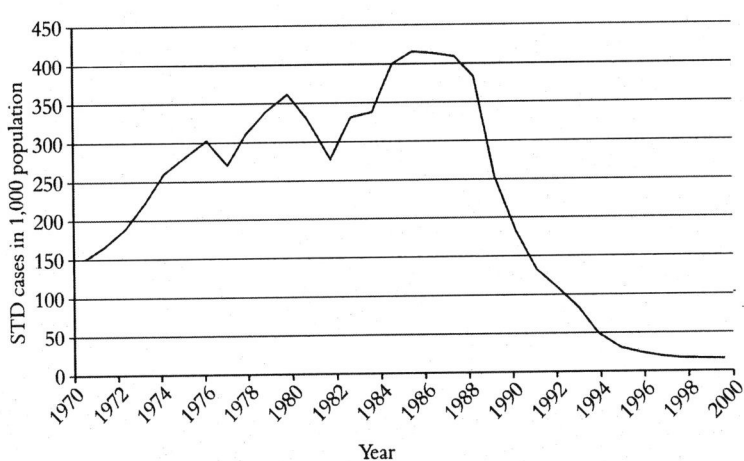

Source: CDC, Ministry of Public Health, Thailand.

Figure 4.5
HIV Prevalence among Young Thai Men
Entering the Royal Thai Army: 1989–2000

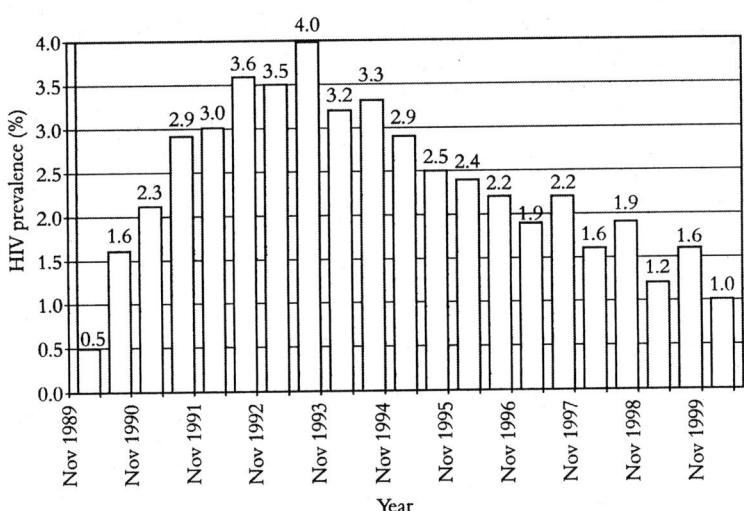

Source: CDC, Ministry of Public Health, Thailand.

The economic benefit of the programme is very obvious (UNAIDS/ MOPH 2000). The prevention of 260,000 STI cases per year in government clinics alone has resulted in saving of over 70 million baht a year, the amount that would have to be spent on STI drugs for patients. The amount saved is higher than the investment of 60 million baht used for the yearly procurement of condoms. This calculation does not include the saving of billions of baht that would have to be used to buy drugs for opportunistic infections and antiretroviral therapy if the 2 million HIV infections were not prevented.

In addition to health and economic benefits, the implementation of the 100 per cent condom use programme in Thailand has had many positive impacts on Thai society:

1. Sex work is decriminalised. The acceptance of the programme by the authorities is indirectly a sign of acceptance of sex work in the society. Although it is illegal in all countries in Asia, the authorities seem to accept the existence of the business as long as it does not spread HIV to the general population.

   Although prostitution is illegal in Thailand, the government's measures to solve the problem were mainly demand-and-supply reduction strategies, which were unable to control the existence of the sex business. The 100 per cent condom use programme utilises the 'harm reduction' strategy, and is found to be very effective in reducing health and social consequences resulting from sex work.

   Acceptance of the 100 per cent condom use programme by the Thai government does not mean sex work is legal. Sex business owners, pimps, customers and/or parents of sex workers will be arrested if one of the following conditions is detected: (a) managing a sex business involving a child (or so-called juvenile sex worker aged under 18); (b) forcing a woman to be chained or beaten to sell sex; and (c) the business involves an illegal immigrant. It should also be noted that under the current Prostitution Act revised a few years ago, sex workers will no longer be punished. Sex business owners, pimps, customers and parents of the sex workers will be the target of the punishment.

2. The programme promotes multi-sectoral collaboration and the role of non-health sectors, particularly the local administration

authority, the police and the business sector to work together in the fight against the HIV/AIDS epidemic.

3. The programme provides benefits to all sectors of society. It is a win-win strategy in the fight against HIV/AIDS. For example, (a) sex business owners get the same or higher level of income when, although with the same level of business as before, they have to incur less expenditure for STI care for their employees; (b) sex workers themselves get the benefit of the high level of income with very low or even no risk of acquiring STI and HIV; (c) clients of sex workers and their family members are free of HIV infection; (d) the health sector has a lower workload with regard to HIV/STI services; and (e) the province benefits from low prevalence of both HIV and STI in the general population.

4. Condom use is accepted as an important tool in preventing an HIV epidemic in the country. In general, many governments feel reluctant to promote condom use because of social and cultural reasons. However, the advantages of prevention of HIV and STI has changed the perception of governments, leading to a greater acceptance of condom promotion in their country.

5. The 100 per cent condom use programme does not place responsibility on sex workers. The people who take responsibility for ensuring condom use are the owners of the places. While sex workers can move to other locations very easily, sex establishments cannot. Therefore, owners themselves have to protect their own businesses by making sure that their workers use condoms in all sexual encounters. Since the nationwide implementation of the programme in 1991, there has not been a single case of an establishment being sanctioned. All owners are willing to participate in the programme because of the benefits they receive from it.

There is almost no negative side effect of the programme. Although it may not be effective in freelance type of sex service, it does not mean that the programme is not efficient. Additional strategies should be identified and implemented to cope with such situations. However, most sex services in Asia are of the establishment type, making it very suitable for many countries in the region.

Implementation of the
Programme in Other Asian Countries

Cambodia

In 1998, with the support of the WHO Western Pacific Regional Office, a 100 per cent condom use programme was piloted in Cambodia in a tourist province, Sihanoukville. The project has been very successful (WHO Western Pacific Regional Office 2001, 2002). Recent data from behavioural surveillance and STI prevalence studies in Cambodia confirm the initial observations of rapid impact on condom use and reduction of STI transmission. The behavioural surveillance survey in 1999 showed a significant trend in increasing condom use among both brothel-based sex workers and their clients. Among brothel-based sex workers condom use increased from 53.4 per cent in 1998 to 78.1 per cent in 1999. Treatment of STIs among sex workers brought down the incidence of syphilis from 9 per cent in 1998 to 1.8 per cent in 2000. The government of Cambodia is expanding the programme to cover the whole country. On 14 October 1999 the prime minister of Cambodia, Hun Sen, called upon the officials of the Royal Government and governors of all provinces and municipalities in the country to 'efficiently apply the 100 per cent condom use programme countrywide'.

The Philippines

The project was started in two cities (Angeles City and General Santos) in 1999. It was planned to expand to more sites in 2002.

Myanmar

A special project on the 100 per cent condom use strategy developed by the National AIDS Programme was approved by the Ministry of Health to be implemented in four cities: Bago, Pyay, Kawthoung and Tachilek. Financial support has been provided by UNAIDS South-East Asia and Pacific Inter-country Team (SEAPICT) through the United Nations Theme Group on HIV/AIDS. Wider expansion of the programme is currently under way in 10 other communities.

Vietnam

Two projects were initially developed by the Ministry of Health to implement the 100 per cent condom use strategy in two pilot sites: Ha Long Bay and Can Tho. The programme was subsequently expanded to Ha Tay, Thanh Hoa and Dong Nai. It is planned to cover all 21 provinces.

China

The 100 per cent condom use strategy is piloting in two sites in China (Wuhan in Hubei province, and Jiangsu in Jingjiang province). Two more provinces (Hunan and Hainan) are also starting the project.

Indonesia

In Indonesia the 100 per cent condom use programme was started in two sites: Jayapura and Merauke in Irian Jaya province.

Mongolia

The 100 per cent condom use approach was started in 2002 in Mongolia in Darkhan, a city close to the Russian border.

India, Bangladesh and Laos have shown an interest in the programme, but have not yet started any activity. The Dominican Republic, a country in Central America, has also reported implementation of the Thai approach.

Key Elements for Success

The following important lessons emerge from the experiences of the 100 per cent condom use programme in Thailand:

1. **Political commitment is needed at both national and local levels:** The strong national commitment increases programme participation by local government authorities, and they subsequently are able to engage the owners and managers of sex establishments in the programme. The adoption of a national policy of 100 per cent condom use coupled with aggressive efforts to enlist

the aid of provincial governors set the framework for active programmes at the local level and for using existing health and police infrastructures to ensure programme participation by sex establishments throughout the provinces.

2. **STD care and condom promotion synergistically support one another in such a programme:** The 100 per cent condom use programme has resulted in rapid reduction of STIs in almost every province in the country. At the same time, using existing sources of STD care to evaluate the programme has provided positive feedback, indicating that the efforts are making a difference. These synergistic interactions contribute in the expansion of both condom promotion and STI care efforts in the provinces, and help build support for the two programmes.

3. **Multi-sectoral cooperation among various sectors, including the involvement of the police and entertainment owners:** While some enforcement may be helpful in launching the programme, multi-sectoral cooperation is more effective for ensuring sustainability. The governor's backing and police cooperation clearly moved some establishment owners to participate in the early stages, and almost no sanctions have been applied. All concerned parties participated in the programme because of the obvious benefits that every sector obtained from its implementation.

4. **Certain sex work situations are favourable for the implementation of the 100 per cent condom use approach:** The 100 per cent condom use approach in Thailand works well because of the ability of local authorities to convince and prevail upon the owners of sex establishments. It would not be possible if the sex business was unorganised or existed in the form of street work.

5. **Adequate supply of good-quality condoms for the programme:** The MOPH and some related organisations supplied condoms to users at no cost as part of the national family planning programme, which began more than 30 years before the AIDS epidemic began. There are two main suppliers of condoms in the country, the MOPH supplying free condoms through its disease prevention and family planning infrastructure, and the private sector (chemists and various convenient stores) selling condoms to users through the market mechanism. The availability and accessibility of condoms has greatly facilitated the implementation of the programme.

6. **Integration of the programme into existing infrastructure:** The programme in its current form in Thailand is quite sustainable because it is well integrated within the existing health structures with a division of responsibility to avoid overburdening any one unit. This has also reduced the need for extensive special budgeting for the local health authorities beyond the provision of free condoms.

Conclusions

The inability of various strategies to control sexually-transmitted infections in sex workers in Thailand led to the implementation of a 100 per cent condom use programme in sex establishments with astounding success. The key elements for the success of the programme were a strong political commitment at both national and local levels; multi-sectoral cooperation among various sectors, including the involvement of the police and entertainment owners; adequate supply of good-quality condoms for the programme; and integration of the programme into existing infrastructure. The programme has brought down rates of STI as well as HIV prevalence. Many other countries have initiated efforts to replicate it as a major strategy to contain the spread of the HIV pandemic.

Finally, the 100 per cent condom use programme has received quite a lot of attention in the last few years. Over a thousand leads can be observed by just a single Internet search. Many of these provide information and discussions on the implementation and success of the 100 per cent condom use programme in Thailand and other countries implementing it.

[R] E F E R E N C E S

Boonchalaksi, Wathinee, Aphichat Chamratrithirong and **Philip Guest** (1998). 100 percent condom programme and the decline of sexually-transmitted diseases (STDs) in Thailand. Unpublished report, Institute for Population and Social Research, Mahidol University, Nakhon Pathom, Thailand.

Chamratrithirong, Aphichat, Varachai Thongthai, Wathinee Boonchalaksi, Philip Guest, Churnrutai Kanchanachitra and **Anchalee Varangrat** (1998). *The success of the 100% condom promotion programme in Thailand: Survey results of the evaluation of the 100% condom promotion programme* (IPSR Publication No. 238). Institute for Population and Social Research, Mahidol University, Nakhon Pathon, Thailand.

Rojanapithayakorn, W. and **R. Hanenberg** (1996). The 100 per cent condom programme in Thailand. *AIDS*, 10(1), 1–7.

UNAIDS/Ministry of Public Health (MOPH) (2000). *Evaluation of the 100% condom programme in Thailand* (UNAIDS case study). Geneva: UNAIDS.

UNAIDS/WHO (2003). *AIDS epidemic update*. December.

WHO Western Pacific Regional Office (2000). *100% condom use programme in entertainment establishment*. Manila: WHO.

——— (2001). *Controlling STI and HIV in Cambodia: The success of condom promotion*. Manila: WHO.

——— (2002). *Monitoring and evaluation of the 100% condom use programme in entertainment establishments*. Manila: WHO.

Management and Control of Sexually-Transmitted Infections and Their Implications for AIDS Control in South-East Asia | 5

Heiner Grosskurth and Gurumurthy Rangaiyan

Sexually-transmitted infections represent a major public health problem in developing countries worldwide. Nearly 50 million STIs occur annually in South-East Asian countries. Incidence of curable STIs in these countries varies from 7 to 9 cases per 100 women in the reproductive age (WHO 1997). Genital herpes infection, a treatable but incurable viral STI, is also highly prevalent at least in some Asian populations (Bogaerts et al. 2001). In addition, among women, non-sexually-transmitted reproductive tract infections (RTIs) such as bacterial vaginosis are very common, with reported prevalences of up to 47 per cent in the general population (Garg et al. 2001; Joesoef et al. 2001; Mathew et al. 2001).

Some countries in Asia currently face major STI epidemics. In a study from Cambodia, among women seeking antenatal care and other reproductive health services, 5 per cent suffered from cervical STI, 4 per cent from syphilis and 5 per cent were already HIV infected. Among policemen and military personnel, 6 per cent were found to have gonococcal or chlamydial urethritis, 4 per cent syphilis and 13 per cent HIV infection (Ryan et al. 1998). In China, surveillance data suggest that the incidence of syphilis increased about 20 times from 1989 to 1998, whilst the incidence of gonorrhoea tripled over the same period (X.S. Chen et al. 2000). All the ingredients for a major HIV epidemic are present in these countries, and substantial efforts are required to prevent such a disastrous development.

According to the *World Development Report 1993*, the burden of disease in women of childbearing age caused by STIs (without HIV infection) and RTIs is the second highest of all groups of diseases, surpassed only by maternity-related disorders (World Bank 1993). Medical complications and economic consequences rather than the acute infections make STI an important public health problem for women and their offspring. The complications include acute and chronic pelvic inflammatory disease, infertility, puerperal sepsis, ectopic pregnancy, miscarriage, stillbirth, preterm delivery, low birth weight and severe congenital infections (Laga 1994; Wasserheit 1989).

The public health importance of STIs has risen even more since it has been known that STI influences propagation and spread of HIV (Box 5.1).

Box 5.1
STI and HIV

STI increase:
Sexual transmission of HIV
Susceptibility to HIV
Infectiousness of HIV+ve cases
Shedding of HIV
Risk of acquisition

Whilst good case management of STIs and RTIs should be provided at the individual level at all times, the effective control of STI in early HIV epidemics, particularly among high-risk behaviour groups and bridging populations where STI prevalences are high, has the potential to prevent the generalisation of these epidemics, and is therefore of paramount importance (White et al. 2002). This is precisely the epidemiological situation that currently still prevails in most parts of Asia, including China and India, its most populous countries.

Case Management

Appropriate case management for STI comprises brief history, physical examination, correct diagnosis, early and effective treatment, health education to achieve good treatment compliance and sustainable risk reduction, and effective partner notification (Adler et al. 1998; WHO 2001).

Approaches to STI Diagnosis

There are three distinct approaches to arrive at an STI diagnosis: clinical, laboratory based and syndromic diagnosis.

The clinical approach attempts to arrive at a specific diagnosis based on clinical examination and to treat the assumed aetiology. This traditional approach has been widely used by care providers without access to laboratory services. However, many studies have demonstrated that the sensitivity and specificity of this strategy is low even in the hands of experienced providers (Holmes and Ryan 1999). For example, in a study from South Africa, clinicians diagnosed correctly only about one-third of men with chancroid and 10 per cent of patients with mixed aetiologies (Dangor et al. 1990). In a similar observation from China, 12 of 106 cases of syphilis were incorrectly classified as herpes genitalis, and did not receive the correct treatment (Wang et al. 2002). The clinical approach should, therefore, be abandoned.

The laboratory-based aetiological approach tries to identify the organism responsible for the symptoms a patient presents. A number of obstacles make this approach largely inappropriate for many areas in South-East Asia. Sufficiently equipped laboratories do not exist in rural communities and many smaller towns, and even in urban areas where they exist, quality control systems are often insufficient (WHO 2001). For some STIs, such as *Chlamydia trachomatis* infection, available tests are expensive, sophisticated or too insensitive.

The syndromic approach is based on the diagnosis of the syndrome, and deliberately does not attempt to identify the underlying aetiology. A syndrome is defined as a combination of symptoms and easily recognisable signs. Important STI/RTI syndromes are genital ulcers in men and women, urethral discharge syndrome in men, painful testicular swelling in men, vaginal discharge in women, lower abdominal pain in women and inguinal adenopathy (buboe) in men and women. Each STI/RTI syndrome can be caused by a variety of aetiological agents.

The syndromic approach to case management implies that all major likely aetiological causes of the presenting syndrome are treated simultaneously at the place and time of first contact of the patient with the health sector. This approach has been promoted by the World Health Organisation for more than a decade (WHO 1991).

Advantages of Syndromic STI/RTI Case Management

Delays in the initiation of treatment are avoided in syndromic management as patients do not need to wait for laboratory results. Second, because all major possible causes of STI/RTI syndromes are covered, cure is usually achieved early on. These advantages are important from a public health perspective: onward transmission is reduced, complications are prevented, clients are satisfied and their confidence in the health system strengthened.

The increased costs due to over-treatment of aetiological agents (that are not present in a particular patient) are outweighed by savings on laboratory costs. In a study of 1,500 hypothetical STI patients with different syndromes using decision-theory analysis, it has been demonstrated that both clinical and laboratory-based case management would cost two to three times as much as the syndromic approach (WHO 1993).

The treatment of STIs can be standardised with the help of algorithms, thus enabling paramedical staff to treat them effectively in areas where physicians are not available. The WHO has published a complete set of syndromic management algorithms and recommendations for the selection of drugs (WHO 2001). Syndromic case management thus allows STI treatment services to be integrated within the existing primary care system. The validity and the operational feasibility of this approach and its cost-effectiveness in reducing new HIV infection have been demonstrated in studies in Asia and elsewhere (Chilongozi et al. 1996; Djajakusumah et al. 1998; Grosskurth et al. 2000; Hong et al. 2002).

The effectiveness of specific algorithms depends on the correct choice of drugs to be included. The WHO has emphasised that the recommended algorithms should not be applied blindly, but have to be adapted to the specific local epidemiological and anti-microbial sensitivity pattern (WHO 2001). It is, therefore, essential that countries monitor these patterns and that algorithms are constructed based on sound surveillance data. Each country should have at least one reference clinic and laboratory that have access to primary care STI/RTI patients, and large countries require more than one such sentinel site. Unfortunately, this essential requisite is often lacking.

A study conducted at rural child health/family planning clinics in Bangladesh has recently demonstrated the importance of this principle. Women who presented with vaginal discharge were examined to identify the causative agents of their complaints. Only about 30 per cent of the 320 participating women had detectable infections, most of which were caused by bacterial vaginosis and candidiasis. Cervical infections due to *Neisseria gonorrhoeae* and *Chlamydia trachomatis* were found in only three women. The application of the unadapted WHO algorithm that is presently in use in Bangladesh would lead to a high rate of over-treatment, and almost 90 per cent of programme costs would be spent on uninfected women. In addition, women diagnosed as having an STI are potentially exposed to matrimonial conflicts or even violence. Clearly, local adaptation of the algorithm is required, and this particular case should take other causes for abnormal vaginal discharge, such as potential side effects of contraceptive use, into consideration.

Disadvantages of the Syndromic Approach

Not rarely, physicians who are familiar with the classical diagnostic principle, whereby treatment should always be based on a precise diagnosis, have difficulties in accepting a method they perceive as 'unscientific' (Kumar et al. 1995) or 'Third World medicine'. However, few procedures recommended in the context of disease management in developing countries are based on so much careful research as the syndromic management of STI (Chilongozi et al. 1996; Grosskurth et al. 2000; Mayaud et al. 1997).

The main problem, however, lies in the management of cervical infections due to *Neisseria gonorrhoeae* (NG) and *Chlamydia trachomatis* (CT). Because NG and CT are the most dangerous infective agents of the female reproductive tract, and because they occasionally present as vaginal discharge, their treatment is often included in algorithms for the management of the vaginal discharge syndrome. Unfortunately, these infections are usually asymptomatic, and seem to cause clinical symptoms in less than 15 per cent. Such algorithms have a high sensitivity because all genuine cervical infections will be treated, but a very low specificity, as many women will be treated unnecessarily. For example, in a study from Bangladesh, 97 per cent of women were unnecessarily treated (Bogaerts et al. 1999). On the other hand, the sensitivity would be zero if the treatment of NG and CT were not included in the algorithm.

An attempt to overcome this problem has been made through the introduction of a risk assessment step into algorithms for the management of vaginal discharge syndrome, hoping that this would increase the algorithms' specificity for NG and CT infection without losing much sensitivity (Mayaud et al. 1998; WHO 2001). Risk assessment refers to parameters known to be associated with an increased risk of cervical infection. Questions are, for example, asked about the age of the patient (for example, less than 21 years), about marital status (unmarried; new partner in the previous three months), about the number of partners during the recent past, recent use of condoms and whether the partner himself has a discharge or ulcer. The validity of this approach has been evaluated in a variety of settings, but the results are not at all encouraging, unfortunately. Whilst the specificity of this approach is often higher than 90 per cent, its sensitivity in detecting cervical infections ranged only from 5 to 46 per cent in studies from India, Myanmar and Tanzania (Department of Health, Myanmar and Population Council 2002; Mayaud et al. 1998; Vishwanath et al. 2000).

Rapid Diagnostic Tests for the Detection of STI

A final solution to this dilemma will only be found once inexpensive, simple and accurate diagnostic tests for the detection of cervical infections become available. Such tests should be suitable for use in primary care facilities and provide an immediate result (Peeling 2001). Although there are currently over 40 such test kits, some of which are now commercially available, there is so far very little information on the efficacy of their use in primary health care (PHC) settings, and little data on their effectiveness (sensitivity, specificity, etc.) and utility when applied in developing countries.

A programme has been launched recently by the WHO Special Programme for Research and Training in Tropical Diseases (WHO/TDR) to address this issue. The programme, called the Sexually Transmitted Diseases Diagnostics Initiative (SDI), promotes the development and evaluation of rapid tests for the detection of gonorrhoea, *Chlamydia* infection and syphilis at PHC level in developing countries.

STI Control at Population Level

Good case management is essential, but without a bundle of other measures it is insufficient to control STI in populations. This becomes evident when the chain of events is considered that leads to infection and from there to possible cure, as visualised in Figure 5.1. This model is adapted from a similar one originally developed by Marc Piot for tuberculosis control.

Figure 5.1
Piot's Model on STIs

Only a small proportion of individuals with STIs in a population reach effective treatment services, and an even smaller proportion will become and remain cured. This model also shows the various potential points for STI interventions. Although effective STI services are important, the greatest effect may actually be achieved through interventions directed to the upper parts of the cascade, particularly if focused on groups exposed to high-risk behaviours.

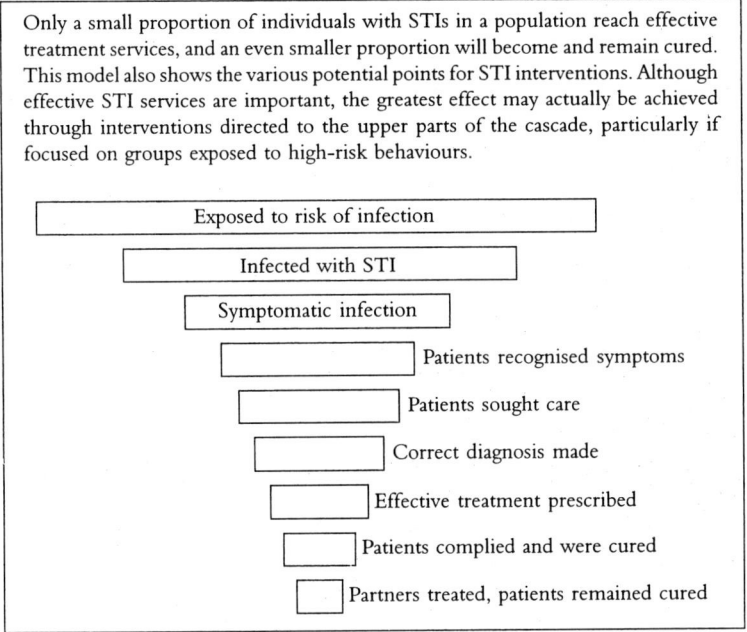

The model can also be used to systematically consider the options available for STI control (Adler et al. 1998). These are:

- primary prevention of STIs in those who are not (yet) infected;
- screening for individuals with asymptomatic infections;
- screening for patients with symptomatic but neglected STIs;
- improvement of treatment-seeking behaviour;
- improvement of STI treatment services; and
- improvement of partner notification and treatment.

In many countries STI control programme planners traditionally focused on the last steps of the cascade, neglecting the initial ones, although these obviously determine the epidemiological situation. As argued above, the impact of STI control programmes on the HIV epidemic will be particularly strong if they are directed towards high-risk behaviour groups and bridging populations. STI and HIV rates among sex workers in Asia are often very high. For example, the prevalences of gonorrhoea were 39 per cent, 32 per cent, 36 per cent and 24 per cent among sex workers from Cambodia, Papua New Guinea, Bangladesh and Indonesia respectively (Joesoef et al. 1997; Mgone et al. 2002; Rahman et al. 2000; Ryan et al. 1998). STI control among sex workers and their clients is clearly a priority in all these populations.

The enormous effect that can be achieved if well-designed interventions are directed towards primary prevention has been demonstrated in Thailand. Regular voluntary screening of sex workers for STI is known to reduce the rate of infection, and is well accepted by the target population. In a study from Abidjan, the capital of Ivory Coast, monthly clinical STI screening and treatment of sex workers including condom promotion led to a sustainable decline of STI and to a steep reduction in the incidence rate of new HIV infections from 16.3 to 5.3 per 100 person-years (Ghys et al. 2002). Such services should be offered in a voluntary and non-coercive manner, which in turn requires that sex work is at least tolerated if not legalised, so that women are not afraid of using these services.

Campaigns to improve the treatment-seeking behaviour for STI care are also important. In many cases patients do not recognise symptoms and delay treatment for many months (Aggarwal et al. 1998). Occasionally genital discharge syndromes are so highly prevalent that discharge is perceived as a physiological expression of sexual maturity rather than as a sign of an infection.

In high-risk groups, because of the high proportion of asymptomatic cervical infections, it may be justified to combine good STI treatment services for symptomatic patients with regular presumptive treatment. This strategy has been employed successfully in several mining communities of South Africa. Sex workers were given a directly observed treatment of 1 g azithromycin for bacterial STI at monthly intervals, regardless whether they had STI symptoms or not. This intervention led to a two- to four-fold decline of various STI among both sex workers themselves and among the male mining population within the same community (Steen et al. 2000).

Screening programmes in general populations to detect asymptomatic Chlamydia infection have been introduced in some industrialised countries (Mangione-Smith et al. 1999). Such programmes are expensive and may not be feasible under the prevailing conditions in developing countries. However, this may change once rapid diagnostic tests become available. Regular screening of pregnant women for latent syphilis is known to be feasible and highly cost effective (Hira et al. 1990). Integration of effective STI treatment services into the primary care system has been shown to substantially reduce STI *and* the rate of new HIV infections in the general sexually active population in a randomised trial from Mwanza, Tanzania (Grosskurth et al. 2000).

An alternative option would be to treat the entire sexually active population in areas with high STI prevalence. This concept has been evaluated in the population-based trial from Rakai district, Uganda (Wawer et al. 1999). Interestingly, the intervention resulted in a substantial reduction of some STIs, but had no impact on the rate of new HIV infections. Another community-based HIV intervention trial with two intervention arms, recently completed in neighbouring Masaka district, Uganda, found that improved STI services led to a reduction in infection and that a behavioural intervention resulted in an increase of condom use. However, again, none of these interventions was able to reduce the rate of new HIV infections in this setting (Kamali et al. 2001). This is possibly because of the level and intensity of the HIV epidemic in this area.

The Herpetic Connection

A comparative analysis of populations and risk factors from two high and two low HIV prevalence cities in Africa showed that two factors were significantly associated with a high HIV prevalence: a lack of circumcision in men and a high prevalence of genital herpes (Weiss et al. 2001). In South Africa, herpes simplex virus-2 (HSV-2) infections are now the leading cause for genital ulcers (C.Y. Chen et al. 2000), and this was also the case in the Rakai trial population mentioned above (Wawer et al. 1999). Herpetic ulcers enhance HIV acquisition in HIV-negative persons, and are a source of HIV shedding in HIV-infected individuals. Treatment of herpetic ulcers reduces HIV shedding.

On the other hand, HIV infection increased both the shedding of HSV-2 in genital fluids and the frequency of recurrence of herpetic lesions in HSV-2-infected persons (C.Y. Chen et al. 2000). The sexual transmission of genital herpes does not only occur in the presence of herpetic ulcers, but frequently also through asymptomatic carriers (Casper and Wald 2002). Advanced HIV infection also increases the duration and the size of herpetic lesions. The two infections seem to enhance each other, thus forming a vicious circle that drives populations deeper and deeper into the HIV epidemic.

All this has several consequences. First, national AIDS control programmes in South-East Asia should gather data on the prevalence of HSV-2 infections in general populations and high-risk groups. This will enable them to detect sub-populations that are particularly vulnerable to the HIV epidemic and to launch targeted behavioural and biomedical interventions that aim to prevent local epidemics.

Second, it is obvious that STI/HIV control programmes directed at bacterial STIs will have only limited effects in areas with high incidence of genital herpes. Interventions to reduce the incidence of herpes would be important. Recent studies have demonstrated that consistent condom use can protect against herpes acquisition (Casper and Wald 2002).

Third, at present most syndromic treatment algorithms for genital ulcers do not include an option to provide patients who have herpetic lesions with anti-herpetic therapy through antiviral drugs such as acyclovir or valacyclovir. This policy should be reconsidered for populations with high HIV prevalences, and high incidences and prevalences of herpetic ulcers.

And, last, a trial to determine the effectiveness of anti-herpetic suppressive therapy (provided to HSV-infected persons) on the incidence of HIV infection among sex workers and their clients should be seriously considered. The results will be highly relevant to AIDS control policies, as the impact of such an intervention on HIV transmission is potentially enormous in populations with high HSV-2 prevalences and still low or moderately advanced HIV epidemics. The same would apply to trials of vaccines against HSV infection. Unfortunately, such vaccines are not yet available, and their development should be another top priority.

Responses to STI in South-East Asia

Until the advent of the HIV epidemic in the region and for several years thereafter, the public health response to STI in South-East Asia was weak or almost invisible in most countries, although some had national STI control programmes for more than two or three decades, for example, Thailand and India (Limpaphayom 1996; NACO 2002). These programmes focused on case management of STIs, thus mainly employing a clinical rather than a public health approach. In response to the advancing HIV pandemic, all countries in South and South-East Asia established national HIV/AIDS programmes, which usually also comprised an STI control component. However, national responses have not been uniform with respect to intensity or success. For example, there is a wide variation in the level of political commitment, the adequacy of funding and the coverage achieved within countries. In some countries, however, comprehensive control programmes have been launched and can be considered successes. Thailand and Cambodia have shown that strong government commitment, early and adequate responses with substantial funding, and targeted interventions can have a tangible effect on the STI and HIV epidemics (Limpaphayom 1996). For example, in Thailand, the incidence of STI reportedly decreased from 7.85 per 1,000 population in 1986 to 2.07 in 1992 (ibid.). The policy documents of most national AIDS control programmes in the region include some STI control components, but no country has a central task force with the executive powers required to mount a national STI control programme with all its required components, including systematic intervention planning, drug supply, training, supervision, monitoring and evaluation. Such comprehensive programmes with certain vertically organised components are clearly desirable in the face of the accelerating HIV epidemics that most countries in the region are presently confronted with.

There is also little international coordination of control efforts. Systematic surveillance of anti-microbial resistance development for important aetiological agents such as *Neisseria gonorrhoeae* is not in place in the region. Whilst gonococcal resistance is monitored in some places (Divekar et al. 1999; Lesmana et al. 2001; Rahman et al. 2002), these efforts seem to be isolated rather than coordinated. A systematic monitoring programme such as the one in the WHO's Western Pacific Region (Tapsall 2000) is still to be established.

Monitoring and Evaluation of STI/RTI Case Management Services

While sound recommendations for the effective case management of STIs and RTIs at a peripheral level as described above have been widely promoted in South-East Asia over the last 10 years or so, evaluations show that reality is quite sobering. For example, in a study from Chennai, India, 84 per cent of 108 private physicians reported that they treated STI patients based on a clinical aetiological diagnosis (Mertens 1998). The treatment prescribed was effective in only about 12 to 20 per cent of the time, depending on the prevailing syndrome. In only 30 per cent of the consultations was condom use promoted, and only 1 per cent of the patients actually received condoms. Health education was given to only 12 per cent of patients, and only 27 per cent were asked to refer their partners for treatment.

In 1998 one of the authors was asked to evaluate four STI control projects in India. The evaluation showed that effective case management was in place in 12 clinics, which were all part of a centrally coordinated project. In all of these a standardised set of syndromic flowcharts was used and was easily available on the desk of all clinicians. There was regular supervision, and aetiologies were monitored at larger intervals. However, in another nine clinics run by other projects, physicians claimed to use syndromic case management, but in reality some sort of clinical diagnosis was made, and a broad variety of treatment regimens given of which only about 60 per cent were likely to be effective. Good planning, training, monitoring, supervision and regular critical feedback are all essential ingredients to ensure the effectiveness of STI treatment.

In South-East Asia most STI and RTI patients seek help from private providers rather than from the public sector. National programmes and professional organisations need to make a major effort to ensure the adoption of up-to-date case management procedures to STI care by these providers. Most patients may not even reach clinically skilled and certified providers. Instead, they seek care from pharmacies and private providers without formal training who provide a huge variety of allopathic drugs. During such consultations ineffective drugs are often provided, health education is almost never given, and partner notification is rarely encouraged (Benjarattaporn et al. 1997; Tuladhar et al. 1998). Regular campaigns to educate the public (and providers) may improve this unfortunate situation.

Clearly, in many parts of Asia there is a need to evaluate existing services and to use the results for interventions aiming to improve these services. The WHO developed a set of 'prevention indicators' (called PI 6 and PI 7) that can be used in health facility surveys to evaluate the quality of service with respect to clinical management and health promotion (Mertens 1998; WHO 1994).

REFERENCES

Adler, M., S. Foster, H. Grosskurth, J. Richens and H. Slavin (1998). Sexual health and care: Sexually transmitted infections—Guidelines for prevention and treatment. Occasional paper, DFID Health and Population, London.

Aggarwal, A.K., R. Kumar, V. Gupta and M. Sharma (1998). Community based study of RTIs among ever married women of reproductive age in a rural area of Haryana, India. *Journal of Communicable Diseases*, 31(4), 223–28.

Benjarattaporn, P., C. Lindan, S. Mills, J. Barclay, A. Bennett, D. Mugrditchian, J. Mandel, P. Pongswatanakulsiri and T. Warnnisorn (1997). Men with sexually-transmitted diseases in Bangkok: Where do they go for treatment and why? *AIDS*, 11(Supplement 1), S87–95.

Bogaerts, J., J. Ahmed, N. Akhter, N. Begum, M. Rahman, S. Nahar, M. Van Ranst and J. Verhaegen (2001). Sexually-transmitted infections among married women in Dhaka, Bangladesh: Unexpected high prevalence of herpes simplex type 2 infection. *Sexually Transmitted Infections*, 77(2), 114–19.

Bogaerts, J., J. Ahmed, N. Akhter, N. Begum, M. Van Ranst and J. Verhaegen (1999). Sexually-transmitted infections in a basic health care clinic in Dhaka, Bangladesh: Syndromic management for cervicitis is not justified. *Sexually Transmitted Infections*, 75(6), 437–38.

Casper, C. and A. Wald (2002). Condom use and the prevention of genital herpes acquisition, *Herpes*, 9, 10–14.

Chen, C.Y., R.C. Ballard, C.M. Beck-Sague, Y. Dangor, F. Radebe, S. Schmid, J.B. Weiss, V. Tshabalala, G. Fehler, Y. Htun and S.A. Morse (2000). Human immunodeficiency virus infection and genital ulcer disease in South Africa: The herpetic connection. *Sexually Transmitted Diseases*, 27(1), 21–29.

Chen, X.S., X. Gong, G. Liang and G. Zang (2000). Epidemiologic trends of sexually-transmitted diseases in China. *Sexually Transmitted Diseases*, 27(3), 138–42.

Chilongozi, D.A., C.C. Daly, L. Franco, N.G. Liomba and G. Dallabetta (1996). Sexually-transmitted diseases: A survey of case management in Malawi. *International Journal of STD and AIDS*, 7(4), 269–75.

Dangor, Y., R. Ballard, F.L. Exposto, G. Fehler, S.D. Miller and H.J. Koornhof (1990). Accuracy of clinical diagnosis of genital ulcer disease. *Sexually Transmitted Diseases*, 17(4), 184–89.

Department of Health, Myanmar and Population Council (2002). *Reproductive tract infections in Mandalay clinics, Myanmar: A cross-sectional prevalence and cost-analysis study*. Bangkok: Population Council.

Divekar, A.A., A.S. Gogate and L.K. Shivkar (1999). Association between auxotypes, serogroups, and antibiotic susceptibilities of *Neisseria gonorrhoeae* isolated from women in Mumbai, India. *Sexually Transmitted Diseases*, 26(6), 358–63.

Djajakusumah, T., S. Sudigdoadi, K. Keersmaekers and A. Meheus (1998). Evaluation of syndromic patient management algorithm for urethral discharge. *Sexually Transmitted Infections*, 74(Supplement 1), S29–33.

Garg, S., P. Bhalla, N. Sharma, R. Sahay, A. Puri, R. Saha, P. Sodhani, N. Murthy and M. Mehra (2001). Comparison of self-reported symptoms of gynaecological morbidity with clinical and laboratory diagnosis in a New Delhi slum. *Asia-Pacific Population Journal*, 16, 75–92.

Ghys, P.D., M.O. Diallo, V. Ettiegne-Traore, K. Kale, O. Tawil, M. Carael, M. Traore, G. Mah-Bi, K.M. De Cock, S.Z. Wiktor, M. Laga and A.E. Greenberg (2002). Increase in condom use and decline in HIV and sexually-transmitted diseases among female sex workers in Abidjan, Cote d'Ivoire, 1991–98. *AIDS*, 16(2), 251–58.

Grosskurth, H., E. Mwijarubi, J. Todd, M. Rwakatare, K. Orroth, P. Mayaud, B. Cleophas, A. Buve, R. Mkanje, L. Ndeki, A. Gavyole, R. Hayes and D. Mabey (2000). Operational performance of an STD control programme in Mwanza region, Tanzania. *Sexually Transmitted Infections*, 76, 426–36.

Hira, S.K., G.J. Bhat, D.M. Chikamata, B. Nkowane, G. Tembo, P.L. Perine and A. Meheus (1990). Syphilis intervention in pregnancy: Zambian demonstration project. *Genitourinary Medicine*, 66(3), 159–64.

Holmes, K.K. and C. Ryan (1999). STD care management. In K.K. Holmes, P.H. Sparling, P. Mardh, S. Lemon, W. Stamm, P. Piot and J. Wasserheit (eds.), *Sexually Transmitted Diseases*. New York: McGraw-Hill.

Hong, S., C. Xin, Y. Qianhong, W. Yanan, X. Wenyan, R. Peeling and D. Mabey (2002). Pelvic inflammatory disease in the People's Republic of China: Aetiology and management. *International Journal of STD and AIDS*, 13(8), 568–72.

Joesoef, M.R., M. Linnan, Y. Barakbah, A. Idajadi, A. Kambodji and K. Schulz (1997). Patterns of STDs in female sex workers in Surabaya, Indonesia. *International Journal of STD and AIDS*, 8(9), 576–80.

Joesoef, M.R., A. Karundeng, C. Runtupalit, J. Moran, J. Lewis and C. Ryan (2001). High rate of bacterial vaginosis among women with intrauterine device in Manado, Indonesia. *Contraception*, 64(3), 169–72.

Kamali, A. et al. (2001). Preliminary results of the Masaka HIV intervention study. Oral presentation at a technical consultation on STI case management. WHO, Geneva.

Kumar, B., S. Handa and G. Dawn (1995). Syndromic management of genital ulcer disease: A critical appraisal. *Genitourinary Medicine*, 71(3), 197.

Laga, M. (1994). Epidemiology and control of sexually transmitted diseases in developing countries. *Sexually Transmitted Diseases*, 21(Supplement 1), S45–50.

Lesmana, M., C.I. Lebron, D. Taslim, P. Tjaniadi, D. Subekti, M. O. Wasfy, J.R. Campbell and B.A. Oyofo (2001). In vitro antibiotic susceptibility of *Neisseria gonorrhoeae* in Jakarta, Indonesia. *Antimicrobial Agents and Chemotherapy*, 45, 359–62.

Limpaphayom, K. (1996). Status of STD screening, diagnosis and treatment in Thailand: Issues in management of STDs in family planning setting workshop proceedings, http://www.jhpiego.org/pubs/STD/stdproc.htm.

Mangione-Smith, R., J. O'Leary and E. McGlynn (1999). Health and cost-benefits of chlamydia screening in young women. *Sexually Transmitted Diseases*, 26(6), 309–16.

Mathew, R., J. Kalyani, R. Bibi and M. Mallika (2001). Prevalence of bacterial vaginosis in antenatal women. *Indian Journal of Pathology and Microbiology*, 44, 113–16.

Mayaud, P., F. Mosha, J. Todd, R. Balira, J. Mgara, B. West, M. Rusizoka, E. Mwijarubi, R. Gabone, A. Gavyole, H. Grosskurth, R. Hayes and D. Mabey (1997). Improved treatment services significantly reduce the prevalence of sexually-transmitted diseases in rural Tanzania: Results of a randomised controlled trial. *AIDS*, 11(15), 1873–80.

Mayaud, P., E. Uledi, J. Cornelissen, G. ka-Gina, J. Todd, M. Rwakatare, B. West, L. Kopwe, D. Manoko, H. Grosskurth, R. Hayes and D. Mabey (1998). Risk-scores to detect cervical infections in urban antenatal clinic attenders in Mwanza, Tanzania. *Sexually Transmitted Infections*, 74(Supplement 1), S139–46.

Mertens, T. (1998). Observations of sexually-transmitted disease consultations in India. *Public Health*, 112(2), 123–28.

Mgone, C., M. Passey, J. Anang, W. Peter, T. Lupiwa, D. Russell, D. Babona and M. Alpers (2002). HIV and other STIs among female sex workers in two major cities in Papua New Guinea. *Sexually Transmitted Diseases*, 29(15), 265–70.

National AIDS Control Organisation India (NACO) (2002). http://naco.nic.in/vsnaco/nacp/program/prog2.htm.

Peeling, R.W. (2001). The public health impact of rapid STI diagnostics: Promises and challenges. Symposium at the International Congress of Sexually Transmitted Infections, 24–27 June.

Rahman, M., A. Alam, K. Nessa, A. Hopssain, S. Nahar, D. Datta, S. Khan, R. Mian and J. Albert (2000). Etiology of STI among street-based female sex workers in Dhaka, Bangladesh. *Journal of Clinical Microbiology*, 38(3), 1244–46.

Rahman, M., Z. Sultan, S. Monira, A. Alam, K. Nessa, S. Islam, S. Nahar, Shama-A-Waris, S. Alam Khan, J. Bogaerts, N. Islam and J. Albert (2002). Antimicrobial susceptibility of *Neisseria gonorrhoeae* isolated in Bangladesh (1997 to 1999): Rapid shift to fluoroquinolone resistance. *Journal of Clinical Microbiology*, 40(16), 2037–40.

Ryan, C.A., O. Vathiny, P. Gorbach, H. Leng, A. Berlioz-Arthaud, W. Whittington and K. Holmes (1998). Explosive spread of HIV-1 and sexually-transmitted diseases in Cambodia. *Lancet*, 351, 1175.

Steen, R. et al. (2000). Evidence of declining STD prevalence in a South African mining community following a core-group intervention. *Sexually Transmitted Diseases*, 27(1), 1–8.

Tapsall, L.W. (2000). Surveillance of antibiotic resistance in *Neisseria gonorrhoeae* in the WHO Western Pacific Region, 1998: The WHO Western Pacific Gonococcal Antimicrobial Surveillance Programme. *Communicable Disease Intelligence*, 24(1), 1–4.

Tuladhar, S., S. Mills, S. Acharya, M. Pradhan, J. Pollock and G. Dallabetta (1998). The role of pharmacists in HIV/STD prevention: Evaluation of an STD syndromic management intervention in Nepal. *AIDS*, 12(Supplement 2), S81–87.

Vishwanath, S., V. Talwar, R. Prasad, K. Coyaji, C. Elias and I. de Zoysa (2000). Syndromic management of vaginal discharge among women in a reproductive health clinic in India. *Sexually Transmitted Infections*, 76(4), 303–6.

Wang, Q.Q., D. Mabey, R. Peeling, M. Tan, D. Jian, P. Yang, M. Zhong and G. Wang (2002). Validation of syndromic algorithm for the management of genital ulcer diseases in China. *International Journal of STD and AIDS*, 13(7), 469–74.

Wasserheit, J. (1989). The significance and scope of reproductive tract infections among third world women. *International Journal of Gynecology* and *Obstetrics*, Supplement 3, 145–68.

Wawer, M.J. et al. (1999). Control of sexually-transmitted diseases for AIDS prevention in Uganda: A randomised community trial. *Lancet*, 353(9152), 525–35.

Weiss, H.A., A. Buve, N.J. Robinson, E. Van Dyck, M. Kahindo, S. Anagonou, R. Musonda, L. Zekeng, L. Morison, M. Carael, M. Laga and R.J. Hayes (2001).

Study group on heterogeneity of HIV epidemics in African cities: The epidemiology of HSV-2 infection and its association with HIV infection in four urban African populations. *AIDS*, 15(Supplement 4), S97–108.

White, R., K. Orroth, E. Korenromp, R. Bakker, M. Wambura, D.F. Serwadda, J. Whitworth, R. Gray, H. Grosskurth, D. Habbema and **R. Hayes** (2002). Effects of population characteristics on the impact of STD/HIV control strategies. Oral presentation at the 14th International AIDS Conference, Barcelona (abstract MoOrD1087).

WHO (1991). Management of patients with sexually-transmitted diseases. Report of a WHO Study Group, World-Health-Organ-Tech-Rep-Ser., 810, pp. 1–103.

———— (1993). Analysis of the cost-effectiveness of approaches to STD control. Informal Technical Working Group Meeting on STD activities in GPA, background paper No. 4, WHO/GPA, Geneva, February.

———— (1994). Global programme on AIDS: Protocol for the assessment of STD case management through health facility surveys. WHO GPA/TCO/SEF/94.1, Geneva.

———— (1997). Reproductive health in Southeast Asia region. WHO-Regional Office of SE Asia, http://www.hsph.harvard.edu/grhf/Sasia/suchana/0628/whoregional/html.

———— (2001). Guidelines for the management of sexually-transmitted infections. WHO/HIV_AIDS/2001.01,WHO/RHR/01.10, Geneva.

World Bank (1993). *World Development Report 1993: Investing in Health*. New York: Oxford University Press.

6

THE '3 BY 5' INITIATIVE: CHALLENGES AND OPPORTUNITIES FOR ASIA

Jai P. Narain and Charles F. Gilks

The human immunodeficiency virus is the leading cause of death among adults in the world (WHO 2003a). AIDS, if untreated has a case fatality rate that approaches 100 per cent. It has devastated families and societies, and caused untold suffering in the most heavily burdened regions. In hard-hit areas, including some of the poorest parts of the world, HIV has reversed gains in life expectancy registered in the last three decades of the 20th century. According to the World Bank, AIDS could lead to economic collapse in Africa by destroying human capital over three generations, especially killing young adults at their prime; decreasing quality of childrearing, resulting in children dropping out of school; and finally children of AIDS victims being less able to raise their own children and to invest in their education.

Besides having enormous health and economic impact in Africa and parts of Asia, HIV also fuels other epidemics of global concern—most notably tuberculosis, which has become a leading cause of death not only among people living with HIV, but also among their HIV-negative family members and contacts. But AIDS is not the same everywhere. Access to effective prevention and treatment, and consequently the fates suffered by individuals infected with HIV, vary widely. People living with HIV who benefit from the latest medical developments can hope to lead normal lives in many respects. The use of combination chemotherapy with antiretroviral (ARV) agents improves survival and renders AIDS a chronic and treatable disease (Figure 6.1).

Thus, while many people with AIDS living in the industrialised and some middle-income countries can lead normal lives, where deaths

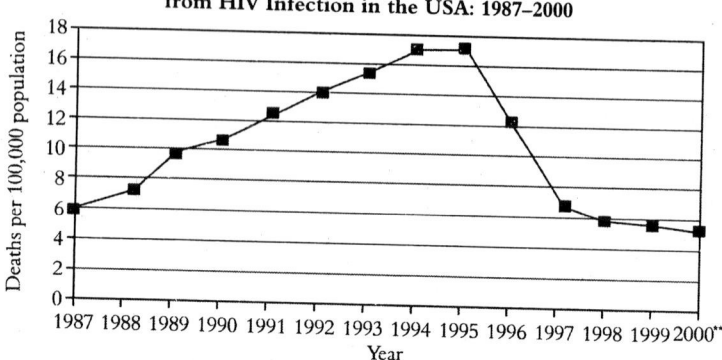

Figure 6.1
Trends in Age-adjusted* Rate of Death
from HIV Infection in the USA: 1987–2000

Source: Centres for Disease Control and Prevention.
Notes: *Using the year 2000 US standard population; **Preliminary mortality data for 2000.

due to AIDS have declined over the past years thanks primarily to their access to antiretroviral treatment (ART), in developing countries on the other hand HIV remains a death sentence and those with AIDS die within a year. This treatment gap between developed and developing countries, between the haves and the have-nots, is inequitable and unacceptable. Bridging the gap is, therefore, not only a programme necessity but also a moral, ethical and human right imperative.

The HIV/AIDS Epidemic and the Treatment Gap

AIDS was first described in 1981, when previously healthy homosexual men in the United States began falling ill with bizarre opportunistic infections previously unknown among this group but indicative of an acquired immunodeficiency syndrome (hence the acronym AIDS). Similar infections were soon described in Africa, the Caribbean and Europe. AIDS was clearly an epidemic disease. Most of these young people died. Soon the virus now called the human immunodeficiency virus or HIV was identified. By the time accurate HIV testing was available, it was apparent that the virus had already spread silently throughout the world, to every continent and all countries.

The most recent estimates from WHO/UNAIDS show that as of December 2003, 40 million people were living with HIV/AIDS and another 31 million had already died of AIDS worldwide (WHO/ UNAIDS 2003). During 2003 alone, some 5 million people became infected with HIV, and almost 3 million people died of AIDS. Despite remarkable scientific achievements over the past two decades, the virus has continued to spread relentlessly.

Africa is hardest hit where the spread of the pandemic has been accelerated by a variety of factors, including widespread poverty, gender inequality and weak health systems. Africa is home to more than 70 per cent of those currently infected with HIV. Of all AIDS deaths worldwide—28 million at the end of 2002—the majority have also occurred on this continent. Next to Sub-Saharan Africa, Asia is the region where nearly 7 million people are currently living with HIV/AIDS. In 2003, 1 million Asians became infected with HIV and nearly a third of a million died (WHO 2003b).

Of 40 million people currently living with HIV/AIDS worldwide, 6 million urgently need antiretroviral therapy, but fewer than 8 per cent are receiving it. Without rapid access to properly managed treatment, 3 million women, children and men will die every year. In Asia 800,000 people need ART, but only 42,000 are presently receiving it. Only a handful of countries, including Japan, are currently providing universal access to treatment. Elsewhere, patients have to pay full costs of care. Linked to poverty, those most in need of immediate treatment are often the least likely to receive it. By scaling up ART, this human toll and the accompanying social and economic devastation can be averted.

Scaling Up Antiretroviral Therapy: The Rationale

The huge shortfall in ART for AIDS in many resource-poor countries is inequitable and unacceptable. Delivering treatment for HIV/AIDS in the developing world is necessary if the international community is to live up to commitments on human rights, the Millennium Development Goals and the Declaration of the United Nations General Assembly on HIV/AIDS.

Over the past few years two international developments have had profound implications for national AIDS programmes and in showing that scaled-up delivery of ART in resource-poor settings, once thought impossible, could be made a reality. First, the prices of antiretroviral drugs have dropped sharply, triggered by a landmark announcement made by Cipla of India in 2001 that it would offer combination treatment to Africa through MSF at only US$ 350 per patient per year compared to US$ 10,000–15,000 in the United States. Second, experiences from Brazil (Figure 6.2) and Thailand show that implementation and delivery of ART as a part of national programme is feasible and sustainable (Marins et al. 2003; Tassie et al. 2003).

Figure 6.2
Distribution of PCP, Toxoplasmosis and
Tuberculosis in Reported AIDS Cases in Brazil: 1981–2001

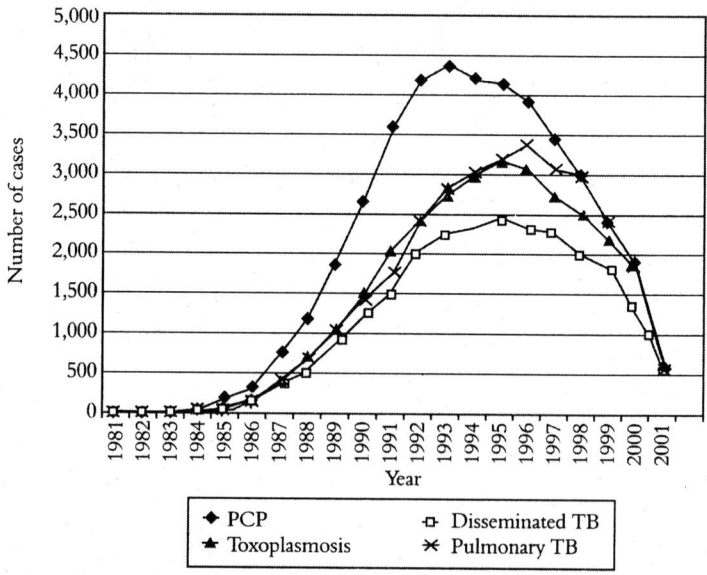

Source: MOH Brazil, Barcelona AIDS Conference, 2002.

Moreover, there is now a growing worldwide political mobilisation, led by people living with HIV/AIDS, affirming treatment as a human right. The World Bank has channelled increased funding into HIV/AIDS. New institutions such as the Global Fund to Fight AIDS, Tuberculosis and Malaria have been launched, reflecting an exceptional level of political will and unprecedented resources for the HIV/AIDS battle. This unique combination of opportunity and political will backed up by unprecedented financial resources must now be seized with urgent action.

The '3 by 5' Initiative ██ 111

The '3 by 5' Initiative

On 22 September 2003 Lee Jong-wook, director-general of WHO joined with the executive director of UNAIDS and executive director of the Global Fund to Fight AIDS, Tuberculosis and Malaria to declare failure to provide access to antiretroviral drugs to be a global health emergency (WHO 2003c). In response, WHO and its partners launched the 'Treat 3 million by 2005' ('3 by 5') Initiative. Given the proven feasibility of treating people living with HIV/AIDS in industrialised and developing countries, a global target of treating 3 million people with antiretroviral therapy by the end of 2005 is considered a necessary, achievable target on the way to the ultimate goal of universal access to ART for everyone who requires it. The target represents only 50 per cent of those who will need antiretroviral treatment, including 400,000 in Asia. Reaching the '3 by 5' target demands new commitment and a new way of working across the global health community. Countries are on the front lines of the struggle, but they cannot succeed alone. Intensive, collaborative mobil-isation linking countries, multilateral organisations, bilateral agencies, communities and the non-state sector is required (Kasper et al. 2003).

Focus on treatment in no way undermines or compromises HIV prevention or management of opportunistic infections. Prevention will remain central to all HIV interventions. Indeed, universal access to ART for those needing treatment according to medical criteria opens up ways to accelerate prevention in communities in which more people may want to know their HIV status. As HIV/AIDS becomes a disease that can be both prevented and treated, attitudes will change, and denial, stigma and discrimination will rapidly be reduced. Rolling out effective HIV/AIDS treatment is the single activity that can most effectively energise and accelerate the uptake and impact of prevention. Under '3 by 5', this will occur as part of a comprehensive strategy linking treatment, prevention, care and full social support for people affected by HIV/AIDS. Such support is critical—both to ensure adherence to ART and to reinforce prevention.

Fighting HIV/AIDS has implications for the entire health sector. The impact of HIV/AIDS both directly and indirectly undermines the performance of national health systems. An ART scale-up should be used as an opportunity to further strengthen health system capacities at the country level that would have ensured sustainability of the national response. Successful implementation of '3 by 5' will accelerate the attainment of the Millennium Development Goals (MDG) for HIV/AIDS, as well as associated health and development MDGs. The WHO is consulting intensively with national authorities and relevant international partners, including the World Bank, to ensure the coordination of efforts.

The Goal

The goal of the initiative is for the WHO, UNAIDS and its partners to support countries make the greatest possible contribution to prolonging the survival and restoring the quality of life of individuals with HIV/AIDS. This will advance towards the ultimate goal of universal access to antiretroviral therapy to those in need of care as a human right and within the context of a comprehensive response to HIV/AIDS.

The Target

By the end of 2005 3 million eligible people in developing countries who need it will be receiving effective ART. The target for Asia is 500,000, with an overall goal in the long term of universal access as human right.

Guiding Principles

The WHO adheres to a set of principles and values related to this initiative:

1. **Urgency:** Immediate action is required to avert millions of needless deaths. The HIV/AIDS treatment emergency demands new resources, swift redeployment of resources, streamlining of institutional procedures and a new spirit of goal-focused teamwork.
2. **Added value:** Recognising that ART will reduce suffering, prolong life and improve quality of life will also enhance HIV prevention activities and ultimately lead to the overall strengthening of the health system.
3. **Integrated approaches:** ART will become an integral part of the comprehensive HIV/AIDS package, where prevention is individually linked to care, and will usually be delivered as an integral component of health care, down to the primary level.
4. **Partnership building:** Involvement of key stakeholders and partners from the government and non-governmental sector, civil society to people living with HIV as well as international organisations and donor agencies are crucial for an ART scale-up.

5. **Treatment as a human right:** The initiative will advance the United Nations' goal of promoting human rights as codified in the Universal Declaration of Human Rights, as expressed in the WHO Constitution in seeking the attainment of the highest possible standards of health, and clarified in the Declaration of Commitment of the United National General Assembly Special Session on HIV/AIDS in 2001. Under '3 by 5', special attention will be given to protecting and serving vulnerable groups in prevention and treatment programmes. The initiative will make special efforts to ensure access to ART for people who risk exclusion because of economic, social, geographical or other barriers.

The WHO Strategy

The WHO's strategic framework for emergency scaling up of antiretroviral therapy contains 14 key strategic elements. These elements fall into five categories, the pillars of the '3 by 5' campaign. These include: global leadership, strong partnership and advocacy; urgent, sustained country support; simplified, standardised tools for delivering antiretroviral therapy; effective, reliable supply of medicines and diagnostics; and rapidly identifying and reapplying new knowledge and successes.

1. **Global leadership, alliances and advocacy:** The most vital work towards the '3 by 5' target will happen in countries and communities, but global alliances and advocacy will be crucial enablers. UNAIDS has driven the global advocacy effort and catalysed growing international determination to respond to the HIV/AIDS crisis, including in the area of treatment access. Working within UNAIDS and alongside other partners, the WHO will step forward and fully exercise its specific responsibility for the health sector, above all in advocating for treatment.
2. **Urgent, sustained country support:** The success of ART programmes depends on coordinated, scaled-up country action. Countries must drive the process of expanding HIV/AIDS treatment, and their specific needs and capacities will shape strategies and determine scaling-up activities. The WHO has significant opportunities to lend concrete support to these processes The WHO will provide implementers with essential technical and policy advice and tools, and will cooperate with countries at every stage in designing and implementing national plans to scale up

ART. Countries have demonstrated their demand for active collaboration with the WHO by responding to the declaration of the global health emergency on 22 September 2003. Immediately following the declaration, more than 20 countries aligned their national goals to the global emergency and requested collaboration with the WHO and partners, including visits by WHO '3 by 5' emergency missions.

3. **Simplified, standardised tools for delivering ART:** Rapidly scaling up antiretroviral therapy requires user-friendly guidelines to help health workers identify and enrol people living with HIV/AIDS, deliver therapy and monitor results. Providing these guidelines and updating them as new information comes in is a central part of the WHO's role.

4. **Effective, reliable supply of medicines and diagnostics:** The viability of ART programmes and the lives of people living with HIV/AIDS depend on a reliable, efficiently managed supply of quality medicines and diagnostics procured at a sustainable cost. The WHO recognises the importance of drug procurement and supply management for scaling up antiretroviral therapy and of the challenges many countries and providers face in this area. For this reason, a key component of the WHO '3 by 5' strategy is the establishment of an AIDS Medicines and Diagnostics Service (AMDS).

5. **Rapidly identifying and reapplying new knowledge and successes:** The most successful organisations are those that have valued and applied experimentation, innovation and real-time learning with rapid diffusion. The many challenges surrounding the scaling up of ART require a robust programme to consistently learn, document, share and act.

The South-East Asia Regional Framework for Action at Country Level

In the South-East Asia region (SEAR) nearly 6 million people are living with HIV/AIDS, making it the second most affected region in the world after Sub-Saharan Africa. Four countries bear an overwhelming majority of the HIV/AIDS burden in the region, namely, India (4,580,000), Thailand (670,000), Myanmar (200,000) and Indonesia (130,000).

Approximately 800,000 people living with HIV/AIDS (PHAs) in the region are in immediate need of ART. In line with the global '3 by 5' target, the South-East Asia Regional Office (SEARO) of the WHO has proposed a target of getting 400,000 people on ART by the end of 2005. Currently, only 40,000 PHAs in SEAR are on it. Thus, a 10-fold scale-up of ART coverage is required by 2005. In this regard, the most important countries in the region include India, Thailand, Myanmar and Indonesia, which together constitute 98 per cent of the burden. The ART gap also needs to be bridged. During mid-2003, WHO/SEARO conducted a rapid assessment of country preparedness for scaling up ART, which showed that the HIV/AIDS burden as well as the ART gap is largest in India, followed by Myanmar and Indonesia (Table 6.1).

Table 6.1
Estimated HIV Prevalence and Antiretroviral
Treatment Needs in the South-East Asia Region

Country	HIV prevalence	Total number of people needing ART	Number of people on ART in 2003	Proposed WHO target by 2005	Treatment gap (number on treatment and WHO target)
Bangladesh	13,000	1,800	5	900	895
Bhutan	<100	–	–	–	–
Democratic People's Republic of Korea	n/a	–	–	–	–
India	4,580,000	600,000	13,000	300,000	287,000
Indonesia	130,000	18,400	500	9,200	8,700
Maldives	100	–	–	–	–
Myanmar	330,000	25,000	1,000	15,000	14,000
Nepal	60,000	8,000	250	4,000	3,750
Sri Lanka	4,800	680	25	340	315
Thailand	670,000	98,000	23,000	48,000	25,000
Timor Leste	n/a	–	–	–	–
Total (approx.)	6,000,000	750,000	40,000	375,000	335,000

Source: HIV/AIDS Programme, WHO/SEARO, 2003.

Thailand currently has the largest number of people on ART in the region and is already making commitments to achieve the global target by 2004 with universal coverage by 2005. It has considerable practical experience to build upon. Elsewhere, India recently (30 November 2003) committed to providing ART free to 100,000 patients over one year starting April 2004 in six high-prevalence states. Myanmar,

Indonesia and Nepal are also fully committed to the provision of ART within the framework of the '3 by 5' Initiative. The initial findings from '3 by 5' emergency missions to India, Indonesia and Myanmar showed that despite a sea change in political commitment, apart from Thailand, most other countries will need considerable preparedness, particularly in terms of capacity building of health services, for delivery of ART.

In order to address the key challenges faced by member countries for scaling up ART coverage and ensuring quality of services, SEARO has prepared a regional strategy that provides a framework for action at the country level for implementing the '3 by 5' Initiative. The strategy has been discussed and endorsed at a three-day meeting (19–21 November 2003) with national AIDS programme managers of the member countries (WHO 2003d), as well as by the SEAR core group consisting of clinicians, ART experts, programme managers, essential drugs experts, NGOs, PHAs, donors, and WHO and other UN staff (22–23 November 2003). Recognising that scaling up of ART will be a part of the comprehensive care package for people living with HIV/ AIDS without compromising on basic HIV prevention strategies and reaffirming that enhanced HIV prevention and care efforts should be maintained and utilised further to strengthen national health system capacities, the regional strategy consists of the following five core elements for action at the country level. The strategy emphasises that unless all the five elements are in place, in a geographic area ART should not be initiated.

1. Mobilising political and financial commitment.
2. Building capacity of health services to deliver ART (including expansion of voluntary counselling and testing facilities, strengthening laboratory capacity particularly for CD4 enumeration, and training of health care workers both in the public and private sector).
3. Ensuring uninterrupted supply of antiretroviral drugs and diagnostics.
4. Mobilising community, including involvement of PHA networks for use of ART and for ensuring treatment adherence.
5. Monitoring and evaluation, and operational research.

One of the crucial elements is ensuring treatment adherence because of the lifelong nature of treatment and the risk of rapid emergence of ARV resistance in case of irrational and inappropriate use of the treatment. Innovative approaches are needed to enhance adherence to ART and achieve adherence rate of at least 95 per cent. Strategies could include minimising pill counts and dosage frequencies by preferentially using combination pills on once or twice daily basis. A number of fixed dose combinations containing two or three ARV drugs are currently marketed that can be used twice a day. Other approaches that might facilitate adherence include enlisting the assistance of family or community members to support or even observe patients taking their medications on a regular and timely basis; extensive counselling and patient education; and directly observed therapy where health care workers, NGOs or social workers could play the role of treatment observers.

In order to track if the strategy is implemented as planned, examples of monitoring and evaluation indicators and targets can be used, which could include:

1. indicators of political commitment, that is, ART as a national policy;
2. indicators of ART implementation (process), that is, number of health workers trained, VCT facilities established;
3. indicators of ART implementation (output or coverage), such as number of patients registered for treatment, number or proportion of administrative areas such as districts with established ART services; and
4. indicators of quality (outcome), or proportion of patients with changed CD4 levels, proportion returning to work, etc.

Challenges and Opportunities

Several opportunities exist that provide optimism that the '3 by 5' target is feasible. The most important opportunity is the marked decline in ARV drug prices and the enhanced political commitments both at national and international levels. The South-East Asia region is home to some of the world's leading manufacturers of affordable generic drugs, including ARVs, who are expected to play a key role not only in making ARVs available at affordable prices for the developing world but also in ensuring that the '3 by 5' Initiative is achievable. Four countries in the region—India, Thailand, Indonesia and Bangladesh—are domestic manufacturers of various life-saving medicines that are not protected by a product patent in their territories. India and Thailand are already producing ARVs that are allowed within the countries' intellectual property laws. Generic drugs manufactured in India and Thailand, in addition to being used nationally, are also being exported to several African countries like Nigeria, Kenya, Ethiopia, Zambia and Senegal as permitted under the intellectual property laws of those countries. India is emerging as a major manufacturer of affordable ARV drugs that will benefit AIDS patients the world over. Several Indian pharmaceutical companies including Cipla, Ranbaxy, Hetero, Aurobindo and Matrix are taking the lead in pulling down the prices of AIDS drugs at the global level. The remarkable reduction in the prices of ARVs were triggered by a breakthrough announcement made about two years ago by Cipla in India that it would offer through the NGO Medecins Sans Frontieres (MSF) combination ARV therapy to patients in Africa for only US$ 350 per patient per year. More recent developments on pricing are even more encouraging, with large guaranteed orders companies in India and South Africa seeing a price below US$ 150 per patient per year as achievable.

In addition to reducing drugs prices, other opportunities for achieving the '3 by 5' target include the availability of large NGO and PHA networks, enormous scope for public–private partnerships and excellent examples of programme scale-up as in Thailand.

Several challenges exist. Drug prices as well as prices of diagnostics such as CD4 are still too high and beyond national capacities in many resource-poor countries. Health services in most countries are still weak, highlighting the need for staffing and capacity building at the national and state levels in order to enable it to deliver antiretroviral treatment. The '3 by 5' Initiative represents an opportunity to strengthen health systems so everyone benefits.

Denial, stigma and discrimination are still common in much of the region, undermining efforts to put in place an effective prevention and care services, particularly at the community level. As a result, those at risk and those requiring the services do not come forward to use the very services meant for them. Most people who are marginalised or are vulnerable do not access VCT services and do not know their HIV status. Wide-scale treatment will catalyse improvements in attitude and banish denial. Prevention remains the bedrock of interventions. If properly implemented, prevention activities will be synergised by ART. The initial key is wider use of counselling and testing services; the final challenge is that sufficient resources are not yet available in many countries to enable them to substantially scale up ART. Therefore, substantial additional resources must be mobilised from various sources in order to take the initiative forward.

In the SEAR, the WHO has set up a regional '3 by 5' core group with membership representing national AIDS programmes, clinicians with expertise in ART, laboratory experts, essential drugs specialists, as well as representatives of the UN and donor agencies. The core group met for the first time in November 2003 with the mandate of advising on strategy development and supporting implementation at the country level. In addition, an in-house working group on HIV/AIDS and '3 by 5' has been established in the WHO regional office to mainstream new initiatives into various WHO programmes.

To assist building capacity in the member countries, various initiatives have been taken, including development of a simplified treatment guidelines, inter-country training on HIV/AIDS clinical management including ART, and on voluntary counselling and testing, as well as on diagnosis of HIV-associated opportunistic infections. The first training on CD4, which is an entry point for initiating treatment and monitoring treatment outcome, was held in December 2003. Plans are under way to establish ARV resistance surveillance in a systematic manner.

In the area of advocacy and resource mobilisation, the WHO in the region has briefed national AIDS programme managers on '3 by 5' during their annual meeting, which focused almost entirely on the subject. The opportunity was taken to develop consensus on regional strategy, which provides a framework for action at the country level. Most countries, including India, have started using this framework for planning ART strategy in the respective countries. The '3 by 5' Initiative was discussed at meetings of health ministers and of health secretaries of the region. WHO missions visited India, Indonesia, Myanmar and Nepal. In India the team deliberated with the National AIDS Control Organisation on the steps for operationalising the policy decision made by the health minister on 30 November 2003 that the government of India will provide free ART through government health facilities in the six high-burden states, starting 1 April 2004.

Recognising that implementation of '3 by 5' requires massive investments in training, national capacity building and resources for ARV drugs, the WHO regional office has been assisting countries in resource mobilisation, including through the Global Fund to Fight AIDS, TB and Malaria. Availability of substantial additional financial and human resources would be necessary to move forward in closing the HIV treatment gap and for meeting '3 by 5' targets at the country level. This ambitious

'3 by 5' target does indeed present numerous challenges, but with united action it can be achieved. In declaring lack of access to ARV treatment to be a global health emergency, the WHO is fully committed to providing accelerated, intensified support to countries to tackle critical barriers to scale up, including to help build a critical mass of highly competent and skilled staff to expand national capacity for ARV delivery and to advocate for funding by working with UNAIDS and other partners. Achieving the '3 by 5' target requires not only funding for drugs, but a massive investment in training and for strengthening health services in countries. Health systems strengthening will benefit both ARV delivery and the delivery of other health services.

Conclusions

The HIV/AIDS epidemic is a global emergency and calls for an emergency response. In addition to scaling up and sustaining effective AIDS prevention and care interventions, supplementary efforts are needed to meet the objectives and targets set by the '3 by 5' Initiative. The fight against HIV/AIDS cannot be won unless the global health community immediately responds to the need for AIDS treatment similar to the way it responds to other emergencies. The WHO has committed itself to confronting this global health emergency with urgent measures. The days of a 'business as usual' approach to AIDS are over.

Significantly increased resources are needed to tackle pressing public health problems, including HIV/AIDS. The new '3 by 5' initiative not only forces us to look at the AIDS challenge with a different perspective calling for substantial additional efforts, but also offers opportunities to strengthen the health system and ensure sustainability in the long run.

Confronting AIDS more boldly will enable a strengthening of primary health care, based on the principles laid out at Alma-Ata in 1978. But achieving this objective will demand greater investments in health from international donors and from countries themselves. Sufficient knowledge and resources exist to prevent the majority of new HIV infections and deaths now occurring. Through better use of existing resources and by bringing new resources to bear on a novel and growing problem, the WHO will work in an emergency mode in support of countries to redress inequalities of access to proven therapies. If conducted properly, this emergency response can generate sustained advances. Investing in prevention equity and improved access to care will bring multiple benefits, including a narrowing of the inequalities, both social and medical, that threaten the fragile peace and stability of the global community.

R EFERENCES

Kasper, T. et al. (2003). Demystifying antiretroviral therapy in resource-poor settings. *Essential Drugs Monitor,* 32, 20–21.

Marins, J.R. et al. (2003). Dramatic improvement in survival among adult Brazilian AIDS patients. *AIDS,* 17(11), 1675–82.

Tassie, J.-M., E. Szumilin, A. Calmy and **E. Goemaere** (2003). Highly active antiretroviral therapy in resource-poor settings: The experience of Medecins Sans Frontieres. *AIDS,* 17(13), 1995–97.

WHO (2003a). *World health report: Shaping the future.* Geneva: WHO.

——— (2003b). *HIV/AIDS in Asia and the Pacific region.* Manila: WHO Regional Office for South-East Asia and Regional Office for Western Pacific.

——— (2003c). WHO declares failure to deliver AIDS medicines a global health emergency. *Bulletin of the World Health Organization,* 81(10), 776.

——— (2003d). Report of the national AIDS programme managers' meeting, November 2003. WHO Regional Office for South-East Asia, New Delhi.

WHO/UNAIDS (2003). *AIDS epidemic update,* December.

7

DRUG-RELATED HIV IN SOUTH AND SOUTH-EAST ASIA

Swarup Sarkar, Anindya Chatterjee and Anne Bergenström*

The Continuing Spread of Drug-related HIV in the Asia Region

According to data on reported injecting drug use and injecting-related HIV globally in 170 countries, 134 countries had reported injecting practices, leaving 36 that were yet to report any injecting drug use by mid-2000 (Needle et al. 2000). Only 20 out of the 134 injecting countries have not reported HIV among injectors (ibid.).

As is evident from Figure 7.1, most countries in Asia have reported both injecting drug use and HIV among IDUs.

Trends in Injecting Drug Use and Outcome in the South and South-East Asia

Following presence of indigenous opium dependence in countries surrounding the Golden Triangle and the Golden Crescent, heroin epidemics have been common in most South-East Asian countries from the 1960s onwards, with major epicentres in Thailand, Myanmar and Malaysia (Poschyachinda 1993), and in South Asia in Afghanistan, Pakistan and India since the 1980s (Stimson 1993). Wide availability of drugs plays a major role in fuelling a dual epidemic of drugs and HIV (Sarkar et al. 1997), and countries that produce injectable drugs soon become trafficking countries as well as transit countries, quickly report injecting practices (Stimson 1993) and HIV among IDUs (Beyrer et al.

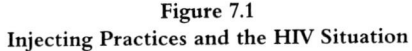

Figure 7.1
Injecting Practices and the HIV Situation

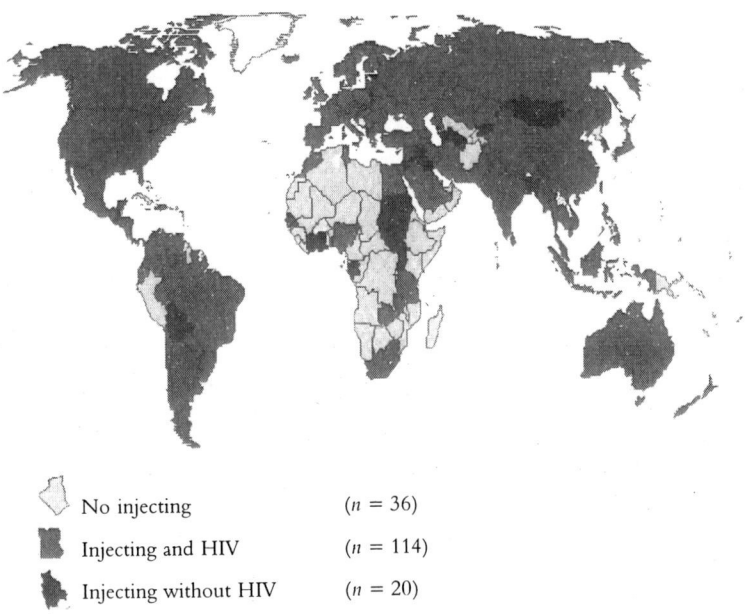

No injecting   ($n = 36$)

Injecting and HIV   ($n = 114$)

Injecting without HIV   ($n = 20$)

2000). Literature in the last decade indicates that once the injecting habit is established, diminishing supply of drugs by itself does not reduce injecting practices. In fact, reduction of the availability of an injectable drug (for example, smokable heroin) or impurity of injectable drugs often leads to injecting on a large scale (Centre for Harm Reduction 1999) because drug-dependent persons continue to maintain their body requirement through alternate supplies via another drug or by increasing the efficiency of the drug through the injecting route. In some areas of South Asia heroin smoking has been replaced by over-the-counter buprenorphine, and by amphetamine-type substances in Thailand and in the Philippines. It will be of interest to observe whether reduction of opium cultivation in Afghanistan will lead to further increase in injecting in the region.

Asia being the epicentre of world's heroin production, it is not surprising that IDUs in the region were among the first populations to be affected by HIV (MAP 2001). Between 1 and 10 per cent of adults in South and South-East Asia have acquired HIV through IDU

(Needle et al. 2000). Except Cambodia and major parts of India, the HIV epidemic began among the injecting population, in Thailand, Myanmar, China, Malaysia, Vietnam, north-eastern India, Nepal and very recently in Indonesia. Although in many of these countries drug trafficking can result in capital punishment, drugs continue to be both widely available and used.

Countries frequently report very rapid rise of HIV prevalence among injectors once the first case of HIV is notified. A classical case is Manipur in the north-east of India where no HIV was reported during 1986 to 1989, when over 1,200 injectors were tested (Naik et al. 1991). However, from the first reported case of HIV among injectors in 1989, HIV prevalence rapidly increased to 54 per cent within six months (Sarkar et al. 1993).

A similar dramatic rise in HIV prevalence has been reported in other Asian countries including Thailand (Nelson et al. 2002), China (Yu et al. 2002), Vietnam (Quan et al. 2000), Nepal (Oelrichs et al. 2000), Myanmar (Lwin et al. 1999), Malaysia and more recently Indonesia (MAP 2001). While Malaysia and Thailand report overall HIV prevalence rates lower than 50 per cent among IDUs, it has reached as high as 80 per cent in four countries: Myanmar, Vietnam, China and Manipur in India (Rhodes and Stimson 1998). In Vietnam HIV prevalence among IDUs ranges from 0 to 89.4 per cent in different provinces, with IDUs accounting for an estimated 89 per cent of all HIV cases (Quan et al. 2000). In China an estimated 3 to 3.5 million persons inject drugs (Reid and Costigan 2002), and in new HIV outbreak areas an increase of HIV-1 prevalence from 8 to 42 per cent was reported within a year (Yu et al. 2002). In Nepal HIV seroprevalence among IDUs has also been explosive, with an increase from 0 to 40 per cent between 1995 and 1997 (Oelrichs et al. 2000). Although Bangladesh is still a low-prevalence country, a 2.5 per cent HIV prevalence level has been reported among buprenorphine injectors (Jenkins et al. 2001), and hepatitis C rates have been reported at 67 per cent in some areas (Azim et al. 2002), indicating considerable HIV vulnerability among IDUs.

Heterogeneity is inherent to the HIV epidemic and frequently a national HIV seroprevalence represents a skewed picture. Disturbingly high HIV prevalence rates have been reported in epicentres of drug-related IDU in certain cities, states and provinces in Asia, while the overall national HIV seroprevalence rates are usually lower. For example, while the national seroprevalence rate among IDUs in China is

12 per cent, HIV seroprevalence has reached 86 per cent among IDUs in some areas (Zheng et al. 1997).

Unfortunately, most countries do not initiate HIV prevention interventions aimed at drug users before HIV seroprevalence rates have reached 50 per cent or above in the drug user population. In low HIV prevalence countries, surrogates of HIV, such as hepatitis C and B, which are mostly attributed to sharing of needles in these settings, have been reported with alarming seroprevalence rates. Pakistan is an example where a baseline survey carried out in 1999 indicated 89 per cent of IDUs to be infected with hepatitis C, while none of them tested positive for HIV (UNDCP and UNAIDS 1999). In Japan HCV antibodies were reported among 75 per cent of the 47 IDUs tested (Ichimura et al. 1995). These two countries illustrate classical cases of high level of HIV vulnerability faced by drug users, yet interventions aimed at drug users are scarce. Nevertheless, in view of preventing an HIV epidemic among them, it is at this point in time that quality interventions should be implemented as a matter of priority. Once HIV is introduced among IDUs, prevalence frequently increases in an explosive manner and the benefits of early interventions are lost, as has recently been experienced in Indonesia (MAP 2001).

Aside from an increased risk of HIV, other frequent outcomes associated with injecting via contaminated equipment or unregulated dose of drug include excess mortality due to infection and overdose. Unfortunately, systematic data on the incidence of these two outcomes are not available in most Asian countries.

Heterosexual Spread of HIV from IDUs to Partners and Mother-to-Child Transmission

The need for a large-scale intervention among the IDU population has often been questioned because of the notion that HIV among injectors would not lead to a generalised heterosexual epidemic (Chin 2001). This belief has been reinforced by the presence of two separate subtypes of HIV B and E respectively among IDUs and heterosexual population in a study published from Thailand in early 1990s (Weniger et al. 1994). However, recent data from Manipur, north-east India, show that HIV prevalence among spouses of HIV-positive injectors increased from 5 to 45 per cent over a period of five years (Panda et al. 2000). One per cent prevalence of HIV among the general population is a high level of infection and indicates large-scale heterosexual spread. In two north-eastern states of India, Manipur and Nagaland, 1 per cent prevalence has been reported among antenatal clinic women in the absence of any other significant risk factor or behaviour except an IDU partner or ex-partner (Sarkar et al. 1993). High level of heterosexual HIV spread in predominantly injecting settings has also been reported in Myanmar (Lwin et al. 1999). Thus, it is evident that non-drug-using sexual partners of IDUs are at considerable risk of HIV. Furthermore, should the woman also inject drugs, she is at an even greater risk of HIV (Klee 1996). Thus, epidemiological data indicate that heterosexual transmission is taking place from HIV-positive injectors to their sexual partners and through mother-to-child transmission (Needle et al. 2000).

Recent HIV sub-type studies set up specifically to address this question demonstrate that HIV sub-types C and E have been responsible for heterosexual spread in Manipur (Panda et al. 1998, 2000). Sub-type studies from other countries including China (Chen et al. 1999; Kato et al. 1999), Vietnam (Nerurkar et al. 1996, 1997) and Thailand (Panda et al. 1998) also establish preponderance of non-B HIV sub-types like HIV E among injectors and heterosexuals in all Asian countries.

Both epidemiological data and sub-type studies indicate that heterosexual spread is occurring from injectors to their sexual partners, transmission that could act as a catalyst for a large-scale generalised epidemic. Yet scarce attention has been given to focused HIV interventions of IDUs and their female partners to prevent future spread of HIV in the general population in South and South-East Asia.

Women Drug Users and HIV

Globally as well as in Asia, women drug users have received considerably less attention, and the majority of the studies have been conducted on males. In most societies drug use is viewed at odds with expected behaviour by women and drug-using women are likely to experience even greater stigmatisation compared with their male counterparts. Frequently women drug users exchange sex for drugs or money to sustain their drug habit or livelihood for themselves and their children (Panda et al. 2001). There are fewer treatment services that cater specifically to drug-using women (Klee 1996), and experiences in other countries indicate that women appear less inclined to access services attended by a predominantly male clientele (Ford and Lisa 2001).

Studies in South and South-East Asia show that women account for between 5 and 10 per cent of the total drug injecting population (WHO

International Collaborative Group 1994). Although drug-use-related HIV in India is viewed as a problem among men, one study found 57 per cent of female drug users to be HIV positive (Panda et al. 2001). In one city in Bangladesh 6 to 14 per cent of street-based and brothel-based sex workers reported injecting drug use (MAP 2001). Yet few studies have examined drug-related HIV among female drug users beyond monitoring prevalence of sexually-transmitted infections, HIV, reproductive tract infections, hepatitis B or C, injecting behaviour and practice of sex work. HIV prevention aimed at female partners of IDUs has remained a difficult behaviour change issue to address and there have been no systematic gender-specific efforts to implement HIV prevention interventions for this group in Asia. In view of the high HIV prevalence rate among female IDUs, there is an urgent need to design and implement focused interventions, including peer outreach for female drug users and sexual partners of drug-using men, whether drug users themselves or not. Such interventions need to consider the context in which women live, as many women drug users depend on sex work for their livelihoods (Panda et al. 2001; Waver et al. 1996).

Critical Issues Relating to Interventions among IDUs

In spite of successful demonstrations of HIV interventions for drug users in Asia, current interventions are unlikely to be effective due to several factors. Implementation of effective policies and strategies early on in the epidemic can keep HIV at significantly low levels even in presence of injecting practices (Loxley 2000), and the incidence of HIV can be reduced (Peters et al. 1998), showing thereby that prevention of drug-related HIV is feasible. Characteristics of effective HIV prevention interventions include early introduction of intervention (ideally before HIV is reported among the IDU population), availability of needle and syringe exchange programmes (NSP), and drug treatment programmes such as methadone substitution and outreach with active partnership by the drug user community. Creation of a supportive policy and legal environment that tolerates such interventions in the community is crucial as is the decriminalisation of NSP. A multi-country study of 36 countries conducted by the WHO showed that the above elements of interventions either reduce incidence of HIV or maintain a very low prevalence of HIV among the IDU population (United Nations 2000; WHO International Collaborative Group 1994). Unfortunately, success reported in various parts of the world in terms of declining frequency of injecting and sharing of injecting equipment, as well as a decrease in HIV incidence among IDUs (Des Jarlais et al. 1998; Stimson 1995; Wodak 1999) has not been achieved in most Asian countries for a variety of reasons.

First, although in most countries the HIV epidemic can be traced to drug-related risk behaviour, interventions for the drug user population have been implemented too late. Second, the effectiveness of these interventions is constrained due to ineffective strategy, poor quality or inadequate resources. Finally, the interventions are frequently implemented with insufficient coverage to result in the desired impact.

An example of a country that is yet to implement harm reduction programmes is Thailand, which is otherwise the most successful country in Asia in terms of a large-scale national HIV prevention programme. The progression of the epidemic in Thailand has been well documented (Tarantola et al. 1999). The epidemic begun with the steep rise of HIV among the IDU population, followed by an epidemic among the commercial sex worker (CSW) population, STD clinic attendants and finally antenatal women, representing the general population. The HIV response in Thailand has been phenomenal, with political support being a key determinant of success, leading to $1.32 per capita of investment per year (highest in Asia) and adoption of a policy of 100 per cent condom use, resulting in a decline of HIV prevalence among sex workers, STD clinic attendants (Nelson et al. 1996) and sero-stabilisation among antenatal women. The notable exception has been the IDU population in which the prevalence of HIV has increased from 32 per cent in 1995 to 50 per cent in 2000 (Reid and Costigan 2002) (Figure 7.2).

The ongoing increase in HIV seroprevalence among IDUs can be attributed to the fact that programmes known to be effective for this population, such as outreach, NSP, drug treatment and an enabling environment, have not been institutionalised in the large-scale national HIV programme in Thailand. While drug treatment programmes have been operationalised with limited to moderate coverage, outreach, NSP or a conducive policy environment have not been the practice except in small project sites on a limited scale.

Implementing Interventions that are Effective

Studies from the region have shown that frequently adopted strategies of reduction of drug supply, enforcement of prohibitive laws and incarceration or forced detoxification programmes as means of HIV

Figure 7.2
HIV Prevalence in Four Sub-groups in Thailand: 1989–2001

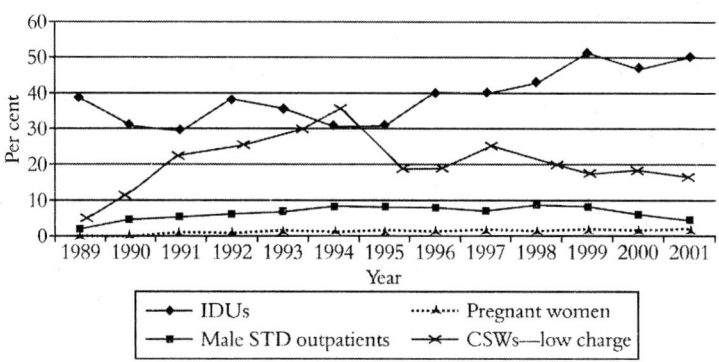

Source: Ministry of Public Health, Thailand.

prevention interventions are of limited success (Reid and Costigan 2002). In fact, criminalisation of drug use and possession of needles and syringes have been associated with an increase in needle sharing (Reid and Crofts 2000), thus making drug users even more vulnerable to HIV. Abstinence-oriented treatment approach has remained the most popular therapeutic approach (Abdul-Quader et al. 1999), with almost no efficacy in public health terms in view of the reported relapse rates of over 90 per cent among drug users who have been through detoxification at a deaddiction centre. Similarly, HIV intervention programmes restricted to awareness and IEC (information, education and communication) to promote knowledge on modes of HIV transmission combined with awareness raising on methods of cleaning injecting equipment and promotion of non-sharing of needles are of limited effectiveness (Sarkar et al. 1995). On many occasions drug users continue to share injection paraphernalia despite a very high level of HIV knowledge.

Frequently, the first HIV intervention drug users are subject to is an awareness programme including information on the transmission modes with the assumption that IEC will lead to behaviour change. In spite of considerable literature on behaviour change theories and findings from India (Sarkar et al. 1995), Bangladesh (Jenkins et al. 2001), Nepal (Family Health International, personal communication) and Pakistan (UNDCP and UNAIDS 1999) that awareness alone does not result in behaviour change among drug users, most interventions for this population in South Asia continue to be awareness focused. South-East Asia is no exception as the majority of the countries are implementing HIV interventions focused on drug users mostly through IEC and awareness without provision of effective services (see Table 7.1).

Efforts to reduce the supply of drugs may sometimes result in increased injecting behaviour and vulnerability to HIV. The ecological association between intensified activities of seizure for smokable heroin and arrests of drug users and increase in the proportion of injectors among drug users seeking treatment in detoxification has been documented in Kolkata (Panda et al. 1998) and Dhaka (unpublished data, CARE Bangladesh). Switching to injecting drug use has also been associated with stringent narcotic control laws in many parts of the developing world. In recent times reduced supply of injectable heroin (white sugar) or smokable heroin by intensified customs and excise procedures has led to large-scale switch from smoking to injecting of over-the-counter painkillers or buprenorphine injection in South Asia.

Based on a probability of 1 per cent risk of acquiring HIV from sharing an infected needle or syringe and three sharing partners in a setting with 80 per cent of injectors being HIV positive, a new injector may sero-convert within 500 days and the incidence of new HIV infections remains high (Samson et al. 1999). In order to maintain low HIV incidence in such a scenario, all efforts must be undertaken to reduce the number of HIV-positive persons from joining the sharing pool.

Provisions of drug treatment by non-injecting routes such as methadone or buprenorphine may be one such procedure. In spite of large-scale drug-related HIV epidemics experienced by many countries in the region, such measures have not been fully explored. The majority of Asian countries do not yet offer appropriate drug treatment services for the injecting population (see Table 7.1). Operational research is required to examine the impact of reintroduction of presently extinct government-run opium outlets or similar services on HIV among IDU in high-prevalence settings in South Asia.

Another HIV prevention intervention, voluntary counselling and testing (VCT) for HIV has been shown to be an effective intervention to reduce risk behaviours with non-primary partners among mainstream heterosexual relationships (Voluntary HIV-1 Counselling and Testing Efficacy Study 2000) and among discordant couples (Allen et al. 1992). Role of VCT among marginalised populations, such as sex workers, men who have sex with men or drug users is less clear (Allen et al. 1992; Sarkar et al. 1996). Apart from the limited role of individual interventions in drug-related HIV prevention, one-to-one VCT for HIV

Table 7.1
Drug Treatment Services for the Injecting Population in Asia

Country	Estimated number of IDUs	HIV prevalence among IDUs(%)*	Substitution	NSP	Both	Coverage of IDUs**
High prevalence						
Cambodia	No data	No data	No	No	NA	–
Myanmar	150,000–250,000	96.0	No	No	NA	Limited outreach
Thailand	100,000–250,000	54.0	Yes	No	No	Limited
Moderate prevalence						
India	100,000 (5 cities)	80.0	Yes	Yes	Yes	Low
Malaysia	200,000	30.0	No	No	NA	Limited outreach
Nepal	20,000	50.0	Yes	Yes	Yes	Low
Papua New Guinea	No data	No data	No	No	NA	–
Pakistan	180,000	0.0	No	No	NA	Limited outreach
Vietnam	50,000	89.0	No	Yes	No	Low
Low prevalence						
Afghanistan	No data	No data	No	No	NA	–
China (excluding Hong Kong)	3–3.5 million	85.7	Yes	Yes	Yes	Low
Bangladesh	20,000–25,000	2.5	No	Yes	No	Low
Bhutan	No data	No data	No	No	–	–
Brunei Dar es Salaam	No data	No data	No	No	NA	–
Hong Kong (HKSAR, China)	12,600	No data	Yes	Yes	Yes	Moderate
Indonesia	Over 1 million	53.0	No	Bali pilot	No	Low
Japan	150,000–500,000	2.1	No	No	NA	–
Lao People's Democratic Republic	No data	No data	No	No	NA	Low
Republic of Korea	No data	0.0	No	No	NA	–
Maldives	No data	No data	No	No	NA	–
Mongolia	No data	0.0	No	No	NA	–
Philippines	10,000–400,000	1.0	No	Cebu city	NA	Low
Sri Lanka	6,000	No data	No	No	NA	–
Taiwan	60,000	No data	No	No	NA	–

Sources: Baqi et al. (1998); Chen et al. (2001); Hussain (2000); Ichimura et al. (1995); MAP (2001); Oh and Choe (1999); Quan et al. (2000); Reid (2001); Reid and Costigan (2002); Schwebke et al. (1998); Singh and Crofts (1993); WHO and Department of Health (2000); Zheng et al. (1997).

Notes: *Highest rate reported.
**Coverage by either NSP, substitution or peer outreach.
Low = <10%; moderate = 10–50%; high = >50%.

remains costly, and it is difficult to deliver intervention for a large population that would require such services. The future challenge involves in not only designing appropriate VCT services that are effective for the drug user population, but also in making them acceptable and accessible.

Late Implementation of Interventions

The interventions mentioned earlier are either not initiated in the first place or are implemented considerably late, by which time HIV prevalence has already reached a significant level among the IDU population and possibly among their partners (Table 7.2). Unfortunately, evidence of injecting practices alone or HIV among IDUs does not institute enough priority for prevention of HIV in this population and therefore the window of opportunity for early prevention has closed in many countries. An example of this is Indonesia, which was until recently considered a low-prevalence country for HIV, until HIV prevalence among IDUs increased to 40 per cent in Jakarta and 53 per cent in Bali (MAP 2001). Indonesia has over 1 million IDUs (Reid 2001), but is yet to introduce large-scale harm reduction programmes for drug users. The example of Pakistan has been provided earlier where HIV interventions are yet to be introduced on a large scale despite very high prevalence of hepatitis C among injectors (UNDCP and UNAIDS 1999).

Table 7.2
Examples of Late Introduction of Effective Intervention Programmes in Some Asian Countries

Country	Year High HIV prevalence	Intervention
Bangladesh	1998	1998
India	1989	1993
China	1990	1997
Vietnam	1990	1994
Myanmar	1988	–
Malaysia	1994	1998

Large-scale implementation of interventions, which directly address HIV prevention among the drug user population such as NSP and methadone substitution, are scarce in Asian countries experiencing explosive drug-related HIV epidemics. By end of 2001 only a minority of countries had implemented nationwide NSP and/or methadone and other substitution treatment programmes. For example, although Thailand has introduced a methadone programme with moderate coverage, there is still no NSP. In India, China and Vietnam, where HIV prevalence levels have crossed 80 per cent in some areas, NSP or drug treatment programmes only reach a small proportion of the number of estimated IDUs, which in case of China has been estimated at over 3 million. Only Bangladesh and Hong Kong (before it became a Special Administrative Region of the People's Republic of China) had implemented such programmes while HIV prevalence was still below 5 per cent.

In all other countries such scientifically demonstrated programmes were introduced after HIV prevalence rates had already reached 40 per cent among injectors. Some countries, including Myanmar, have not introduced any NSP or substitution treatment even though the prevalence has reached 96 per cent among IDUs in certain districts. Similarly, despite reports of a large number of IDUs in Taiwan, Japan and Pakistan, large-scale NSP and methadone substitution is yet to be implemented. In the remaining countries, including Cambodia, with one of the highest rates of adult HIV prevalence in the region, actual data on the numbers of IDUs are not available.

Coverage of the Drug User Populations with HIV Interventions

Public health impact is rarely achieved in the absence of large-scale programmes. Introduction of a programme alone is not enough to create an impact unless the coverage of the target population is optimum. Therefore, in the context of HIV interventions, a high level of coverage of target populations is crucial for effectiveness of national HIV/AIDS programmes (Binswanger 2000). In most countries of South and South-East Asia the coverage of IDU populations through programmes that directly address HIV vulnerability, including needle exchange, drug treatment and outreach has remained below 10 per cent (see Table 7.1).

Nepal is the first South Asian country where a needle exchange programme was introduced while HIV prevalence was still less than 1 per cent among injectors. Similarly, a drug treatment programme was introduced at an early stage of the HIV epidemic in Delhi, India, when HIV prevalence was very low. Yet the prevalence increased to 45 per cent recorded in a clinic-based cross-sectional study (Luke Sampson, personal communication), demonstrating that early introduction of harm reduction strategies alone is not a sufficient condition for maintaining low HIV incidence over time. In Delhi less than 10 per cent of the IDU population has been covered by the intervention, clearly pointing to the importance of a high level of coverage if anticipated impact is to be achieved. The most important challenge for effective HIV interventions in Asia is the issue of coverage, which is likely to remain in the coming years.

Partnership with the Drug User Community

In terms of efficacy of behaviour change communication and HIV prevention interventions, the following three issues are well established. First, it has been shown that repeated contacts need to be made by outreach programmes to reinforce the same messages of behaviour change if the desired impact is to be achieved. Second, knowledge of HIV alone does not change behaviour unless means of behaviour change are made available, including clean needles, injecting equipment and condoms. Third, previous experience shows that targeted HIV programmes, outreach and services are unlikely to be accepted by drug users unless they are involved at an early stage in the designing and implementation of the programmes aimed at their communities. Peer outreach as a means of HIV prevention intervention, in other words, outreach implemented by members of the drug user community for HIV prevention, is one example of such a partnership. In one study it has been shown that not more than 50 per cent of the estimated drug user population in the city could be reached by a conventional 'legal approach' consisting of a detoxification programme and individual counselling. When street-based peer education was initiated, with bleach distribution combined with an IEC HIV education programme, 80 per cent of the target population was reached within six months (Hangzo et al. 1997).

Over one decade of experience shows that empowerment of marginalised populations plays a great role in HIV intervention among other high-risk groups such as men who have sex with men, sex workers and drug users. Community organisations run by members of the drug user community, linking of the HIV prevention programme with other services and decriminalisation are essential programmatic components of successful HIV prevention interventions for this population.

Resources and a Supportive Policy Environment: Endorsement of Interventions by Political Leaders

As is the case with many public health programmes in general, insufficient resources have been allocated for HIV prevention interventions aimed at drug-dependent populations in a majority of Asian countries. Even in countries where linkage services do not exist and basic structures for social services are unavailable, cost of a drug user intervention, including peer education, NSP, condoms and primary health care at the project level has not been higher than $36 per person per year (Sarkar 2000). To date, most Asian countries have allocated resources for HIV at less than $1 per capita per year with the notable exception of Thailand. In some countries the total resources allocated for HIV interventions in all target sub-populations would not even meet the treatment and prevention needs of drug users. Furthermore, cost–benefit analyses show that maximum benefit can be obtained when interventions are focused among highly vulnerable populations in the stages of early and concentrated epidemic (before HIV epidemic becomes generalised), such as drug-dependent persons (Ainsworth and Over 1997). Unfortunately, the majority of the overseas development aid for developing countries has remained unavailable for programmes such as NSP or drug treatment due to restrictions by donor governments or agencies. Substitution programmes, including oral substitution such as buprenorphine, remain costly and few efforts have been made to reduce the cost of these drugs compared to progress made in price reduction of condoms and antiretroviral treatment.

Policies relating to behaviour change and risk reduction are crucial for successful HIV prevention interventions aimed at IDUs. Such policies include legalisation of sales and possession of injecting equipment, and enabling NSPs to be implemented. In addition, environmental changes are required for enabling drug-dependent persons to lead meaningful lives as well as to practise and sustain safer behaviours, including safer sex. It is frequently a difficult choice for decision makers to justify resources for drug user interventions when basic health care amenities are scarce. Therefore, the role of the politicians is crucial in terms of endorsing drug-related programmes, including NSP and drug treatment, which are still perceived as 'controversial' despite scientific evidence in support of their effectiveness.

Peer outreach programmes run by current or ex-drug users are frequently perceived as undesirable in localities where these are implemented. Yet an enabling micro- and macro-level environment is a prerequisite for implementation of successful HIV prevention programmes, although the importance of environmental factors on the effectiveness of HIV prevention interventions is frequently overlooked. Finally, the challenge lies in implementing scientific yet 'controversial' interventions, and in this context the role of the policy makers is crucial.

Conclusion

Even after two decades of drug-related HIV epidemics in Asia, an extremely limited coverage of the IDU population with HIV prevention programmes has so far been achieved. Furthermore, an unfavourable policy and legal environment, and absence of essential enabling conditions for the drug-using population, combined with a lack of comprehensive and strategic approach render the benefits of current HIV prevention efforts restricted only to a few drug users in Asia. The rapidly spreading drug-related HIV epidemic in Asia requires synergy and coordination among international agencies and governments, particularly the health and law departments. A multi-disciplinary approach is necessary to plan a comprehensive mix of strategies for drug and HIV prevention measures, and to ensure quality and coverage of these interventions. Increased resources and genuine partnerships with drug user communities as well as the creation of a supportive policy environment and social context is necessary to enable IDUs bring about and sustain changes in drug use and the behaviours that put them at risk for HIV.

N OTE

* The views expressed by the authors are their own, and do not represent those of their institutions.

R EFERENCES

Abdul-Quader, A.S., D.C. Des Jarlais, A. Chatterjee, A.E. Hirky and S.R. Friedman (1999). Interventions for injecting drug users. In Gibney et al. (eds.), *Preventing HIV in developing countries: Biomedical and behavioral approaches.* New York. Plenum Press.

Ainsworth, M. and M. Over (1997). *Confronting AIDS: Public priorities in a global epidemic.* Washington, DC: World Bank.

Allen, S. et al. (1992). Effect of serotesting with counselling on condom use and sero-conversion among HIV discordant couples in Africa. *British Medical Journal*, 304, 1605–9.

Azim, T., J. Bogaerts, D.L. Yirrell, A.C. Banarjea, M.S. Sarker, G. Ahmed, M.M. Amin, A.S. Rahman and A.M. Hussain (2002). Injecting drug use in Bangladesh: Prevalence of syphilis, hepatitis, HIV and HIV subtypes. *AIDS*, 4(16), 121–23.

Baqi, S. et al. (1998). HIV antibody prevalence and associated risk factors in sex workers, drug users and prisoners in Sindh, Pakistan. *Journal of Acquired Immune Deficiency Syndromes and Human Retrovirology*, 18, 73–79.

Beyrer, C., M.H. Razak, K. Lisam, J. Chen, W. Lui and X.-F. Yu (2000). Overland heroin trafficking routes and HIV-1 spread in South and South-East Asia. *AIDS*, 14, 75–83.

Binswanger, H.P. (2000). Scaling up HIV/AIDS programs to national coverage. *Science*, 288, 2173–76.

Centre for Harm Reduction (1999). *Manual for reducing drug-related harm in Asia.* Melbourne: Centre for Harm Reduction, Burnet Centre for Medical Research and Asia Harm Reduction Network.

Chen, J.W., L.Y. Liu and L.Y. Nancy (1999). Molecular-epidemiological analysis of HIV-1 initial prevalence in Guangxi, China. *Zhonghua Liu Zing Bing Xue Za Zhi* (Chinese Journal of Epidemiology), 20(2), 74–77.

Chen, Y.M.A. et al. (2001). Temporal trends and molecular epidemiology of HIV infection in Taiwan from 1988 to 1998. *Journal of Acquired Immune Deficiency Syndromes*, 26(3), 274–82.

Chin, J. (2001). The epidemiology of HIV/AIDS in Asia and policy implications for IDU populations. Paper presented at the 12th International Conference on the Reduction of Drug Related Harm, New Delhi, 1–5 April.

Des Jarlais, D.C., K. Choopanya, P. Millson, P. Friedman and S.R. Friedman (1998). The structure of stable seroprevalence HIV-1 epidemics among injecting drug users. In G.V. Stimson, D. Des Jarlais and A. Ball (eds.), *Drug injecting and HIV infection: Global dimensions and local responses.* London: University College London Press.

Ford, C. and L. Lisa (2001). Are UK substance misuse services failing women? Paper presented at the 12th International Conference on the Reduction of Drug Related Harm, New Delhi, 1–5 April.

Hangzo, C.Z., A. Chatterjee, S. Sarkar, G.T. Zomi and A.S. Abdul-Quader (1997). Reaching out beyond the hills: HIV prevention among the injecting drug users in the north-eastern state of Manipur. *Addiction*, 92(7), 813–20.

Hussain, A.M.Z. (ed.) (2000). Report on the sero-surveillance and behavioural surveillance of STD and AIDS in Bangladesh 1998–99. Government of Bangladesh/ UNAIDS, June.

Ichimura, H., O. Kurimura, I. Tamura, I. Tsukue, H. Tsuchi and **T. Kurimura** (1995). Prevalence of blood-borne viruses among intraveneous drug users and alcoholics in Hiroshima, Japan. *International Journal of STD and AIDS*, 6(6), 441–43.

Jenkins, C., H. Rahman, T. Saidel, S. Jana and **A.M. Hussain** (2001). Measuring the impact of needle exchange programs among injecting drug users through the National Behavioural Surveillance in Bangladesh. *AIDS Education Prevention*, 5, 452–61.

Kato, K.S. et al. (1999). Genetic similarity of HIV type 1, subtype E in a recent outbreak among injecting drug users in northern Vietnam to strains in Guangxi province of southern China. *AIDS Research and Human Retroviruses*, 15, 1157–68.

Klee, H. (1996). Women drug users and their partners. In Sherr, Hankins and Bennett (eds.), *AIDS as a gender issue: Psychosocial perspectives*. London: Taylor and Francis.

Loxley, W. (2000). Doing the possible: Harm reduction, injecting drug use and blood borne viral infections in Australia. *International Journal of Drug Policy*, 11(6), 407–16.

Lwin, T., R. Mra, K.T. Aye, K. Oo, S. Thein and **K. Moe** (1999). HIV transmission in sexual partners of persons with HIV/AIDS attending the Infectious Diseases Hospital, Yangon. *Southeast Asia Journal of Tropical Medical Public Health*, 30(2), 251–56.

Monitoring the AIDS Pandemic (MAP) (2001). The status and trends of HIV/ AIDS/STI epidemics in Asia and the Pacific, MAP, Melbourne, 4 October.

Naik, T.N., S. Sarkar, H.L. Singh, S.C. Bhunia, Y.I. Singh, P.K. Singh and **S.C. Pal** (1991). Intravenous drug users: A new high-risk group for HIV infection in India. *AIDS*, 5(1): 117–18.

Needle, R.H., A. Ball, D.C. Des Jarlais, C. Whitmore and **E. Lambert** (2000). The Global Research Network on HIV Prevention on Drug-using Populations (GRN) 1998–2000: Trends in the epidemiology, ethnography, and prevention of HIV/AIDS in injection drug users. Paper presented at the Third Annual Global Research Network Meeting on HIV Prevention in Drug-using Populations, Durban, July.

Nelson, K.E. et al. (1996). Changes in sexual behaviour and decline in HIV infection among young men in Thailand. *New England Journal of Medicine*, 335, 297–303.

Nelson, K.E., S. Eiumtrakul, D.D. Celentano, C. Beyrer, N. Galai, S. Kawichai and **C. Khamboonruang** (2002). HIV infection among young men in northern Thailand, 1991–1998: Increasing role of injection drug use. *Journal of Acquired Immunodeficiency Syndromes*, 29(1), 62–68.

Nerurkar, V.R., H.T. Nguyen, W.-M. Dashwood, P.R. Hoffman, D.M. Morens, A.H. Kaplan, R. Detels and **R. Yanagihara** (1996). HIV-1 subtype E in commercial sex workers and injection drug users in southern Vietnam. *AIDS Research and Human Retroviruses*, 12(9), 841–43.

Nerurkar, V.R., H.T. Nguyen, C.L. Woodward, P.R. Hoffman, W.-M. Dashwood, H.T. Long, D.M. Morens, R. Detels and **R. Yanagihara** (1997). Sequence and phylogenetic analyses of HIV-1 infection in Vietnam: Subtype E in commercial sex workers and injection drug users. *Cellular and Molecular Biology*, 14, 959–68.

Oelrichs, R.B., I.L. Shrestha, D.A. Anderson and **N.J. Deacon** (2000). The explosive human immunodeficiency virus type 1 epidemic among injecting drug users of Kathmandu, Nepal, is caused by a subtype C virus of restricted genetic diversity. *Journal of Virology*, 74(3), 1149–57.

Oh, M. and **K. Choe** (1999). Epidemiology of HIV infection in the Republic of Korea. *Journal of Korean Medical Science*, 14(5), 469–74.

Panda, S., L. Bijaya, N. Sadhana Devi, E. Foley, A. Chatterjee, D. Banerjee, T.N. Naik, M.K. Saha and **S.K. Bhattacharya** (2001). Interface between drug use and sex work in Manipur. *National Medical Journal of India*, 14(4), 209–11.

Panda, S., A. Chatterjee, S.K. Bhattacharya, B. Manna, P.N. Singh, S. Sarkar, T.N. Naik, S. Chakrabarti and **R. Detels** (2000). Transmission of HIV from injecting drug users to their wives in India. *International Journal of STD and AIDS*, 11(7), 468–73.

Panda, S., S. Sarkar, S.K. Bhattacharya, R. Detels and **S. Chakrabarti** (1998). HIV-1 in injecting-drug users and heterosexuals. *Lancet*, 352(9123), 241.

Peters, A., T. Davies and **A. Richardson** (1998). Multi-site samples of injecting drug users in Edinburgh: Prevalence and correlates of risky injecting practices. *Addiction*, 93(2), 253–67.

Poschyachinda, V. (1993). Drugs and AIDS in Southeast Asia. *Forensic Science International*, 62(1–2), 15–28.

Quan, V.M., A. Chung, H.T. Long and **T.J. Dondero** (2000). HIV in Vietnam: The evolving epidemic and the prevention response, 1996 through 1999. *Journal of Acquired Immune Deficiency Syndrome*, 25(4), 360–69.

Reid, G. (2001). The challenges and activities responding to the drug user situation in Bali, Indonesia. *National AIDS Bulletin*, 14(5), 28–30.

Reid, G. and **G. Costigan** (2002). Revisiting 'The Hidden Epidemic': A situation assessment of drug use in Asia in the context of HIV/AIDS. Centre for Harm Reduction and the Burnet Institute, Melbourne, January.

Reid, G. and **N. Crofts** (2000). Rapid assessment of drug use and HIV vulnerability in Southeast and East Asia. *International Journal of Drug Policy*, 11, 113–24.

Rhodes, T. and **G.V. Stimson** (1998). Community intervention among hidden populations of injecting drug users in the time of AIDS. In M. Bloor and F. Wood (eds.), *Addictions and Problem Drug Use*. London: Jessica Kingsley.

Samson, L., S. Panda, F. Mesquita, A. Ball and **S. Sarkar** (1999). Harm reduction for drug-related HIV in developing countries. Paper presented at the 10th International Conference on the Reduction of Drug-related Harm, Geneva.

Sarkar, S. (2000). Harm reduction in the developing countries: Next decade (Plenary). Paper presented at the 11th International Conference on the Reduction of Drug Related Harm, Jersey, 9–13 April.

Sarkar, K., S. Panda, N. Das and **S. Sarkar** (1997). Relationship of national highway with injecting drug abuse and HIV in rural Manipur, India. *Indian Journal of Public Health*, 41(2), 49–51.

Sarkar, S., A. Chatterjee, C.B. McCoy, A.S. Abdul-Quader, L.R. Metsch and **R.S. Anwyl** (1996). Drug use and HIV among youth in Manipur. In C.B. McCoy, L.R. Metsch and J.A. Inciardi (eds.), *Intervening with drug involved youth*. Thousand Oaks: Sage Publications.

Sarkar, S., N. Das, S. Panda, T.N. Naik, K. Sarkar, B.C. Singh, J.M. Ralte, S.M. Aier and S.P. Tripathy (1993). Rapid spread of HIV among injecting drug users in north-eastern states of India. *Bulletin of Narcotics*, 45(1), 91–105.

Sarkar, S., S. Panda, K. Sarkar, C.Z. Hangzo, L. Bijaya, N.Y. Singh, A. Agarwal, A. Chatterjee, B.C. Deb and R. Detels (1995). A cross-sectional study on factors determining unsafe injecting practices including HIV testing and counselling among injecting drug users of Manipur. *Indian Journal of Public Health*, 39(3), 86–92.

Schwebke, J.R., T. Aira, N. Jordan, P.E. Jolly and S.H. Vermund (1998). Sexually transmitted diseases in Ulaanbaatar, Mongolia, *International Journal of STD and AIDS*, 9(6), 354–58.

Singh, S. and N. Crofts (1993). HIV infection among injecting drug users in northeast of Malaysia, 1992. *AIDSCare*, 5(3), 273–81.

Stimson, G.V. (1993). The global diffusion of injecting drug use: Implications for human immunodeficiency virus infection. *Bulletin of Narcotics*, 45(1), 3–17.

——— (1995). AIDS and injecting drug use in the United Kingdom, 1987–93: The policy response and the prevention of the epidemic. *Social Science Medicine*, 41(5), 699–716.

Tarantola, D., P.R. Lamptey and R. Moodie (1999). The global HIV/AIDS pandemic: Trends and patterns. In Gibney et al. (eds.), *Preventing HIV in developing countries: Biomedical and behavioral approaches*. New York: Plenum Press.

United Nations (2000). Preventing the transmission of HIV among drug abusers. United Nations, September.

UNDCP and UNAIDS (1999). Baseline study of the relationship between injecting drug use, HIV, and Hepatitis C among male injecting drug users in Lahore. UNDCP and UNAIDS, Islamabad.

Voluntary HIV-1 Counselling and Testing Efficacy Study (2000). Efficacy of voluntary HIV-1 counselling and testing in individuals and couples in Kenya, Tanzania, and Trinidad: A randomised trial. *Lancet*, 356 (9224), 103–13.

Waver, M.J. et al. (1996). Origins and working conditions of female sex workers in urban Thailand. *Social Science Medicine*, 42, 453–62.

Weniger, B.G., Y. Takebe, C.Y. Ou and S. Yamazaki (1994). The molecular epidemiology of HIV in Asia. *AIDS*, 8 (Supplement 2), S13–28.

WHO and Department of Health (2000). Consensus report on STI, HIV and AIDS epidemiology: Philippines. Manila: WHO Regional Office for the Western Pacific.

WHO International Collaborative Group (1994). Multi-city study on drug injecting and risk of HIV infection. Document WHO/PSA/94.4, WHO, Geneva.

Wodak, A. (1999). Fifteen years of HIV prevention among injection drug users in Australia. In *1999 global research network meeting on HIV prevention in drug-using populations: Second annual meeting report*. Atlanta, Georgia: Global Research Network.

Yu, X.F., W. Liu, J. Chen, W. Kong, B. Liu, Q. Zhu, F. Liang, F. McCutchan, S. Piyasirisilp and S. Lai (2002). Maintaining low HIV type 1 end genetic diversity among injection drug users infected with a B/C recombinant and CRF01_AE HIV Type 1 in Southern China. *AIDS Research and Human Retroviruses*, 18(2), 167–70.

Zheng, X., J.P. Zhang and S.Q. Qu (1997). A cohort study of HIV infection among intravenous drug users in Ruili and two other counties in Yunnan province. *Zhonghua Liu Xing Bing Xue Za Zhi*, 18(5), 259–62.

HIV/AIDS AND SEXUALLY-TRANSMITTED INFECTIONS IN THAILAND: LESSONS LEARNED AND CHALLENGES AHEAD | 8

Anupong Chitwarakorn

The first case of AIDS in Thailand was reported in September 1984, followed by sporadic cases until 1987. Early cases were generally confined to homosexual males. This was followed by an outbreak of HIV infection among injecting drug users (IDUs) in Bangkok in late 1987 (Phanuphak et al. 1989; Uneklabh and Phutiprawan 1988; Vanichseni et al. 1989). The first wave of HIV infection among IDUs was followed by the detection of high prevalence of HIV infection among female sex workers in Chiang Mai, the northern province of Thailand in 1989 (Division of Epidemiology 1989). The virus then spread to their clients in 1989–90, with the result that heterosexual transmission became increasingly important causing the second and third waves of the epidemic (Weninger et al. 1991). Between 1990 and 1991 many provinces reported HIV infection among pregnant women at antenatal clinics, followed by cases of mother-to-child transmission with increasing numbers of infected newborns reported in the following years, giving rise to the fourth and fifth waves of the HIV epidemic (Brown et al. 1994; Weninger et al. 1991).

AIDS Case Reporting

Since 1991 the Thai government has increased the utilisation of the AIDS case reporting system. Health institutions and physicians are encouraged to report specific details of AIDS cases anonymously to the public health authority. As in most countries, under-reporting of AIDS cases remains problematic. Figure 8.1 shows the distribution of reported cases of AIDS by year of diagnosis. The cumulative number of reported AIDS cases (as of 31 October 2002) were 204,448. Over 88.56 per cent of the cases were reported in years 1995–2002.

Figure 8.1
Distribution of AIDS Cases and Deaths in Thailand:
September 1984–October 2002

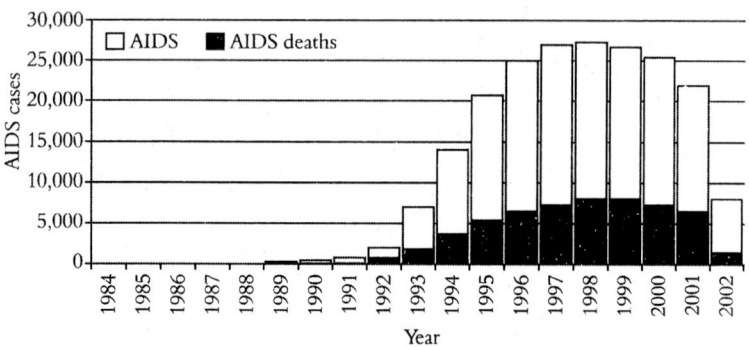

Source: Epidemiology Division, Ministry of Public Health, Thailand.

More than 78.04 per cent of the cases were in the age group of 20 to 39 years, of which 27.08 per cent were in the age group of 25 to 29 years, followed by the age group 30 to 34 years (25.19 per cent), 35 to 39 years (15.36 per cent) and 20 to 24 years (10.41 per cent). The age group 40 to 44 years accounted for 8.18 per cent. Children of less than 5 years of age made up 3.54 per cent. The proportion of reported AIDS cases for males and females in 1995 was 4.5:1. The male and female ratio decreased to 2.83:1 in 1998 and to 1.95:1 in 2001.

Sexual transmission accounted for 83.78 per cent of AIDS cases, while infection among IDUs was responsible for 4.77 per cent. The proportion of vertical transmission or transmission of HIV from infected mothers to child was about 4.42 per cent.

The cumulative number of common opportunistic infections among reported AIDS patients in Thailand during 1984 to 2002 were: *Myco-bacterium tuberculosis* (pulmonary or extra-pulmonary), 57,900 cases (25.0 per cent); *Pneumocystis carinii* (pneumonia), 42,228 cases (18.2 per cent); cryptococcosis, 34,442 cases (14.9 per cent); candidiasis (trachea, bronchi), 10,697 cases (4.6 per cent); and recurrent pneumonia (bacteria), 7,413 cases (3.2 per cent).

Sentinel Seroprevalence Surveillance

The sentinel seroprevalence surveillance system, which consists of sequentially cross-sectional HIV sero-surveys among specific sub-population groups, started in 1989. In 2001 the highest (median) prevalence was among IDUs (50.00 per cent) followed by female direct sex workers (16.56 per cent), male sex workers (9.61 per cent), fishermen (7.30 per cent), female indirect sex workers (5.08 per cent), male STD clients (4.44 per cent) and blood donors (0.30 per cent). The HIV prevalence rate has remained stable among men visiting STD clients for the last eight years, with a small increase to 9 per cent in 1999. However, in the year 2001 this rate dropped to 4.44 per cent. HIV prevalence in pregnant women rose from zero in 1989 to 2.3 per cent in 1995, before falling to 1.5 per cent in 1998. This rate increased again to 1.8 per cent in 1999 and then dropped to 1.37 per cent in the year 2001. HIV prevalence in military conscripts at the national level decreased from 4 per cent in 1993 to 0.5 per cent in the year 2001. Cohort studies in conscripts confirmed the patterns seen at the national level, for example, a 10-fold reduction in incidence had been observed in the north in 1995 when compared to the early 1990s. It was evident that with a strong national response, there was a large decline in new HIV infections. The prevalence rate among intravenous drug users, however, continued to increase from 39 per cent in 1989 to 51 per cent in 1999, but fell 50 per cent in 2001, and is considered one of the major challenges to Thai efforts to control HIV (Figure 8.2).

In the year 2001, from a total population of 61 million, it was estimated by the Thai Working Group on HIV/AIDS Projection that 1,009,748 persons were infected with HIV since the beginning of the epidemic (Thai Working Group on HIV/AIDS Projection 2001). Among these, 344,403 had died and 665,344 were currently living with HIV and AIDS in the country, of which 53,389 would develop serious AIDS illnesses and approximately the same number die of AIDS complications. It was also estimated that 25,790 new infections would occur during that year compared to 142,819 new infections in 1991.

The STI Reporting System

Sexually-transmitted infections (STIs) are not required by law to be reported to health authorities. So the real figures of STI in Thailand are

Figure 8.2
HIV Seroprevalence among Injecting Drug
Users at Treatment Clinics in Thailand: 1989–2001

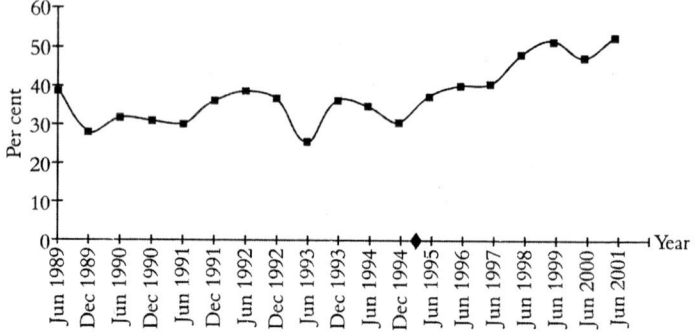

Source: Sentinel Serosurveillance, Division of Epidemiology, Ministry of Public Health, Thailand.

Note: Switching from biannual (June and December) to annual in June since 1995.

not known. Figures are collected from 508 district-level STI clinics through monthly reports. Six major STI reported are syphilis, gonorrhea, non-gonococcal genito-urinary tract infection, chancroid, lymphogranuloma venereum and granuloma inguinale. The only case of granuloma inguinale was reported in 1979 and it was an imported case.

Figure 8.3 shows the reported cases of STI in Thailand between 1967 and 2001. The graph shows a rapid increase in cases of STI from 1967 to 1980. The factors for this initial increase were rapid socio-economic development, enormous industrialisation and migration from rural to urban areas, and changing of sexual behaviour with an expansion of the commercial sex industry. In addition, the resistance to antibiotic of *N. gonorrhoea* with the emergence of the penicillinase-producing strain in 1977 and its rapid increase from 8.6 per cent in 1977 to 42 per cent in 1981 were also responsible (Panikabutra and Suvannamalik 1977, 1991). The temporary drop between 1980 and 1984 was due to the integration of STI services and the reorganisations of the provincial VD clinic from the administration of Department of Communicable Disease Control to the Office of the Permanent Secretary. The dramatic decrease since 1989 has been due to the massive safer sex campaigns, and promotion of condoms and the 100 per cent condom use programme (1989–91) (Rojanapithayakorn and Hanenberg 1996).

Figure 8.3
Reported STD Cases in Men

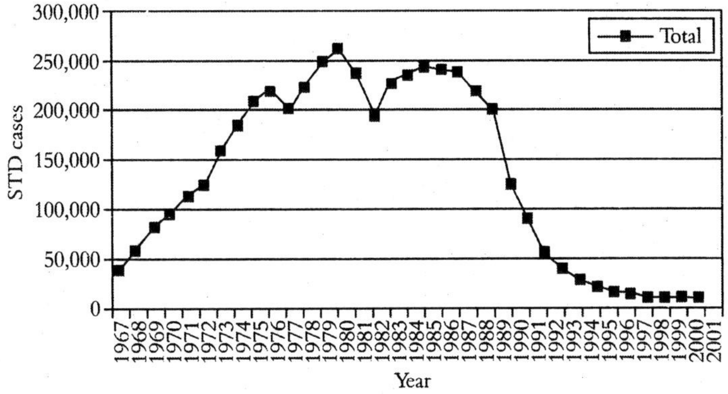

Source: Sentinel Serosurveillance, Division of Epidemiology, Ministry of Public Health, Thailand.

Behavioural Surveillance

The HIV/AIDS risk behaviour surveillance was initiated in 1995 to supplement other HIV/AIDS surveillance systems. The risk behaviour surveillance presented in this chapter is derived from the surveys conducted during 1995–2001 among males (military conscripts, factory workers and students) and females (factory workers, pregnant women and students).

Among the male population surveyed, a significantly lower proportion admitted to have had sex with sex workers in the last 12 months prior to the time of survey (from 48.8 in 1991 to 16.8 per cent in 2001 among military recruits; from 30.6 to 14.6 per cent among factory workers). However, the proportion of those who admitted to have had sex with sex workers always with condom use remained at about 60 per cent for both groups. The condom use rate in casual sex was lower at the average of 30 to 40 per cent. The first age of first sex for both factory men and women was 18 to 19 years and 20 to 21.5 years for pregnant women.

Based on these findings, it is clear that Thailand is still at risk of having another outbreak of HIV among the general population due to the lack of condom use during casual sex. Despite continuous reductions in commercial sex visitation by men, many still engage in casual sex without condoms. The female population surveyed further supports this finding. These results point to the urgent need to improve levels of condom used in casual sex in Thailand.

The National Response to AIDS

The programmatic responses to HIV infections were strongly influenced by available epidemiological, social and behavioural data (Wiput et al. 1998). Basic research and operational research in the social sector and in the fields of epidemiology, economics and medicine have provided valuable inputs to programme development (Figure 8.4).

Figure 8.4
The Three Phases of the Thai National Response to AIDS: 1984–Present

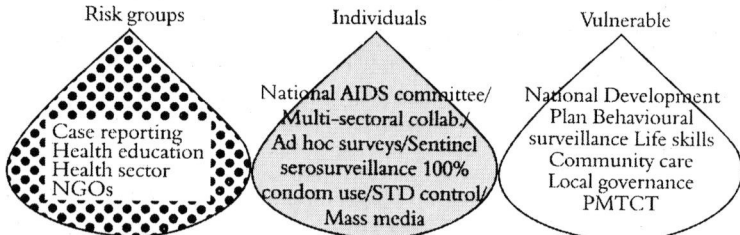

Risk groups   Individuals   Vulnerable

Case reporting
Health education
Health sector
NGOs

National AIDS committee/
Multi-sectoral collab.
Ad hoc surveys/Sentinel
serosurveillance 100%
condom use/STD control/
Mass media

National Development
Plan Behavioural
surveillance Life skills
Community care
Local governance
PMTCT

Phase 1: Health programme   Phase 2: Social programme   Phase 3: Civil society
(1984–90)   (1990–96)   (1997–present)

In response to HIV/AIDS-related issues, Thailand initiated three major strategies. These strategies are categorised into the health, social and holistic phases.

Phase 1: The Health-focused Phase (1984–90)

During the health-focused phase, the AIDS case reporting system was firmly established and strong health education programmes were implemented. The Medium-term Plan for the Prevention and Control of AIDS was implemented during 1989–91, which followed WHO guidelines and emphasised human rights and reducing discrimination. This plan provided a framework for government, NGOs and private initiatives, including measures for programme management, health education, counselling, training, surveillance, monitoring, medical and social care, and laboratory and blood safety control. In January 1990 Prime Minister Chatichai announced the official campaign to control and prevent HIV/AIDS, making HIV/AIDS control a national policy.

This was the first clear-cut government policy stance on AIDS. Government budgetary commitment to combating AIDS also increased significantly.

Phase II: The Socially-focused Phase (1990–96)

The National AIDS Prevention and Control Committee, with the prime minister as chairman, was constituted in 1991. Thai society rapidly expanded its response to HIV/AIDS and a multi-sectoral collaboration was established. All government agencies were provided with funding to implement their own AIDS plan. During this time nearly 300 non-governmental organisations were involved in AIDS prevention, care and support activities throughout the country. This phase was also marked by a dramatic increase in national budget allocations for HIV/AIDS. The supportive political environment of Prime Minister Anand's administration was a decisive factor in keeping the AIDS issue high on government's agenda and this commitment has been sustained by subsequent governments. This was a period of extensive national activity on the HIV/AIDS front. The mass media and the Thai advertising/marketing industry played a vital role in creating awareness for the prevention of HIV/AIDS. Television and radio stations aired HIV/AIDS education spots hourly. Efforts were made to reduce risk in commercial sex through active promotion of condom use between sex workers and their clients. The 100 per cent condom use programme was made national policy in 1991. STD treatment programmes were expanded and strengthened nationwide. Thai NGOs pioneered participatory development of prevention programmes to reach out-of-school youth. Many private firms initiated AIDS education in the workplace, and later the Thai Business Coalition on AIDS was established to promote compassionate workplace policies and workplace prevention efforts. The Thai Red Cross Society (TRCS) established the first anonymous HIV counselling and testing centre, a concept that was then adopted by the Ministry of Public Health (MOPH) for nationwide implementation. The TRCS also supported the formation of the Wednesday Friends Club, the first of many Thai self-supported groups for those living with HIV and AIDS.

Phase III: The Holistic Phase (1997–Present)

In 1995 the National Economic and Social Development Board (NESDB) was entrusted with the formulation of a new National AIDS

Strategic Plan for the period from 1997 to 2001. The planning process was a participatory one, involving concerned agencies from the various sectors, including people with HIV and AIDS. This process took advantage of the extensive experience in HIV/AIDS prevention and care gained in the first decade of the Thai epidemic to decide the most effective approach for the next five years. The plan was also designed to integrate with and share a number of concepts and features with the Eighth National Economic and Social Development Goals in social and economic areas, including HIV/AIDS, children and youth development, labour and social welfare, and cultural development.

The National Plan for Prevention and Alleviation of HIV/AIDS (2002–6)

According to the new five-year plan, which is actually a continuation of the previous one, more emphasis will be placed on the participation of all sectors—private, public and communities—in solving AIDS problems. A holistic approach of management will be utilised, requiring private and public enterprise collaboration aimed at achieving the following:

1. HIV prevalence among the reproductive age population will be reduced to less than 1 per cent by 2006.
2. At least 80 per cent of persons living with HIV/AIDS will have access to quality health socio-economic and education support from the community.
3. Local administrations and community organisations throughout the country will efficiently and continuously plan and carry out the work of HIV/AIDS prevention and alleviation.

The following strategies have been developed through an active participatory mechanism from the stakeholders:

Strategy 1: Developing potential individuals, families, communities and the broader social environment to prevent and alleviate the HIV/AIDS problem.
Strategy 2: Establishing health and social welfare services for the prevention and alleviation of HIV/AIDS.
Strategy 3: Developing knowledge and research for the prevention and alleviation of HIV/AIDS.

Strategy 4: International cooperation for the prevention and alleviation of HIV/AIDS.

Strategy 5: Developing a holistic programme management system to integrate the task of HIV/AIDS prevention and alleviation.

Key Interventions

Promotion of Condom Use

The 100 per cent condom use programme in commercial sex establishments was first established in Ratchaburi province as early as in 1989 (Panikabutra and Suvannamalik 1991), the same year when the first sentinel surveillance was introduced and showed that the prevalence of HIV among direct sex workers was 3.1 per cent. The programme showed an enormous impact among sex workers and their clients, resulting in the decrease of STI among them. In 1999 the programme was adopted in 13 other provinces. In 1991 the National AIDS Control Committee issued a resolution to implement the 100 per cent condom use programme on a national scale. The condom use rate increased from less than 20 per cent in 1989 to above 90 per cent in 1992. It has been well above 95 per cent since then.

Mother-to-Child HIV Transmission Prevention Programme

In early 2000 the Thai MOPH established a national policy on preventing mother-to-child HIV transmission (MOPH 2000a). It was the first resource-poor country to implement such a national programme. The MOPH began supporting the nationwide integration of a prevention of mother-to-child HIV transmission programme into the existing maternal and child health programme. The programme components were: (a) establishment of confidential voluntary HIV counselling and testing in all health care facilities; (b) offering of confidential voluntary HIV counselling and testing to all pregnant women; (c) offering of oral zidovudine (300 mg twice a day) starting from 34 weeks' gestation until labour and 300 mg every three hours during labour for all HIV-seropositive women; (d) offering of oral zidovudine syrup to all infants born to HIV-seropositive women; (e) offering infant formula to substitute breastfeeding until 12 months of age; (f) offering HIV antibody testing to all children born to seropositive women at the ages of 12 and 18 months; and (g) proper medical care and treatment for mothers and children (MOPH 2000b).

The results from the period October 2000 through September 2001 showed that 96.7 per cent women who gave birth in the MOPH hospital had received antenatal care, of whom 93.3 per cent had been tested for HIV. Among women who were tested, 1.3 per cent were seropositive. Among seropositive women 70.1 per cent received prophylactic antiretroviral drugs before delivery and among infants born to HIV-seropositive mothers 88.7 per cent received prophylactic antiretroviral drugs (Amornwichet et al. 2002).

There were several steps—starting from the research results from developing countries, trying to find an affordable regimen, field testing the programme and implementing it—that the Thai MOPH had to take before it could launch its national programme to prevent mother-to-child HIV transmission. Every step has shown to be valuable in identifying a programme that is suitable for the nation.

Access to Care for HIV/AIDS Patients

The development of medical care for HIV/AIDS patients started in 1992 by the National AIDS Committee, which included the treatment for opportunistic infection and antiretroviral drugs. Since 2001 services for the treatment and prophylaxis of common opportunistic infections such as tuberculosis, *Pneumocystis carinii* pneumonia and cryptococcal meningitis have been expanded to be covered by government health insurance. A task force was established to implement a work plan with objectives to: (*a*) ensure the availability of prevention and treatment methods for opportunistic infections at all health care levels; (*b*) enhance information for people with HIV/AIDS (PHA) on available prevention and treatments for opportunistic infections; (*c*) change provider attitudes that discourage AIDS patients from obtaining treatment; and (*d*) develop a well-defined 'package' of health care benefits in the different public insurance schemes for PHA.

In Thailand the majority of PHAs are cared for by family members and supported in some cases by the services of NGOs and community-based organisations (CBO). Capacity building of the communities is being encouraged. This includes the roles of monks in providing psychological support and care for terminally ill patients with AIDS.

Sex Education for the Youth

Generally, HIV infection rates have been naturally high among the age group 15 to 24, not only in Thailand but in several countries. Sexual experience at younger ages is becoming common, along with a lack of awareness of possible HIV/STD infection. As a result, condom use rates can be very low. The Ministries of Education, University Affairs and Public Health together with many NGOs working with the youth have developed effective communication approaches to reach these groups, including sex education in and out of schools.

Voluntary Counselling and Testing (VCT)

VCT is available at nearly all provincial and community hospitals, through the private sector and at selected health centres. It is an entry point for those who seek early clinical management as well as a precautionary measure to prevent the spread of HIV. It can also encourage sexual behaviour change to prevent HIV.

Reduction of Transmission among Injecting Drug Users

Drug treatment programmes have been initiated in Bangkok and five regional drug treatment centres. These centres provide short (21-day) in-patient drug detoxification regimens on a voluntary and involuntary basis. The largest, the Northern Drug Treatment Centre, treats 2,800 to 3,000 drug users per year and includes programmes for opiate addicts, IDUs, alcoholics and those addicted or dependent on other drugs, including amphetamines and anxiolytics. However, it is recognised that IDUs in Thailand still have low access to HIV prevention. New efforts in harm reduction are currently being undertaken.

Vaccine Initiatives

In 1993 the National Plan for HIV/AIDS Vaccine Development was established that catalysed and facilitated the implementation of numerous HIV/AIDS vaccine-related activities. Ten clinical trials of HIV candidate vaccines were conducted in Thailand. In March 1999 the first phase-III efficacy of AIDSVAX B/E gp 120 vaccine was initiated.

Community Responses/Networking

The Thai government has a policy of promoting community response among stakeholders—which includes government, NGOs, PHA and CBOs—potential community leaders and *tambon* (sub-district) administration offices. It aims to strengthen the capacity of these community organisations in implementing prevention, care and support activities at the community level, especially in rural areas. With consideration of sustainability, such partnerships play active roles in HIV/AIDS problems analysis, development of plan of actions for HIV prevention and care, raising community funds, as well as monitoring and evaluation of actions. They have access to their own limited resources from the *tambon* administration offices and are able to seek additional budget from other sources.

Networking of NGOs and PHAs

It is considered that one factor facilitating the success of the national AIDS programme for Thailand is the active roles of PHAs and NGOs. The Thai NGO Coalition on AIDS (TNCA) represents over 300 NGOs working on AIDS throughout Thailand, while the Thai Network of People Living with HIV (TNP+) has a network of over 300 PHA organisations throughout the country. Both networks are represented in the National AIDS Committee. Both TNCA and TNP+ have their own networks in each region of Thailand, with coordinating units in Bangkok. The major objectives of these two networks are to strengthen the capacity of their members in order to effectively respond to community needs as well as identify appropriate strategies for policy development at the national level.

Lessons Learned

In lieu of levels of behaviour change and STD and HIV incidence declines, Thailand has had one of the most effective national responses to the HIV epidemic in the world, noteworthy for its widespread impact. This multi-sectoral, society-wide prevention and care effort has produced major risk reductions and substantially reduced the incidence of HIV and other sexually-transmitted diseases. Yet it has not been a static response—it has evolved and expanded dramatically over time as Thai society came to better understand the underlying causes of the epidemic and its implications for the country's future. As the body of research and experience in prevention and care grew, the response evolved from one rooted in traditional approaches to infectious disease to one emphasising the empowerment of individuals, families and communities to protect and care for themselves. It went from a response driven by a few NGOs and people in the Ministry of Health to one that actively engaged every sector of Thai society and gave everyone a role and a responsibility in responding. It moved from a programme driven from the national level to one that emphasised local involvement at the provincial, district and village level.

Other developing countries can learn much from studying the Thai experience, both its successes and failures, and adapt components of this approach to their own needs. A few important lessons from the material presented here bear emphasis.

1. **Prevention can work and it can work on a national scale, but strong political and financial commitment is needed in a sustained manner.** Thailand is the first country in the developing world where declines in prevalence have been seen on a national level that cannot be attributed to saturation of those at risk, increased mortality among those with HIV or changes in the populations being examined. Prevalence growth in Thailand slowed well before all those at risk were infected, largely due to increase in condom use and reductions in visits to sex workers by Thai men. Thai governments, starting with that of Prime Minister Anand, made a serious political and financial commitment to containing the epidemic, recognising how severely it would damage the country's future if they failed. Subsequent prime ministers have maintained this commitment. Thai society responded with active involvement in prevention and care efforts and widespread behaviour change.

2. **Effective responses require involving all sectors of society in addressing the underlying socio-economic and behavioural roots of HIV transmission.** A major contributor to the Thai programme's impact has been the willingness to alter policies and programmes as knowledge of the extent of risk behaviour grew and the social, economic and cultural roots of the epidemic were exposed. This helped illuminate the role that each sector of society had to play in the response. The subsequent active recruitment of various sectors to participate in the national response allowed the country to move more quickly to a broad-based holistic response emphasising true multi-sectoral involvement and seeking to create enabling environments for risk reduction and care. Another aspect contributing to success in the Thai efforts was the use of multiple simultaneous approach for HIV prevention. With the resources available and the active involvement of the various sectors, each major target population was reached through at least two avenues. For example, sex workers were

approached through peer education, workplace outreach from MOPH health personnel and NGOs, and extensive small media campaigns. Out-of-school youth received workplace education, mass media exposure and community-based peer education. This use of multiple avenues had a synergistic effect in promoting behaviour change and establishing new social norms encouraging safe behaviour. HIV/AIDS risk behaviour surveillance was also a key component in the HIV/AIDS programme. It provided crucial information on trends of risk behaviour over a period of time, information that was essential for proper policy development and planning for HIV/AIDS prevention and control.

3. **Ongoing epidemiological, social and behavioural research and monitoring, and the use of these data in developing policies and programmes to changing conditions are essential to an effective response.** In Thailand an active epidemiological, social and behavioural data collection effort began fairly early in the epidemic. Throughout, these data have been systematically and regularly collected and disseminated. They have been necessary in documenting the spread of HIV, in identifying determinants of risk and determining ongoing prevention directions and needs, and in demonstrating the effectiveness of prevention programme on a national scale. The widespread dissemination of this information, especially to high-level policy makers such as the prime minister and his cabinet, the parliament, national planners and provincial governors, has made it possible to advocate effectively for resources, mobilise political support and financial commitment from the government, and convince society of the need and benefits of responding aggressively. However, at this point in time, many developing countries still rely primarily on passive and potentially biased reporting of AIDS and HIV, which were clearly inadequate to move the early Thai response forward rapidly enough. Until social and behavioural studies became available, the biases in the early Thai HIV/AIDS reporting systems also diverted attention from the more prevalent heterosexual risk behaviour and their determinants that ultimately fuelled the epidemic. Knowledge of the distribution and determinants of risk behaviour is limited in developing countries. Few countries have national data on levels of risk in the general population, making it easier to marginalise HIV/AIDS and treat it as a problem of the

few rather than the many. Countries not basing their responses on a firm foundation of epidemiological and behavioural monitoring will remain focused on limited responses among a few subpopulations and have difficulty in advocating for an effective expanded response.

4. **Early and pragmatic action is needed, especially where there are substantial economic, social or cultural barriers to prevention.** Thailand acted comparatively early, but still not early enough. While behaviour change was already under way when the epidemic hit, had active condom promotion efforts begun two or three years earlier, many of the current infections would have been averted. The country also took a pragmatic approach to HIV prevention and care, building on a strong existing national infrastructure for health and social development, which extended from national to village level. Although commercial sex is illegal, the national programme decided it was more effective to work with those involved than to pursue enforcement actions that would make sex workers less accessible for prevention strategies. Condoms were promoted aggressively, aided in part by the desensitisation of Thai society to condoms. Religious leaders raised no opposition to condom promotion efforts, focusing their efforts instead on care and support activities. There was a willingness to learn from other countries, for example, through policy study tours to heavily affected African countries such as Uganda and Cote d'Ivoire, and through extensive research collaborations. All of these factors contributed to the country's ability to mount a rapid and effective response. Unfortunately, mounting an effective response in some other developing countries may take longer. More limited resources, lack of political commitment, denial of risk behaviours, religious opposition to condom use or public promotion of safer sex, low levels of literacy and lack of development infrastructure can all slow the response and reduce its effectiveness. These barriers to responding will take time to overcome. If countries wait until they see HIV prevalence start to climb before addressing these issues, many will be unable to respond as rapidly as did Thailand. Thus, early preparation to build the needed capacity and reduce existing barriers is essential in those countries. Delays will ultimately be measured in lives lost.

Challenges

Though Thailand has made substantial progress in the fight against AIDS, the national programme still needs to improve its prevention efforts to further reduce incidence and alleviate impact. Some of key strategies will be to:

- Maintain and strengthen the 100 per cent condom promotion programme in sex establishments, both direct and indirect. Condom promotion among casual sex targeted at youth, mobile population, migrants and other groups at risk should also be implemented on a national scale.
- Maintain the current strong national STD prevention and control programme by using rapid diagnosis and treatment, together with appropriate counselling services.
- Strengthen the national programme for the prevention of mother-to-child transmission.
- Strengthen prevention programmes for IDUs.
- Increase accessibility to antiretroviral therapy and quality care services for people with HIV/AIDS.
- Promote research that will provide valuable information on the factors influencing the epidemic and its effective countermeasures.
- Expand partnership in the design, implementation and evaluation of HIV/AIDS-related policies and programmes.
- Increase resources mobilised in support of HIV/AIDS prevention and care.

REFERENCES

Amornwichet, P., A. Teeraratkul, R.J. Simonds, T. Naiwatanakul, N. Chantharojwong, M. Culnane, J.W. Tappero and S. Kanshana (2002). Preventing mother-to-child HIV transmission: The first year of Thailand's national program. *Journal of the American Medical Association*, 288(2), 245–48.

Brown, T., W. Sittitrai, S. Vanichseni and U. Thisyakorn (1994). The recent epidemiology of HIV and AIDS in Thailand. *AIDS*, 8(Supplement 2), S131–41.

Division of Epidemiology (1989). First sentinel surveillance, June 1989. *Weekly Epidemiology Surveillance Report*, 20, 376–89.

Ministry of Public Health (MOPH) (2000a). *National guidelines for the clinical management of HIV infection in adults and children.* Nonthaburi, Thailand: MOPH (Sixth edition).

———— (2000b). *National guidelines for the prevention of mother-to-child HIV transmission and the care for HIV seropositive mother and HIV infected children.* Nonthaburi, Thailand: MOPH.

Panikabutra, K. and **S. Suvannamalik** (1977). Betalactamase producing *N. gonorrhoea* in Bangkok: Report of the first two cases. *Journal of Venereology Group of Thailand*, 4, 24–30.

———— (1991). Penicillinase producing *N. gonorrhoea* and its therapeutic aspect in Bangkok, Thailand. *Journal of Venereology Group of Thailand*, 1, 20–38.

Phanuphak, P., V. Poshyachina, T. Uneklabh and **W. Rojanapithayakorn** (1989). HIV transmission among intravenous drug abusers. Fifth International Conference on AIDS, Montreal, 1989 (abstract TGO 25).

Rojanapithayakorn, W. and **R. Hanenberg** (1996). The 100% condom program in Thailand. *AIDS*, 10(1), 1–7.

Thai Working Group on HIV/AIDS Projection (2001). *Projections for HIV/AIDS in Thailand: 2000–2020.* Bangkok: Karnsana Printing Press.

Uneklabh, C. and **T. Phutiprawan** (1988). Prevalence of HIV infection among Thai drug dependents. Fourth International Conference on AIDS, Stockholm, June (abstract 5524).

Vanichseni, S., K. Planringarm, W. Sonchai, P. Akarasewi, N. Wright and **K. Choopanya** (1989). First seroprevalence survey of intravenous drug users in Bangkok, Thailand. *Thai AIDS Journal*, 1, 75–82.

Weninger, B., K. Limpakarnjanarat and **K. Ungchusak** (1991). The epidemiology of HIV infection and AIDS in Thailand. *AIDS*, 5(Supplement 2), S71–85.

Wiput, Phoolcharoen, Kamnuan Ungchusak, Werasit Sittitrai and **Tim Brown** (1998). *Thailand: Lessons from a strong national response to HIV/AIDS.* Nepal: AIDS Division, Department of Communicable Disease Control, Ministry of Public Health.

9

HIV/AIDS IN INDIA:
PROBLEM AND RESPONSE

Mohammed Shaukat and Salil Panakadan

The first HIV infection in India was detected in 1986. Since then HIV infections and AIDS cases have been reported in all parts of the country. By the end of July 2003, a total of 54,061 AIDS cases had been reported to the National AIDS Control Organisation (NACO) (NACO 2003). Available data from the start of sentinel surveillance to the present indicate a varied picture. Epidemiological analysis of data and reports in India show that the highest number of HIV infections have been reported in Maharashtra and Tamil Nadu, and the highest rates among injecting drug users (IDUs) in the north-eastern state of Manipur (NACO 2001b; Sarkar et al. 2003; WHO Regional Offices for South-East Asia and Western Pacific 2001). Trends indicate two distinct characteristics of the spread of HIV infection: from groups practising risk behaviours to the general population, and from urban to rural areas (NACO 2001b). The predominant mode of transmission is through the sexual route (85 per cent) and another 3 per cent of transmission occurs through injecting drug use, most of them in the north-eastern states. The epidemic in India is really a collection of a number of small and large localised epidemics with their own dynamics and rates of growth, in different groups and parts of the country.

HIV Epidemiology

Trends in HIV epidemiology are monitored through the sentinel surveillance system, which operates through 384 sentinel sites. These sites include 166 sites in sexually-transmitted infections (STI) clinics, 200 sites in antenatal clinics (ANC), 13 sites among IDUs, two sites for sex workers and two sites for men having sex with men (MSM). The data thus collected are analysed to assess trends of HIV prevalence rates among identified risk groups over the years. The population groups and sites are chosen based on information of risk behaviour of various risk groups for HIV infection. The high-risk groups of population include patients attending STI clinics and intravenous drug users, while low-risk population includes women attending antenatal clinics. The whole procedure is 'unlinked anonymous'.

Based on sentinel surveillance data, the HIV prevalence in adult population can be broadly classified into three groups of states in the country (Figure 9.1).

- Group I: Maharashtra, Tamil Nadu, Karnataka, Andhra Pradesh, Manipur and Nagaland, where the HIV infection has crossed 1 per cent or more in antenatal women. These are high-prevalence states.

Figure 9.1
The HIV Epidemic in India: 2002

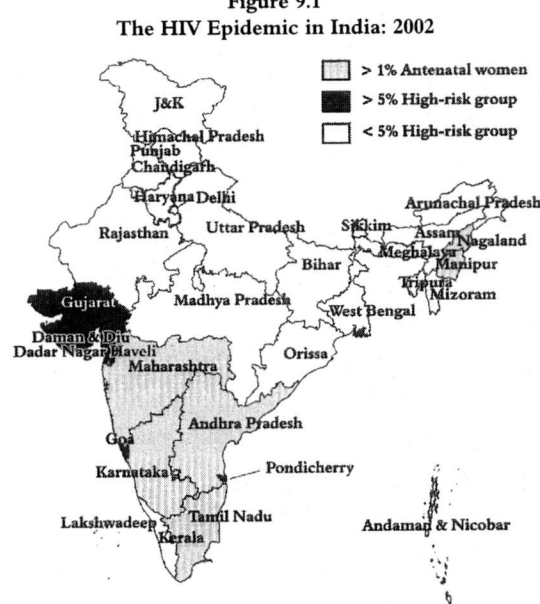

Source: NACO.

- Group II: Gujarat, Goa and Pondicherry, where HIV infection has crossed 5 per cent or more among high-risk groups, but the infection is below 1 per cent in antenatal women.
- Group III: The remaining states, where the HIV infection in any of the high-risk groups is still less than 5 per cent and is less than 1 per cent among antenatal women, constitute the long-prevalence states.

Behavioural surveillance surveys (BSS) show that awareness levels on HIV/AIDS also vary widely among these states. Generally awareness levels are higher in high-prevalence states and lower in low-prevalence states that form a belt across central India, with rural women in these states the most disadvantaged in terms of awareness. Incidence of casual or multi-partner sex also shows wide variations between states. Overall incidence of casual sex in the country was 5.1 per cent. It is the industrially and commercially advanced states in peninsular India that presently show highest rates of infection and risky sexual behaviour (NACO 2001a).

Data from various sentinel sites and other studies in Maharashtra show that over the years HIV infection has increased sharply among commercial sex workers (CSW), rapidly progressing among STI clinic attendees and is steadily spreading in low-risk populations (Figure 9.2) (Brookmeyer et al. 1995; Gangakhedkar et al. 1997; Mehendale et al. 1996). The time lag for HIV infection to spread from high-risk to low-risk

Figure 9.2
HIV Prevalence in Maharashtra

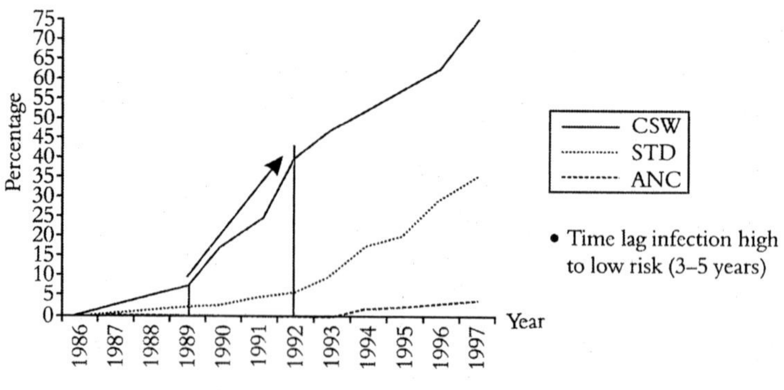

Source: NACO.

groups is between three to five years, as the infection will spread from CSWs to their clients, who act as a bridge population, and then to wives of these clients during this time period.

Among intravenous drug users the infection has spread very sharply in Manipur with HIV prevalence of more than 70 per cent (Figure 9.3). Nagaland also has a similar epidemic.

Figure 9.3
HIV Prevalence among IDUs in Manipur

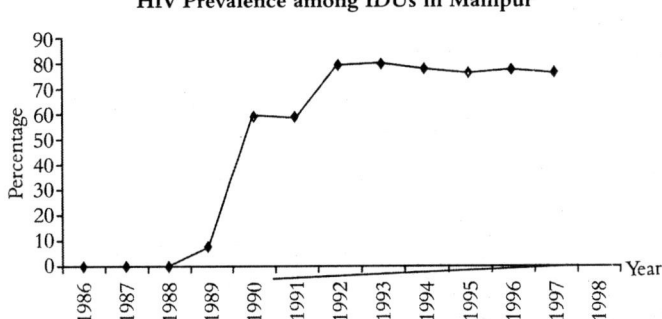

Source: NACO.

The trends of HIV infection among various risk groups of populations in India, reveal that although HIV prevalence is low in a majority of the states, the number of HIV infections are very high. There are wide regional variations in HIV prevalence. There are simultaneous epidemics in certain states, that is, heterosexual epidemic in Maharashtra and Tamil Nadu, and IDU epidemic in Manipur.

AIDS Case Surveillance

Monitoring the HIV/AIDS epidemic is also undertaken through the reporting of AIDS cases. By the end of December 2002, 42,947 AIDS cases were reported to NACO (Figure 9.4). These figures are considered only a fraction of AIDS morbidity as there is widespread under-reporting and under-diagnosis.

Epidemiological analysis of reported AIDS cases reveals that:

1. The disease is mainly affecting people in the sexually active age group. A majority of the patients (85 per cent) are in the age group of 15 to 44 years, thereby making a considerable economic impact to the country (Anand et al. 1999).

Figure 9.4
Epidemiological Analysis of Reported AIDS Cases
(Cumulative Number of AIDS Cases in India): December 2002

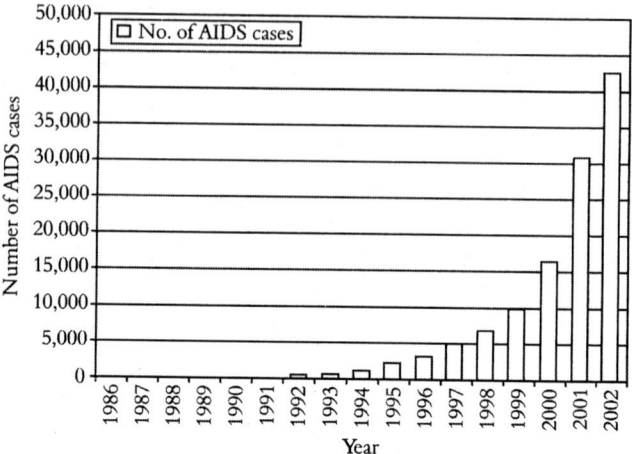

Source: NACO.

2. The predominant mode of transmission of infection in AIDS patients is through heterosexual contact (84.29 per cent). Other modes of transmission are injecting drug use (2.87 per cent), blood transfusion and blood product infusion (2.99 per cent), and others (7.25 per cent) (Figure 9.5).
3. Males account for 74.88 per cent of AIDS cases and females 25.12 per cent. The ratio is 3:1.
4. The major opportunistic infection in AIDS patients is tuberculosis, indicating a possibility of a dual epidemic of TB and HIV in the future (Figure 9.6).

Figure 9.5
Mode of Transmission of AIDS Cases in India: December 2002

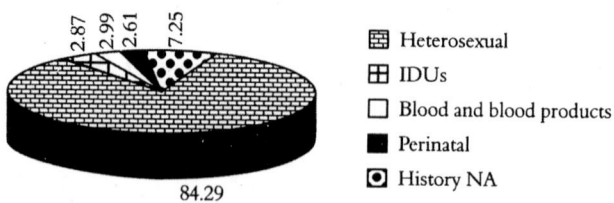

Heterosexual
IDUs
Blood and blood products
Perinatal
History NA

Source: NACO.

Figure 9.6
Major Opportunistic Infections in AIDS Cases in India: December 2002

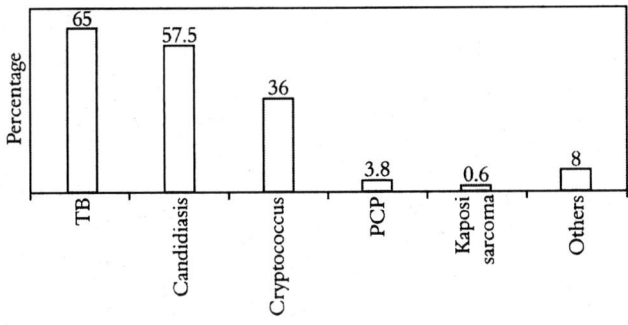

Source: NACO.

AIDS case surveillance data can also supplement the HIV surveillance data in monitoring the epidemic and could contribute to the planning of hospital and home/community-based care for AIDS patients under the programme.

Sexually-transmitted Infections

It is established that the presence of STIs increases the risk of HIV transmissions by three to ten times. Thus, prevention and control of STIs is an integral component of the National AIDS Control Programme. Community-based studies to determine the prevalence of STIs have been designed and are currently in progress. The BSS revealed that awareness about STIs, common symptoms, linkages with HIV, etc. was low across the country, irrespective of whether people lived in urban or rural areas, or were male or female. Self-reported STD prevalence measured as genital discharge or ulcer was 4.6 per cent and about 22 per cent of them went to a government facility for treatment.

The Response

The government of India launched a National AIDS Control Programme in 1987, which concentrated on surveillance, blood safety, and information, education and communication (IEC). A comprehensive five-year strategic plan was launched during 1992–97 with World Bank credit as the National AIDS Control Programme Phase 1. The second phase of the National AIDS Control Programme (NACP-II) was formulated with the two key objectives of reduction of the spread of HIV infection in the country and to strengthen India's capacity to respond to HIV/AIDS on a long-term basis (NACO 1999a, 1999b). Specific objectives of this phase include interventions to change behaviour, especially among high-risk groups through targeted interventions, decentralisation of service delivery through State AIDS Control Societies (SACS), protection of human rights, operational research and management reform. Inter-sectoral collaboration with all government departments, elected representatives of the people, chambers of commerce and industry, community-based organisations and the civil society in general is another feature of this phase.

During the past few years the programme has witnessed a rapid expansion and decentralisation in the country. SACS have been set up in 35 states/UTs and three municipal corporations (Mumbai, Chennai and Ahmedabad). These 38 societies have adequate financial and administrative powers to identify and respond to local needs. SACS operate through the regular health infrastructure and have designated district nodal officers to carry out activities related to prevention and control of HIV/AIDS. Considerable progress has been made in the past few years in implementing quality interventions. Two landmark policies, the National AIDS Prevention and Control Policy and the National Blood Policy, were adopted by the government in 2002. These are expected to be the framework on which the comprehensive national response to the epidemic will be based upon. To facilitate this response, AIDS-related legislation is also on the anvil.

Some of the specific areas of response are discussed here.

Blood Safety

This is one of the unheralded success stories of the programme. From being a non-existent and neglected discipline, blood transfusion services have taken giant strides in the past decade in HIV/AIDS programming. Licensing of all blood banks was made mandatory and professional donation banned. Massive investments were made in infrastructure and training. Over 1,000 blood banks in the government and charitable sector were modernised by the programme. All of them continue to get financial and material support to operate the blood banks. Eighty-two blood component separation facilities were also set up in the country. Testing for all transfusion-transmitted infections has been made mandatory for all blood banks and a strict licensing system has been introduced under the drug and cosmetics rules. Professional blood donation has been phased out since 1998. A National Blood Policy has been adopted by the government and an action plan has been drawn up to implement it. This is expected to usher in a modern blood transfusion service for the country.

Control of Sexually-transmitted Infections

Control of STIs was taken up as a priority activity. Three hundred and seventy-two existing STI clinics were upgraded and 132 new clinics started to function as referral centres. Five regional STI centres were upgraded to conduct training, research, supervision and monitoring. A nationwide facility survey of STD clinics was carried out, which is now being used to plug the gaps in the system. Over 18,000 medical officers from the government health care system and 10,000 private health care physicians were trained in STI case management. The guidelines for syndromic management and treatment of STI were revised and updated, and a training manual prepared by NACO was widely disseminated.

Surveillance

Biological Surveillance

HIV sentinel surveillance through 320 sentinel sites, AIDS case surveillance by adopting standard AIDS case definition in the Indian context and development of information system, and STD surveillance for reporting on both aetiological and syndromic approach are key activities to monitor the progression of HIV/AIDS epidemic in the country.

Behavioural Surveillance

Access to quality data on sexual behaviour of the population is also essential for mounting evidence-based control programmes. A nationwide baseline behavioural surveillance survey was conducted among the general population, bridge and high-risk populations in the country. Findings from these surveys are being used for better programming. Clear differentials between states and groups on various risk practices have been brought out.

Provision of Care, Treatment and Support

In recent times, as an increasing number of people are seeking care for HIV-related illnesses and AIDS, the need for care and support is being increasingly felt. NACO supports the establishment of community care centres, drop-in centres and networks of people living with HIV/AIDS (PLHA). At present 35 community care centres have been funded by the government and these are mainly in the high-prevalence states.

Linkages have been made between HIV care services and the Revised National TB Control Programme to facilitate the free treatment of TB. Treatment of other common opportunistic infections is also provided free in government hospitals. Training manuals and other material for doctors, nurses and counsellors have been developed and are being widely used.

Antiretroviral drugs are being used in the prevention of parent-to-child transmission (PPTCT) programme, in the post-exposure prophy-laxis programme for health care professionals, and also in various health insurance and contributory health care schemes. Since 1 April 2004, free antiretroviral treatment is being provided, to start with, in government hospitals in six high-prevalence states. Development of indigenous vaccine and operational research are the main activities under research priorities of the programme. Efforts are on to develop indigenous vaccines based on sub-type C of HIV.

Promoting Testing through Voluntary Counselling and Testing Centres

VCTCs have been established in order to provide social and psycho-logical support to those affected by HIV. Counselling and testing services are also available to all others who might feel the need for such services, and complete confidentiality is maintained. By June 2003 542 VCTCs were functioning in the country and it is proposed to establish at least one centre in each district of the country.

Preventing Parent-to-Child Transmission

The PPTCT programme offers a combination of low-cost, short-term preventive drug treatment, safe delivery practices, counselling and sup-port, and safe infant-feeding methods. Women consenting to be included in the programme receive prophylaxis, regular antenatal monitoring and supervised delivery. This programme is being implemented in phases, starting with high-prevalence states. In January 2003 the Global Fund to Fight AIDS, TB and Malaria assigned a grant of US$ 100 million for the PPTCT programme. They are also providing funds to scale up

ART and also to implement HIV/TB collaborative programmes in the country.

Learning for Life: School AIDS Education Programme

The school AIDS programme of NACO is a crucial intervention to address schoolgoing youth of the country. It is an innovative effort that offers flexibility to the states to follow models that best suit it in providing peer-driven life skills education to children of classes 9 and 11. It is always implemented through departments of education either directly or through NGOs. The programme focuses on: (a) raising awareness levels about HIV; (b) helping young people resist peer pressure to participate in risky behaviour; and (c) helping develop safe and responsible lifestyles, like abstinence. The programme is presently operational in about 35,000 schools.

NGO Interventions among Vulnerable Populations

The success of the National AIDS Control Programme will depend on the coverage and quality of targeted interventions (TI) that have been launched among the groups that are most vulnerable to HIV infection. Considerable upscaling of the programme in terms of coverage has been taken up in phase II. These interventions are carried out by NGOs as they are best suited to reach these populations, which can often be hard to access and may not necessarily trust the establishment. TIs use innovative approaches based on best practices in the country, combining behaviour change communication, counselling and general health care, including treatment of sexually-transmitted diseases, promotion of condom use and creating an enabling environment that nurtures empowerment. About 735 TIs are being implemented across the country, working among CSWs, truckers, street children, IDUs, MSMs, migrant workers and prison inmates.

Bilateral agencies like the DFID and USAID have supported projects like the Sonagachi project in Kolkata and the APAC project in Tamil Nadu, which have proved to be successful in reducing the risk of transmission among CSWs. The Sonagachi project is considered an example of a 'best practice' intervention the world over, which clearly demonstrates that close involvement and ownership of the project by the community are essential for a sex worker (or any marginalised section) project to succeed (Jana 1998).

Information Education and Communication

Under IEC activities, multimedia campaigns are being taken up. Special communication packages are developed for vulnerable groups like sex workers, IDUs, truckers and street children. Focused radio programmes are broadcast on a regular basis to provide information about prevention and control of HIV/AIDS. Field publicity units, and the song and drama division have taken extensive campaigns in rural areas. AIDS hotlines with the 1097 toll-free numbers have been established in major cities in the country.

Another example of a successful programme for the youth has been the Universities Talk AIDS (UTA) programme, which covered 3.5 million students in 4,044 institutions in the country. This programme was launched in 1991 and implemented by the National Service Scheme (NSS) with assistance from the WHO and NACO. The programme was aimed at reaching all universities and 10+2-level higher secondary schools. Along with a training manual in English (translated into various regional languages), a lot of IEC material was produced for disseminating information to students. The evaluation reports of the UTA programme by the WHO and other professional agencies indicate that the programme was successful in creating awareness about HIV/AIDS and developing a positive attitude towards sex in both boys and girls.

Condom Promotion

Condom supply was organised with the help of Department of Family Welfare. Emphasis was placed on social marketing of condoms. Quality control of condoms was improved and condoms were included in Schedule R of the Drugs and Cosmetic Act. A combination of free distribution and social marketing strategies is being used to make quality condoms available to the general population and high-risk groups.

Family Health Awareness Campaign

The Family Health Awareness Campaign is an innovative public health initiative to create awareness and encourage health-seeking behaviour among rural populations on RTIs and STIs, and to motivate and sensitise field-level health functionaries on the importance of treating such infections. Such a campaign is being organised annually in the entire rural population and in urban slum population in the country. About

226 million target beneficiaries (15 to 49 years) had been covered during the last campaign, out of which 43 million people attended the camps. More than 3.5 million cases were referred from these camps and 1.8 million cases were treated during this campaign in the year 2000.

Monitoring and Evaluation

The second phase of the National AIDS Control Programme in India has a built-in component for monitoring and evaluation (M&E) to ensure that continuous critical information on the course of the epidemic and response is being provided for taking remedial action quickly. This helps in practising evidence-based programming. The main elements of the M&E system are a computerised management information system (CMIS), training of programme management staff, conducting baseline, mid-term and final evaluation, and conducting annual performance reviews (APER).

Conclusion

Just as HIV infection is transcending the boundaries of the high-risk population and spreading into the general populace, prevention and care programmes have also reached a critical phase. The Indian government is fully committed to preventing HIV/AIDS at the initial stage before it emerges as a catastrophic epidemic. It looks at HIV/AIDS prevention and control as a developmental issue with deep socioeconomic implications and not merely a public health issue. It touches all sections of the population, both infected and affected, irrespective of their regional, economic or social status. By following a concerted policy, and an action plan that emerges out of it, the government hopes to control the epidemic and slow down its spread in the general population within the shortest possible time. The government hopes that all participating agencies in the governmental or non-governmental sectors, and international and bilateral agencies will adopt policies and programmes in conformity with this national policy in their effort to prevent and control HIV/AIDS in India.

REFERENCES

Anand, K., C.S. Pandav and L.M. Nath (1999). Impact of HIV/AIDS on the national economy of India. *Health Policy*, 47(3), 195–205.

Brookmeyer, R. et al. (1995). The AIDS epidemic in India: A new method for estimating current HIV incidence rates. *American Journal of Epidemiology*, 142, 709–13.

Gangakhedkar, R.R. et al. (1997). Spread of HIV infection in married monogamous women in India. *Journal of American Medical Association*, 278(23), 2090–92.

Jana, S. (1998). STD/HIV interventions among sex workers in West Bengal, India. *AIDS*, 12 (Supplement B), S101–8.

Mehendale, S. et al. (1996). Evidence of high prevalence and rapid transmission of HIV among individuals attending STD clinics in Pune, India. *Indian Journal of Medical Research*, 104, 327–35.

National AIDS Control Organisation (NACO) (1999a). *The scheme for prevention and control of AIDS (Phase II)* (pp. 2–12). New Delhi: Ministry of Health and Family Welfare.

——— (1999b). *The status of HIV/AIDS*. New Delhi: Ministry of Health and Family Welfare.

——— (2001a). *National baseline general population behavioural survey* (pp. 52–54). New Delhi: Ministry of Health and Family Welfare.

——— (2001b). *The current status and trends of HIV/AIDS epidemic in India* (pp. 1–18). New Delhi: Ministry of Health and Family Welfare.

——— (2003). *AIDS Update*, December, http://naco.nic.in.

Sarkar, Swarup, Anindya Chatterjee and Anne Bergenström (2003). Drug-related HIV in South and South-East Asia. *Journal of Health Management*, 5(2), pp. 277–95.

WHO Regional Offices for South-East Asia and Western Pacific (2001). *HIV/AIDS in Asia and the Pacific*. New Delhi and Manila: WHO.

10

The China HIV/AIDS Epidemic and Current Response

Shen Jie, Liu Kangmai, Han Mengjie and Zhang Fujie

During early 2003 the cumulative number of HIV infections reported in China was 40,560, of which 2,639 had developed AIDS and 1,047 died. According to the Chinese Centre for Disease Control and Prevention, the estimated number of people with HIV/AIDS in China, however, had reached 1 million in 2002. China being a large country and despite having more than 1 million HIV-infected individuals, the overall national prevalence is still less than 0.1 per cent. China is, therefore, classified as a low HIV/AIDS epidemic country. Nevertheless, in recent years the number of people with HIV/AIDS have been rapidly rising and increasingly larger areas are being affected. According to reports, the number of people living with HIV/AIDS (PLHA) has increased significantly since 1985. The cumulative number of HIV/AIDS cases increased by 37 per cent from 1998 to 1999, by 30 per cent from 1999 to 2000, by 37 per cent from 2000 to 2001 and by 32 per cent from 2001 to 2002. These data indicate that the HIV/AIDS situation in China is indeed very serious.

The Changing Epidemic in China

The HIV/AIDS epidemic in China can be described in three phases. During the first phase, from 1985 to 1988, only 19 persons with HIV were reported in the entire country. These cases were geographically dispersed. Most were in the coastal urban areas and among persons of foreign origin or among Chinese returning from abroad. Four haemophilia patients in Zhejiang province were infected with HIV/AIDS from the use of imported contaminated blood products.

The second phase, from 1989 to 1994, was the phase of HIV spread. In October 1989 146 HIV-infected persons were detected in Ruili city, the south-west border city in Yunnan province. The epidemic was mostly focused in local areas within a few cities and counties in Dehong prefecture. Some injecting drug users (IDUs) were found to be HIV-positive in other provinces. Initially, few HIV-infected persons were found among those with sexually-transmitted diseases, among commercial sex workers (CSWs) and repatriated individuals in the country, but their numbers increased every year (Figure 10.1).

During the third phase, from 1995 to the present, reported HIV/AIDS cases increased rapidly. The HIV/AIDS epidemic among IDUs in Yunnan province spread to other prefectures, and rapidly to Xinjiang, Guangxi, Sichuan and other provinces. During the same period a large number of paid blood donors in central China were found to be infected, most of whom were highly mobile and had a high transmission risk. Additionally, HIV/AIDS spread very fast in many areas through sexual transmission among STD patients and CSWs.

Currently, the overall HIV/AIDS epidemic situation can be summarised as follows:

- While HIV prevalence is low nationally, there are clusters where epidemic is increasing rapidly.
- The HIV/AIDS epidemic has not been effectively controlled in the high-risk populations and it has now started to spread to the general population.
- It is felt that China is entering a period where the number of AIDS infections and related deaths is escalating.
- HIV risk factors are extensive, and there is danger of the epidemic spreading more widely.
- In high HIV prevalence areas, the epidemic has resulted in a heavy social and economic burden.

Figure 10.1
The Change in the HIV/AIDS Epidemic Situation in China

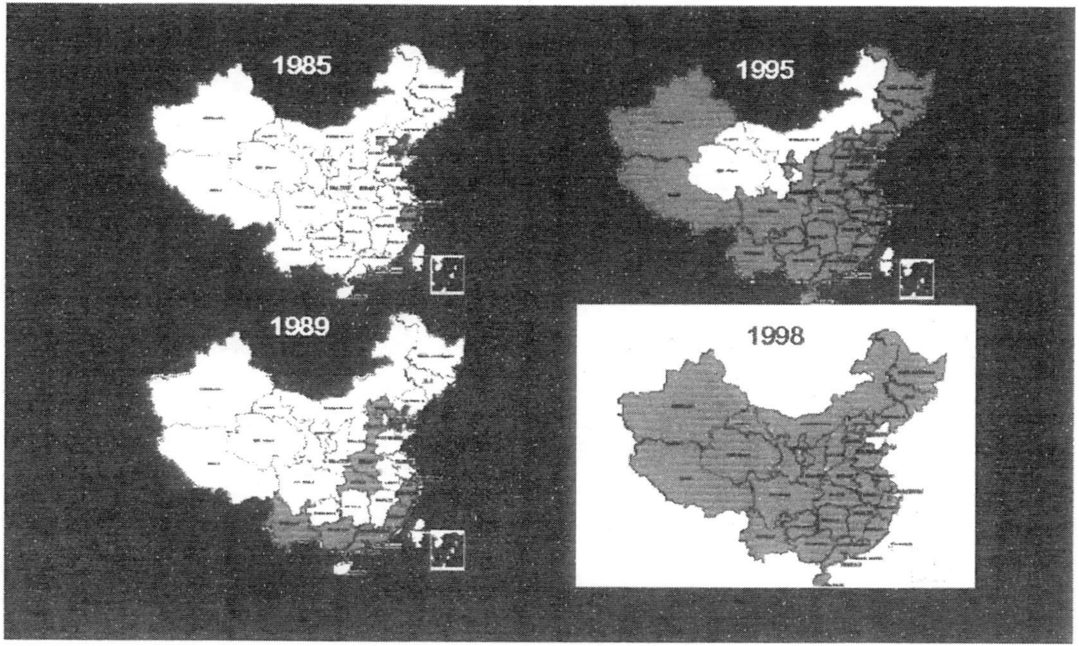

Source: Centre for Disease Control and Prevention, Ministry of Health, China.

Certain characteristics of the HIV/AIDS epidemic in China are discussed.

Low National HIV Prevalence but Clusters of High Prevalence in Certain Groups

According to case reports in China, the number of HIV/AIDS cases has increased significantly since 1995 (Figure 10.2). Since 1999 the annual number of HIV/AIDS cases reported has increased by 30 per cent and has spread to 31 provinces (autonomous regions and municipalities). The HIV infection rate among high-risk groups such as IDUs and CSWs has increased dramatically. Results from surveillance and specific surveys in 2000 and 2002 showed that the HIV prevalence among high-risk groups in previous low-level epidemic areas had gradually increased. For example, at present HIV prevalence among IDUs in some areas of Guizhou is 34.8 per cent. This figure had increased to the high epidemic category in some areas. By the end of 2002 the cumulative number of HIV infections in China was estimated to be 1 million with a prevalence of less than 0.1 per cent among adults (Table 10.1). Although national prevalence is relatively low, China has a huge burden of HIV/AIDS in terms of absolute numbers, and the epidemic has spread geographically.

Table 10.1
Estimated Adult HIV Cases in China

Variable	By 1997	By 1999	By 2001	By 2002
Estimated total HIV/AIDS *	300,000	500,000	850,000	1,000,000
Male/female ratio**	5:1	5:1	4:1	4:1
Estimated total adult HIV/AIDS	289,500	479,000	815,000	960,000
Adult HIV prevalence	<0.03%	<0.05%	<0.08%	<0.10%
Male HIV prevalence	<0.04%	<0.06%	<0.10%	<0.12%
Female HIV prevalence	<0.01%	<0.01%	<0.03%	<0.03%

Sources: * Ministry of Health.
 ** Chinese CDC case report.

The HIV/AIDS burden varies considerably by geographical area, with the epidemic being more severe in certain places and among specific populations (Figure 10.3). For example, Yunnan province has reported a cumulative total of 12,000 HIV infections. Yunnan, Xinjiang, Guangxi, Sichuan, Henan and Guangdong all have reported over 1,000 HIV infections. The main transmission routes are through intravenous drug use and previous sale of blood/plasma.

Figure 10.2
Annual Reported Cases of HIV/AIDS in China: 1985–2002

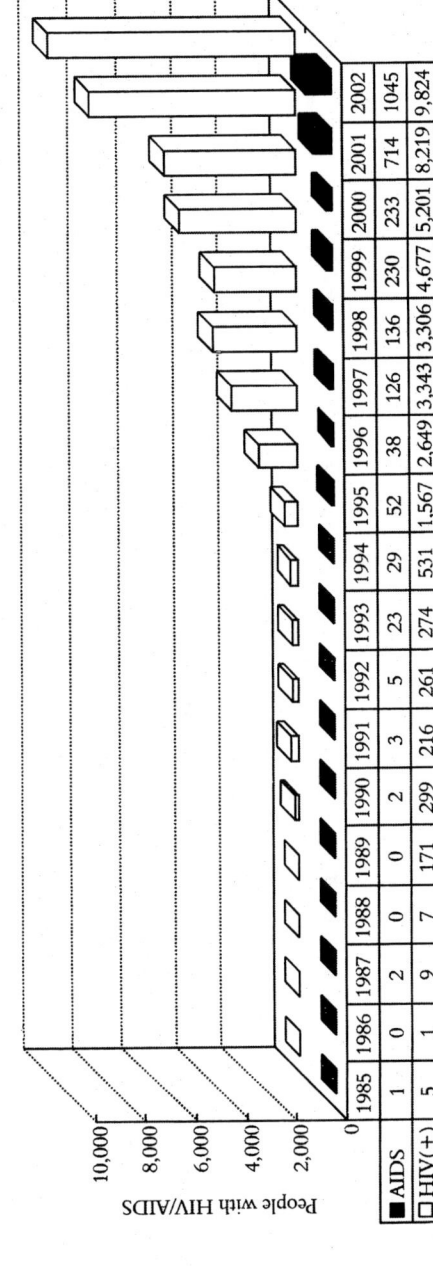

	1985	1986	1987	1988	1989	1990	1991	1992	1993	1994	1995	1996	1997	1998	1999	2000	2001	2002
■ AIDS	1	0	2	0	0	2	3	5	23	29	52	38	126	136	230	233	714	1045
□ HIV(+)	5	1	9	7	171	299	216	261	274	531	1,567	2,649	3,343	3,306	4,677	5,201	8,219	9,824

Source: National Centre for STD/AIDS Control and Prevention (Chinese CDC) Annual HIV/AIDS Case Report.

Figure 10.3
Geographic Distribution of Reported HIV/AIDS
Cases in China: December 2002

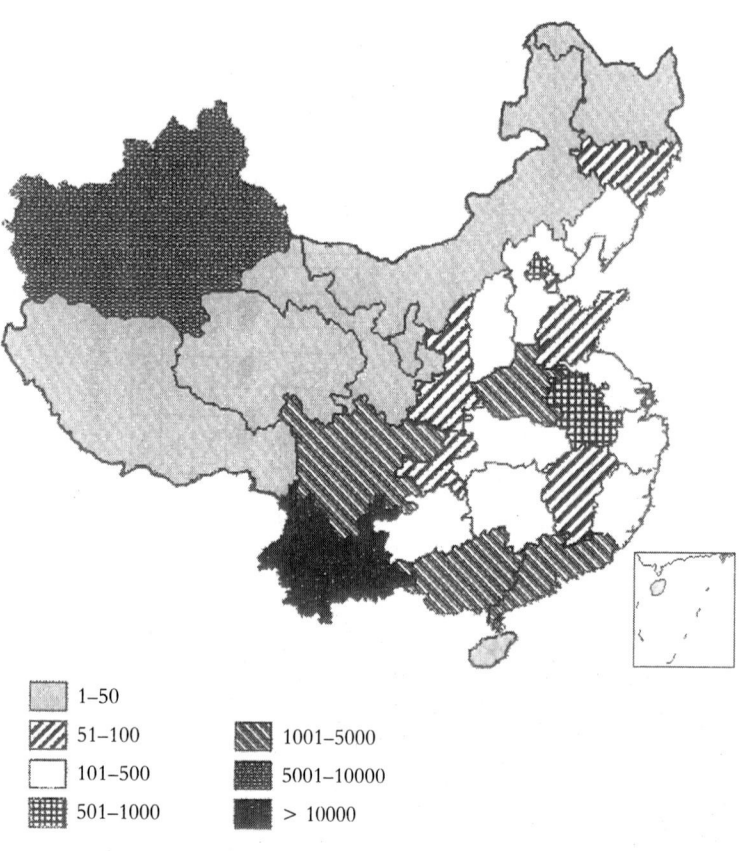

▢ 1–50	
▨ 51–100	▩ 1001–5000
▢ 101–500	▦ 5001–10000
▦ 501–1000	▪ > 10000

Source: Chinese CDC case report, 2002.

High HIV Prevalence among IDUs

During 1989 to 1995 the HIV epidemic among IDUs was reported only in Yunnan province. After 1995 other provinces began reporting HIV infections among IDUs as well. By the end of 2002 all 31 provinces (municipalities and autonomous regions) had reported HIV infections in this high-risk group. According to surveys, HIV prevalence among

IDUs in some regions of Yunnan has reached 80 per cent. In 2001 five of the 24 sentinel sites for IDUs reported a prevalence of more than 10 per cent. HIV prevalence among IDUs is more than 80 per cent in Yining city and Xinjiang province. There are still eight sentinel sites with HIV/AIDS prevalence ranging from 1 to 10 per cent, and another eight sentinel sites with HIV/AIDS-positive individuals.

Data from sentinel surveillance in 2002 indicated that the prevalence of HIV infection reached 78 per cent among IDUs in some areas of Xinjiang; in a few areas of Yunnan province the rate was higher than 50 per cent. In certain areas of Sichuan, Guangxi and Guizhou the prevalence of HIV among IDUs reached 50 per cent, 43.1 per cent and 34.8 per cent respectively. There were seven provinces in China where the rate among IDUs was higher than 10 per cent.

By the end of 2002 nine provinces (municipalities and autonomous regions)—Yunnan, Xinjiang, Guangxi, Guangdong, Sichuan, Hunan, Guizhou, Jiangxi and Beijing—reported a serious HIV epidemic among IDUs (with a prevalence exceeding 5 per cent). The syringe-sharing ratio was found very high among IDUs, and more and more new provinces reported HIV/AIDS in the past several years. Data from surveillance and epidemiological investigations from 2000 to 2002 showed that the prevalence among the high-risk population in the low-epidemic areas has reached to the level of some high-epidemic areas. For example, surveys in Jiangxi, Hunan and Guizhou indicated that the prevalence among IDUs in Jiangxi reached 17.7 per cent in 2000, 34.8 per cent in some areas of Guizhou and 13.9 per cent in Hengyang, Hunan, in 2002. These data indicate that the epidemic situation of HIV/AIDS is very serious among IDUs and there is enormous risk for further transmission (Figure 10.4).

Surveillance Programme in China, 1995–2001

Severe HIV Epidemic among Former Plasma Donors

During 1985 to 1995 farmers from many provinces, especially the central areas of China, were involved in paid blood donation in order to make money. A large number of former blood donors became infected with HIV/AIDS. According to epidemiological investigations, the HIV prevalence among former plasma donors (FPDs) in Henan, Anhui, Shanxi,

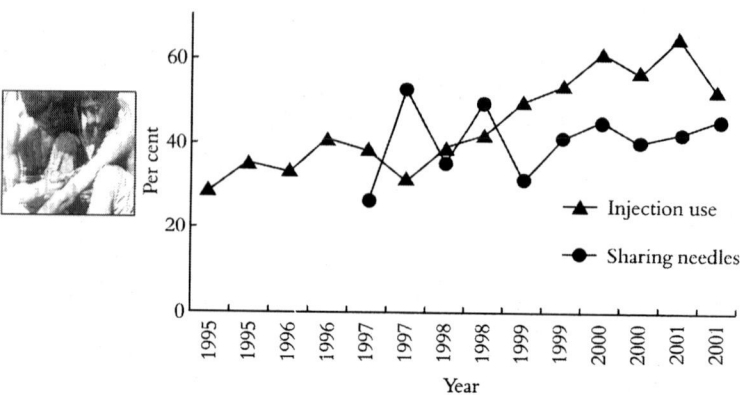

Figure 10.4
Proportion of IDUs and Needle Sharing

Source: Chinese CDC.

Shaanxi, Hubei, Hebei, Shandong and Guizhou provinces reached 60 per cent in some communities. A survey undertaken in 2001 in Henan by the AIDS Prevention and Control Centre of the Ministry of Health (now called the National Centre for STD/AIDS Control and Prevention on the Chinese CDC) showed that 21.6 per cent of the 0- to 60-year-old population were paid blood donors. The proportion of paid blood donors in the 20- to 59-year-old population was 42.8 per cent. In some villages with a large number of FPDs, several hundred villagers were infected with HIV.

Mounting AIDS-related Deaths

There has been a significant increase in the number of HIV/AIDS cases reported in the past few years. According to recent case reports, the cumulative number of AIDS patients are increasing rapidly. The reported number of cases increased by 46.4 per cent from 2001 to 2002, and by 206.4 per cent from 2000 to 2001. According to the annual HIV/AIDS case reports of the Chinese CDC, there were 880 cumulative cases of AIDS and 466 deaths during a 15-year period from 1985 to 2000, and the reported number AIDS cases and deaths in the years 2001 and 2002 were 1,719 and 581 respectively.

HIV/AIDS cases have increased in recent years. In provinces such as Henan and Anhui particularly, there have been a large number of AIDS cases and deaths since 2001. This has not only had a severe impact on individuals and their families, but also affected social stability and development. It is estimated that approximately 200,000 people developed AIDS in the past few years, and 80,000 to 100,000 are presently living with AIDS. AIDS patients usually live for only one to two years after the onset of symptoms without ART. This indicates that China will have mounting numbers of AIDS-related deaths in the coming years.

Spread of HIV/AIDS from High-risk Populations to the General Population

HIV/AIDS transmission in China occurs through various routes—sexual transmission, blood transfusion and from mother to child. Based on reported AIDS cases, the commonest mode of transmission in China is through sharing of contaminated needles and syringes among IDUs. Until December 2002 63.7 per cent of the total reported cases were infected through injecting drug use. The proportion of HIV infections transmitted by unsafe sexual behaviour increased from 5.5 per cent in 1997 to 11.0 per cent at the end of 2002. Results from sentinel surveillance indicate that HIV prevalence among CSWs is increasing. For example, prevalence among CSWs in Guangxi in 1995, 1997, 1999 and 2001 were 0, 0.4, 6.3 and 9.5 per cent respectively. In addition, the investigation showed that premarital HIV/AIDS infection rate was also significant in some areas. In 1997 anonymous, unlinked HIV testing of premarital youth was started in Yining, Xinjiang autonomous region. Results showed a prevalence of 1.72 per cent in 1997. The HIV prevalence in 2001 was 1.14 per cent (and 1.78 per cent among males) in this area. In Yunnan and Xinjiang HIV prevalence among pregnant women in certain areas reached 1.3 per cent and 1.2 per cent respectively, similar to the prevalence among pregnant women in the neighbouring high-burden countries. What is most worrisome is the increase in sexually-transmitted diseases in China since 1986, indicating the increased potential for HIV transmission in the country (Figure 10.5).

While HIV transmission through homosexual behaviour was previously relatively low (accounting for only 0.2 per cent of all cases in 2001), some areas now show a higher prevalence. According to one investigation in Harbin in 2001, HIV prevalence among MSMs was 1 to 3 per cent. In 2001 surveillance among 400 MSMs in Beijing showed the overall infection rate in this group to be about 5 per cent. Enormous dangers of HIV transmission exist in China, and the HIV/AIDS epidemic is spreading from high-risk populations into the general population.

Figure 10.5
Annual Reported STDs in China: 1985–2000

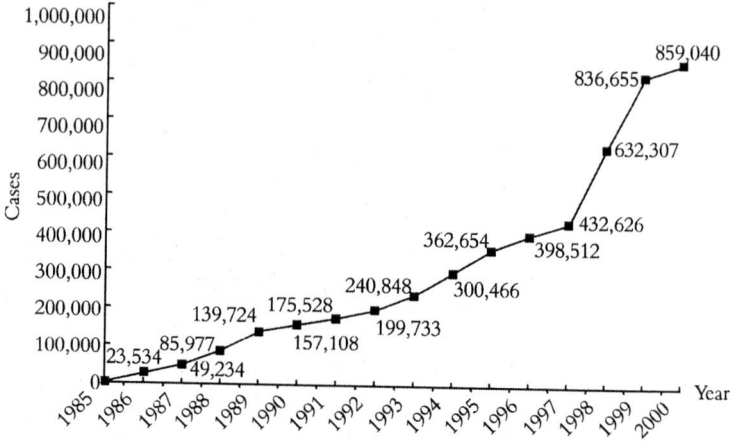

Source: Chinese CDC.

Sex Workers and Low Condom Use

Different kinds of commercial sex services exist in hotels, massage parlours, karaoke halls and bars. Commercial sex is not only found in urban areas, but also in rural areas, remote townships and along the main transportation routes. Commercial sex is illegal in China and the government has established 'Re-education centres' in each province. In these centre, sex workers receive education about morality and the law. For diverse reasons, many women continue to be involved in the sex industry even after their release. Although the proportion of constant condom use has increased gradually among CSWs, the overall figure is still very low. This greatly increases their risk of contracting sexually-transmitted diseases, including HIV/AIDS.

The Social–Economic Impact of HIV/AIDS

The Impact of AIDS on the Macro- and Microeconomy

Although few studies about the social and economic impact of AIDS have been carried out in China, it is evident that the AIDS epidemic has caused a tremendous impact on the social economy of China. The impact on the microeconomy has been mainly in terms of decrease in income and substantial medical costs related to the disease.

With respect to medical costs, the Chinese Academy of Preventive Medicine conducted a retrospective survey in 1999 in two hospitals in Beijing where AIDS patients were treated. The results showed that the annual medical cost for each case was 54,549 Chinese yuan (CNY) (exchange rate of 8 CNY per US$), 87.22 per cent of which was spent on hospitalisation. A further analysis of 29 AIDS patients receiving treatment showed that the average hospitalisation fee per case was 23,231 CNY annually and the cost of outpatient treatment was 16,009 CNY. Patients receiving ARV treatment had an extra expenditure of 23,857 CNY. Recently, however, due to the production and sale of generic ARV drugs, treatment costs for AIDS patients have decreased significantly. Still, the cost of drugs and testing is approximately 20,000 CNY.

According to experts, the number of AIDS patients needing treatment will be 200,000 after five years, 10,000 in the first year, 30,000 in the second, 70,000 in the third, 120,000 in the fourth and 200,000 in the fifth. The costs of ARV treatment alone will be 8.6 billion CNY in five years.

Given that the average age of death for AIDS patients is 35.22 years, the average age of labour for the Chinese people is 60 years and the annual wealth generation of each person is 15,000 CNY, the average economic loss due to each case of HIV/AIDS infection and consequent decrease of wealth generation is about 370,000 CNY. If the number of people living with HIV/AIDS reaches 1 million at the end of 2002, the medical costs due to the increasing number of HIV/AIDS cases and the social and economic loss will be 370 billion CNY. If preventive measures are not effective and the number of HIV/AIDS cases touches 10 million in 2010, the amount will go beyond 3,700 billion CNY.

According to statistics (though incomplete), by the end of 1992, the cumulative expenditure on HIV/AIDS prevention and control in China spent by the central government and international agencies was 30 million CNY. From 1993 to 1998 the Ministry of Health budget for HIV/AIDS prevention and control was 54.9 million CNY. In 1998 the central government increased the annual HIV/AIDS budget to 15 million CNY, and in 2001 the annual AIDS budget increased again to 100 million CNY. In order to deal with the rapid increase of AIDS patients, the government further increased its budget. It is expected that the cost of implementing some of the successful and effective interventions among high-risk target populations over a six-month period would be between 200 and 400 CNY. If China provides interventions to 10 per cent of the number of estimated high-risk individuals, taking into account the cost decrease and other factors when interventions are expanded, the annual budget would be 60 to 120 million CNY. If China were to implement effective interventions nationally, covering at least 60 per cent of the target population, this will require a budget of at least 360 to 720 million CNY.

AIDS-related Social Problems and its Influence on Social Stability

First, the HIV/AIDS epidemic can lead to a large number of children being orphaned. According to a survey among 143 PLHAs in selected parts of China, 16.8 per cent of them had children less than 5 years old who were likely to become orphans. According to experts, if a low-level HIV/AIDS epidemic continues in China, the number of orphans will reach 138,000 by the end of 2010. With a mid-level HIV/AIDS epidemic, there will be 200,000 orphans by the end of 2010. And if China has a high-level HIV epidemic, the number of AIDS orphans would reach 260,000 by the end of 2010.

Second, the HIV/AIDS epidemic will increase the poverty and disparity between the rich and the poor. Most people living with HIV and AIDS in China live in resource-constrained areas where there are few natural resources, where health and education resources are limited, and most people live in poverty. In order to increase incomes, people are more likely to be sell blood or be involved in paid sex, both of which increase the opportunities for the spread of HIV/AIDS. Families affected by HIV/AIDS will have a lower income and higher medical expenditure. These factors will further exacerbate poverty in these areas. A study recently showed that people who have just risen out of poverty and begun to have a steady income returned to poverty because of HIV infection. This disease-induced poverty increases the disparity between rich and poor areas.

In addition, rumours about AIDS may severely impact the social stability and sense of safety, and may lead to panic. For example, in 2000 a local newspaper in the north-east of China published an article regarding some AIDS patients who infused their blood into watermelons, stating that 'it is possible for people to become infected by HIV/AIDS by eating watermelons'. This caused a huge decrease in sales of watermelon and considerable economic loss to producers. At the end of 2001 some AIDS patients threatened the public, creating social confusion in Tianjin, Beijing and Shijiazhuang. Such information was spread, exaggerated and distorted, and finally became a stirring rumour. It caused panic in some regions and seriously disturbed the stability of the local society.

The Goal of China's HIV/AIDS Prevention and Control

Medium and Long-term Goals

China's long-term and immediate goals on HIV/AIDS prevention and control are primarily articulated in the Medium- and Long-term Plan of HIV/AIDS Prevention and Control in China (1998–2010) and the China Action Plan to Contain, Prevent and Control HIV/AIDS (2001–5). The Ministry of Health, together with three other ministries, announced the Medium- and Long-term Plan of HIV/AIDS Prevention and Control in China in October 1998, in which China's overall goals on HIV/AIDS prevention and control were brought forward. This includes setting up a multi-sectoral coordinated STD/AIDS prevention and control system with participation by various sectors of the society under the leadership of the government, spreading knowledge and information on STD/AIDS control and prevention, and ultimately preventing HIV transmission. It was explicitly proposed that 'STD prevalence be steadily decreased and the number of people living with HIV/AIDS be controlled under 1,500,000 by 2010'.

Immediate Goals

China's immediate goals on HIV/AIDS prevention and control are embodied in the 2001–5 Action Plan to Contain, Prevent and Control HIV/AIDS promulgated by the state council of China. This document quantifies and specifies the chief goals in the 1998–2010 Medium- and Long-term Plan of HIV/AIDS Prevention and Control and complements the staged goals in 2002 and 2005 in it. It clarifies the specific objectives that the annual increase of HIV infection and STD be controlled below 10 per cent and HIV infection through clinical blood transfusion be decreased under one per 100,000 by the end of 2005.

Accomplishments in HIV/AIDS Prevention and Control in China

Increased Political Recognition and Commitment by Government

The central gosvernment and the state council are paying serious attention to HIV/AIDS prevention and control in the country. Many significant decisions and related directives have been promulgated.

In 1994 Chen Minzhang, ex-minister of the Ministry of Health, participated in the AIDS Summit in Paris. As the delegate of the Chinese government, Chen Minzhang signed the Paris Declaration and announced China's ongoing political commitment.

In 1996 Peng Peiyun, former Chinese state committee member, presided over the State Council AIDS Coordination Working Mechanism Conference in which delegates from 34 ministries participated. The tasks for HIV/AIDS prevention and control were delegated during the conference.

In October 1996 the National AIDS Prevention and Control Conference was held. Peng Peiyun was present, and addressed the gathering.

Chinese central government leaders are paying serious attention to HIV/AIDS prevention and control. Li Lanqing, ex-vice-prime minister, has listened to AIDS reports and issued important directives. Zhu Rongji, ex-prime minister, specifically listened to the report from the Ministry of Health for HIV/AIDS prevention and control.

Hu Jintao the chairman of the state, and Wen Jiabao, prime minister, have provided significant indications towards HIV/AIDS prevention and control in China.

The Construction of HIV/AIDS Organisations and Systems

In order to prevent the HIV/AIDS epidemic, the central government has established a National Specialists Committee for HIV/AIDS Prevention and Control and the State Council AIDS Coordination Committee. The Ministry of Health HIV/AIDS Coordination Committee was established in 1986, which was converted to a National Specialists Committee for HIV/AIDS Prevention and Control in September 1990. The committee and its four subcommittees advise the Ministry of Health on national laws, regulation and rules, policies, organisation and technical measures for HIV/AIDS prevention and control; provide suggestions related to scientific research, training schemes, research projects for HIV/AIDS control and prevention; review national HIV/AIDS prevention and control programmes; and provide technical guidance for national HIV/AIDS prevention and control activities.

In 1995, recognising that the HIV/AIDS epidemic was worsening, the state council authorised the establishment of the State Council AIDS Coordination Committee. This was then enlarged to cover STDs and AIDS in 1996. The committee, which includes 34 ministries and commissions as well as other relevant departments, defines the responsibilities of each ministry and strengthens the coordination between various departments.

Financial Investments

The principle of government funding as a major resource and fundraising for additional resources through various channels has been established for HIV/AIDS prevention and control. It is required that a central special fund be set up to provide budget for central sectors for carrying out HIV/AIDS prevention and control activities, and for special assistance to difficult areas. The local governments also allocate the investment to meet local needs for HIV/AIDS prevention and control. Investments from social donations and from other countries are also actively pursued to raise resources through various channels. More than half of all 30 provinces (municipalities and autonomous regions) have established special funds for HIV/AIDS prevention and control, which will ensure strengthening of national HIV/AIDS control and prevention.

Between 1998 and 2000 the annual contribution for HIV/AIDS control was 15 million CNY. In 2001 the fund was been increased to 100 million CNY per year and the sum is pledged until 2005. In 2003 the Ministry of Finance began work on an additional 100 million CNY per year from 2003 to 2005. This will be used to improve HIV/AIDS treatment and comprehensive care in the most severely affected areas. In 2001 the State Development and Reform Commission transferred 1.25 billion CNY from national bonds, combined with 1 billion CNY from local governments, to improve basic construction and equipment of blood banks in mid-west China. Nearly, 459 blood banks and stations have been established, reconstructed and enlarged. This investment plays a significant role in the prevention of HIV/AIDS transmission through blood donation and transfusion. In 2002 the State Development and Reform Commission allocated 2.1 billion CNY from national bonds to support the capacity building of the Chinese Centres for Disease Control at the provincial, prefecture and county levels in central and western China.

Investment from local governments has also increased. More than half of all provinces have set up special funds for HIV/AIDS prevention and control. The total contribution by local governments is roughly equal to that of the central government. For example, in 2001 and 2002 the government of Henan allocated the highest financial contribution in China, 14 million CNY per year. Since 2002 Guangdong has secured 10 million CNY each year for HIV/AIDS. There are six provinces that allocated more than 5 million CNY in special funds for HIV/AIDS prevention and control in China in 2002.

Active Involvement of NGOs

In 1993 the China Association of STD/AIDS Prevention and Control and the Chinese Foundation for the Prevention of STD/AIDS were established. This marked a new phase for mobilising Chinese society, especially mass organisations, to take part in the fight against HIV/AIDS. These organisations offer great assistance in coordinating NGOs to carry out activities in raising public awareness, counselling and academic exchanges. Local associations are also established in some provinces and cities.

Since 1996 the China Association of STD/AIDS Prevention and Control has held the annual Chinese NGOs' coordination meetings. Here, more than 20 NGOs joined together and issued the Joint Action Creed for Chinese NGOs taking part in HIV/AIDS prevention and control as the action guideline to fight HIV/AIDS.

Besides mass media education, training, etc., NGOs also have greatly helped in the care and support of people living with HIV/AIDS and in interventions in high-risk populations in recent years. The Chinese government recognised that mass organisations are a pillar of important strength, and have provided powerful support and assistance. Some such mass organisations related to HIV/AIDS control and prevention include the China Association of STD/AIDS Prevention and Control, the Chinese Foundation for the Prevention of STD/AIDS, the Chinese Drug Abuse Control Association, the Chinese Gender Association and the Chinese Drug Rehabilitation Association. These newer emerging associations have joined with some previously established organisations, such as the Chinese Medical Association, the China Preventive Medicine

Association, the All China Trade Union, the All China Women's Federation and the All China Youth League, to form a skeleton network. This network can cover target populations and all sections of society. NGOs have worked as frontline workers and made a significant impact in implementing interventions among high-risk populations in mass media education, care and treatment for people with HIV/AIDS, and mobilising the entire society to take part in HIV/AIDS prevention and control.

Health Education and Public Awareness

It is important to mobilise the entire society to participate in HIV/AIDS control and prevention. The related departments of the state council have established policies and carried out widespread health education activities. At the same time, a series of awareness-raising campaigns are held on and around World AIDS Day on 1 December every year to increase society's understanding of HIV/AIDS, and spread scientific knowledge. The central government also pays attention to this work.

Nearly 1,000 exhibitions about HIV/AIDS have been held in different places since 1998. More than 100 million people have been educated through thousands of educational programmes through TV, radio and other activities nationwide. Numerous educational pictures, leaflets and materials on HIV/AIDS have been developed and used for educational purposes.

Additionally, the Ministry of Health, together with related ministries, has held a series of national and local propaganda activities around 1 December every year. Under the leadership of the local governments, related departments cooperate actively, according to the local situation and carry out all required activities, which are appreciated greatly by the people.

Interventions among High-risk Populations

Intravenous drug use and commercial sex are the main routes for HIV transmission in China. The Ministry of Health and the Ministry of Public Security work closely to control the spread of HIV through drug abuse, drug trafficking and commercial sex, and have carried out pilot studies according to international best practice.

So far a large number of intervention research activities have been carried out among various high-risk populations in China. In 2002, with the support of the WHO, a pilot study to promote 100 per cent condom use was started in Wuhan and other sites. In the same year a pilot project for the social marketing of syringes and needles was conducted in Guangdong province. Drug users are allowed to buy sterile injection equipment at designated pharmacies for harm reduction. Some success has been achieved and experiences gained for further prevention of HIV/AIDS among high-risk populations.

International Cooperation for HIV/AIDS Prevention and Control

China is actively involved in collaborating with both multilateral and bilateral organisations. Through this collaboration, China has gained much support and assistance, both technically and financially. Long and effective partnerships with the WHO, World Bank, DFID, UNDP, UNICEF, UNAIDS and the EU, among others, have been created. According to the National Centre for HIV/AIDS Control and Prevention, there are more than 30 international organisations, countries and regions that have collaborated with China for HIV/AIDS prevention and control. More than 100 international cooperation projects have been carried out. Considerable achievements have been made and projects are being implemented smoothly.

During the past 10 years the Chinese government has collaborated with bilateral and multilateral organisations for technical cooperation. Australia, the United Kingdom, the United States, Germany, Japan, Luxembourg and South Korea, as well as several other countries, are all partners. A significant amount of technical support and assistance have been gained from close cooperation with UN organisations and the World Bank. All multibilateral agencies have provided good support for HIV/AIDS prevention and control in China.

ARV Therapy in China

ARV Treatment in China

At present about 6,000 people are on ARV treatment in China. A small proportion of them bear their expenses themselves, while another small proportion is supported by international cooperation projects. The rest, mainly in Henan, Anhui, Hubei and Shandong province, are receiving free treatment. The treatment results are good. According to a study on the treatment of 3,426 PLHAs in a target county in mid-west China, the proportion of patients whose state of illness has dramatically improved, improved to some extent, remained unchanged or been aggravated was 15.9 per cent, 54.2 per cent, 27.1 per cent and 2.5 per cent respectively. Results from another area, in which 113 people were suitable for ARV treatment, the proportion of patients who have dramatically improved, improved to an extent and not obviously changed was 31 per cent, 42.5 per cent and 21.2 per cent respectively; one patient quit ARV treatment and five died.

The Price of ARV Drugs and Their Availability

Prior to August 2002 the price of ARV drugs in China was quite high because they had to be imported. Through negotiations, GlaxoSmithKline (GSK), Merck & Co., Inc. and Bristol-Myers Squibb Company reduced drug prices by a half to two-thirds in December 2001. The average expense for a patient was reduced from 110,000 to 130,000 CNY to about 35,000 CNY annually. But most of the patients in China still cannot afford the cost, especially those in rural areas for whom ARV drugs are completely inaccessible.

In order to quickly reduce the price of ARV drugs and to increase the availability of the drugs, under the attention of the state council, the Ministry of Health and the State Council Coordinating Committee on HIV/AIDS, active negotiations took place and relevant departments in the state council provided great support. In 2003 the State Development Planning Commission approved the reduction of the retail prices of four kinds of drugs produced by GSK, Merck & Co., Inc. and Bristol-Myers Squibb Company. The State Drug Administration agreed to expedite the registration for imported ARV drugs at first, approving clinical trials, simplifying requests of packaging and accelerating the application processes. The Ministry of Finance, State Administration of Taxation and Customs General Administration exempted the customs and the value-added tax for imported ARV drugs. While the tax rate of customs and value-added tax is 4 to 5 per cent and 17 per cent respectively, after the exemption, the drug price reached 8,000 to 10,000 CNY per person-year.

Domestic pharmaceutical companies are also developing generic ARV drugs. In August 2002 AZT, the first domestically manufactured generic ARV drug, was approved. D4T, DDI and NVP were approved subsequently. At present, the first regimen of domestically manufactured generic drugs is complete and its price is only a tenth that of imported drugs, amounting to about 3,000 CNY for every person-year. The government is trying to reduce prices even further.

In order to resolve the problems of high ARV treatment costs, ARV drugs have been put under the drug list covered within basic medical insurance policies.

To resolve the problem of ARV treatment for PLHAs in under-developed rural areas, 100 comprehensive care demonstration sites focused on treatment and care have been set up. The emphasis is to maximise the benefits of treatment and care in high epidemic areas. Subsidies for drug costs and examination fees are given to AIDS patients. The subsidies vary according to the financial situation of the patients.

At present, the Chinese government is trying its best to provide ARV treatment for more PLHAs through domestic and international financial support.

11

THE AIDS SITUATION IN NEPAL

B.K. Suvedi

Introduction

HIV/AIDS was first reported in Nepal in July 1988. Since then, there has been a gradual increase in the number of cases. In 1994 it was estimated that 5,000 people in the country were infected with HIV/AIDS (Suvedi et al. 1994). However, the most recent estimate (2002) puts the number of HIV-infected persons at around 60,000.

Nepal is considered to be in a 'concentrated epidemic' as HIV prevalence in a few population groups has already exceeded 5 per cent; among sex workers the prevalence is around 17 per cent and among the injecting drug users about 40 per cent. Among the migrant population a prevalence as high as 10 per cent has been noted in some districts of the country. Nepal is, therefore, in a situation of 'transition' towards general epidemic as the bridging population and the factors for rapid transmission of the disease are abundant (Beine 2003; Hannum 1997). The factors considered as major contributors for rapid spread of HIV in the country include poverty, mobility of young people in search of temporary jobs, trafficking of girls for sex work, and low level of awareness on HIV/AIDS and STI (Suvedi 1998). In addition, poor understanding of the epidemic in the general population, gender disparity, and considerable discrimination and stigma associated with HIV all point towards the possibility of an emerging epidemic in the country.

The Epidemiological Situation

Since the first HIV/AIDS case in Nepal, a total of 635 AIDS cases and 159 deaths have so far been reported as of April 2003. This, however, represents a gross underestimation of the real situation because many AIDS cases never come to health facilities and are not diagnosed or reported. Moreover, deaths take place at home.

Of the reported cases, 62 per cent were clients of sex workers, 17.7 per cent were sex workers and 12 per cent injecting drug users. Over the last few years a rapidly increasing trend of infection has been seen among housewives and children. Nearly 93 per cent cases were below the age of 40 years and 62 per cent in the age group 14 to 29 years.

UNAIDS/WHO estimate that in 2002 there were about 60,000 HIV-infected persons in Nepal. This reflects an overall prevalence of 0.57 per cent in the age bracket 15 to 49 years, with an estimated 3,000 deaths per year. The current situation of HIV is summarised in Box 11.1.

Box 11.1
Current Situation of HIV/AIDS in Nepal at a Glance

Estimated number of persons with HIV/AIDS	60,000
Prevalence of HIV among sex workers	3–17%
Prevalence of HIV among injecting drug users	40–68%
Prevalence of HIV among blood donors	0.28–0.48%
Prevalence of HIV among pregnant women	0.2%
Major mode of HIV transmission	Heterosexual

Surveillance among populations with high-risk behaviour has been carried out in Nepal since 1992. This includes HIV surveillance among clients with sexually-transmitted infections (STI) who come to health institutions for treatment. HIV testing is carried out in an unlinked and anonymous manner, which eliminates the possibility of participation bias. At present, six sentinel sites are in operation, located in five regions of the country (Figure 11.1).

The data show no temporal uniformity in the incidence of HIV. An increasing trend is observed in some parts of the country (especially in the far west and mid-west regions), whereas the central and eastern regions of the country show a more or less stable pattern. It is speculated that the high prevalence of HIV in the far and mid-west is due mainly

Figure 11.1
Distribution of HIV Sentinel Sites in Nepal

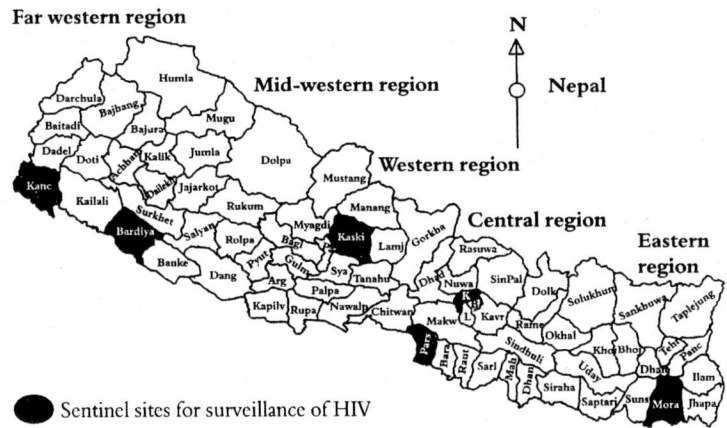

Sentinel sites for surveillance of HIV

Source: National Centre for AIDS and STD Control (NCASC).

to the seasonal mobile population. Besides, high STI rates have also been reported in these regions in the past.

Trends over past four years show that in the western and mid-western sites HIV among STI patients increased from less than 1 per cent in 1998 to more than 3 per cent in 2001. In the eastern and central regions, however, HIV prevalence among STI clients remains less than 0.5 per cent (Figure 11.2).

HIV prevalence among female sex workers has been showing a steady increase from 0.7 per cent in 1992 to 15.7 per cent in 2001 (Figure 11.3). This increase is an area of major concern.

Another finding of great concern in Nepal is the remarkable and explosive increase in HIV noted over the past three to four years among injecting drug users (IDUs) in the country (Figure 11.4). A rapid assessment in 1999 showed that in Kathmandu and other cities up to 50 per cent of IDUs were HIV positive, up from only 1.4 per cent in 1991. The rate in Kathmandu in 2001 was 68 per cent. As seen elsewhere, spread from IDUs to their partners could possibly occur through heterosexual transmission.

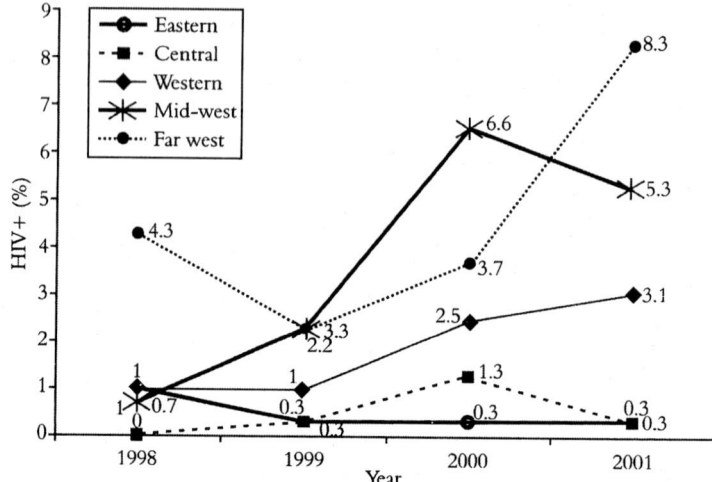

Figure 11.2
Trend of HIV Prevalence among STI Patients:
Data from Sentinel Surveillance Sites

Source: NCASC.

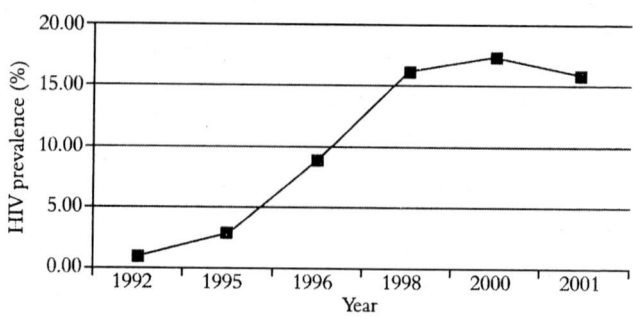

Figure 11.3
HIV Prevalence among Female Sex Workers in Kathmandu

Source: NCASC.

Surveys among migrant populations, however, show rates varying from district to district—the highest rate has been seen in Doti, in far western Nepal.

Tuberculosis has been reported as a frequent infection among HIV-positive people, accounting for about 68.7 per cent of cases. Other

The AIDS Situation in Nepal **195**

Figure 11.4
HIV Prevalence among Injecting Drug Users in Kathmandu

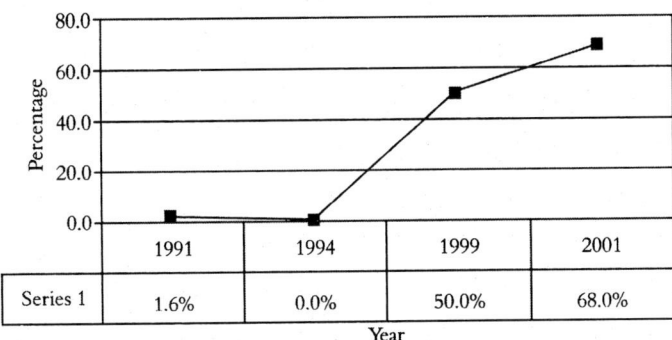

	1991	1994	1999	2001
Series 1	1.6%	0.0%	50.0%	68.0%

Year

Source: NCASC.

common symptoms of HIV-positive status are weight loss (98.4 per cent), fever (95.4 per cent) and diarrhoea (78.7 per cent).

Behavioural Surveillance

Behaviour surveillance has been initiated in the country with three major population sub-groups: sex workers, their clients and injecting drug users. In the intervention areas it has been reported that there is high knowledge of HIV/AIDS and the use of condoms has been increased over few years.

The Nepal Demographic and Health Survey of 2001 showed that knowledge of HIV/AIDS among men (15 to 59 years) was 72 per cent compared to 50 per cent in women (15 to 49 years). However, the knowledge on the means of protection from HIV/AIDS was considerably low in both the groups: 47 per cent among men and 32 per cent among women. This indicates that a more aggressive intervention is needed to raise awareness levels.

Another study carried out among garment industry workers in Kathmandu revealed that the mean age at first sexual intercourse was less than 16 years. In 1991 a knowledge, attitude and practice (KAP) survey among teenagers (12 to 18 years) revealed that 94 per cent of them have heard about HIV/AIDS, but only 74 per cent mentioned that condom can protect against HIV/AIDS. This showed a gap in knowledge and methods of protection.

The impact of HIV/AIDS is still to be seen in a national perspective. However, at the family and community level it is already visible. Impact at family level includes stigmatisation and discrimination, including non-acceptance of HIV-positive persons in the family or community, and marginalising them from getting necessary support and care.

The mean age of death in AIDS cases is 28.8 years, meaning that the younger age group is affected. This is likely to lead to serious socio-cultural and economic impacts in the country.

If effective interventions are not undertaken, it is predicted that there may be a generalised epidemic by the end of the decade, with a prevalence of 1 to 2 per cent estimated in the reproductive age group (15 to 49 years). AIDS then will become the leading cause of death among adults!

National Response

Nepal started HIV/AIDS prevention activities in 1988 with the implementation of a short-term plan, which was followed by a three-year activity. An external review of the programme was carried out in 1992, which recommended initiating medium-term activities in a planned way. This was subsequently carried out for a period of five years (1993–97). During this period, a policy on HIV/AIDS control was brought out and an institution for the execution of HIV/AIDS prevention activities was established—the National Centre for AIDS and STDs Control (NCASC) under the Ministry of Health (NCASC 1995). A high-level National AIDS Coordination Committee (NACC) was established under the chairmanship of the health minister and with representation from various ministries and civil society. The Ministry of Education has incorporated HIV/AIDS and STI into the curriculum of secondary schools, a policy for universal screening of donated blood has been established, and a public–private–NGO partnership initiated for HIV/AIDS prevention.

A Five-Year Strategy for HIV/AIDS Prevention (1997–2001) was initiated in 1997, which has been implemented over the years. However, in recent years the epidemiological situation has changed, especially in high-risk behaviour groups. In addition, Nepal has committed itself to achieving the Millennium Declaration Goals set in 2000 and the United Nations General Assembly Special Session on HIV/AIDS Declaration of Commitment made in June 2001. The Tenth Five-Year Development Plan has identified HIV/AIDS as a cross-cutting issue affecting national development.

A study commissioned in 2000 to assess the situation and response came to the following conclusions:

1. Groups already affected with HIV/AIDS (sex workers and IDUs) must be considered priority for immediate targeted interventions.
2. Other groups such as mobile populations and young people are vulnerable to HIV/AIDS/STI, and appropriate interventions should be designed and implemented for prevention in these groups.
3. The capacity of the institutions involved in Nepal's HIV/AIDS response is weak and interventions have been limited.
4. There is a clear need to develop a national strategy.
5. Political commitment is needed to fight HIV/AIDS.
6. Capacity of the NCASC needs to be strengthened for providing leadership and expertise for the expanded response.
7. There is a need for providing care and support to people living with HIV/AIDS.

Recent Initiatives and Future Actions

Keeping in view the increasing incidence of HIV among high-risk behaviour groups leading to a 'concentrated epidemic', Nepal initiated a special programme in 2001 named the 'Nepal Initiative'. It focused on creating awareness and garnering a high level of commitment, which resulted in formation of the National AIDS Council under the chairmanship of the prime minister. Multi-sectoral representation and representation from the civil society are the major features of this committee, which provides policy directives to the NACC.

Condoms are currently provided free of charge through various outlets. Both public and private sectors are promoting condoms for HIV prevention. Voluntary counselling and testing (VCT) services are so far very limited and need expansion. Support and care to HIV-infected persons is minimal and antiretroviral (ARV) drugs are available only in the private sector. However, major hospitals are providing care to AIDS patients.

In 2002 a national HIV/AIDS prevention strategy was developed covering a period of five years (2002–6) (NCASC 2002). This strategy concentrates its activity on vulnerable populations, and promotes care and support activities for those who are infected/affected by HIV/AIDS. Major 'vulnerable groups' identified in this strategy are sex workers,

IDUs, youths, prisoners and armed forces. A comprehensive approach has been advocated in this strategy (UNAIDS and NCASC 2003).

The National HIV/AIDS Strategy identifies following components for expanded responses for a period of five years (2002–6): (*a*) vulnerable groups, including sex workers and their clients, IDUs, migrant labourers, men who have sex with men, and prisoners; (*b*) young people; (*c*) treatment, care and support; (*d*) measuring changes through surveillance, monitoring and evaluation; and (*e*) expanded response and its management.

Nepal is planning to undertake major interventions targeting the youth and mobile population besides sex workers, their clients and IDUs. ARVs will be made available to HIV-infected persons. VCT centres will be established in major settlements. Information, education and communication (IEC) and behaviour change communication (BCC) will be a major component of future activities. The opportunities and challenges for Nepal in the future are:

1. Expanded response to HIV/AIDS through involvement of various ministers, agencies, NGOs and the private sector.
2. Provision of prophylactic treatment with ARV drugs to pregnant women to reduce mother-to-child (MTC) transmission.
3. Provision of treatment (ARV therapy) to people with HIV/AIDS along with de-stigmatisation.
4. Establishment of VCT centres for providing services to needy people.
5. Initiation of second-generation surveillance, extending the surveillance to pregnant women and IDUs.
6. Multi-sectoral involvement of the corporate and private sector in HIV/AIDS prevention activities.

Since Nepal has already entered a phase of 'concentrated epidemic' with all the potential for a generalised epidemic in the future, there is no room for complacency. Timely and aggressive interventions are the only ways to stop a generalised epidemic. This demands for expanded response, cooperation and coordination from all stakeholders.

REFERENCES

Beine, D.K. (2003). *Ensnared by AIDS: Cultural contexts of HIV/AIDS in Nepal.* Kathmandu: Mandala Book Point.

Hannum, J. (1997). *AIDS in Nepal: Communities confronting an emerging epidemic.* New York: Seven Stories Press.

National Centre for AIDS and STD Control (NCASC) (1995). *HIV/AIDS policy.* Kathmandu: Ministry of Health.

———(2002). *National HIV/AIDS strategy (2002–2006).* Kathmandu: Ministry of Health.

Suvedi, B.K. (1998). Mapping the trend of HIV/AIDS in Nepal. *Journal of the Institute of Medicine,* 21(3&4), pp. 236–42.

Suvedi, B.K., S. Thapa and J. Baker (1994). HIV/AIDS in Nepal: An update. *Journal of the Nepal Medical Association,* 32(111), 224–38.

UNAIDS and NCASC (2003). *HIV/AIDS/STD situation and the national response in Nepal* (Country Profile). Kathmandu: UNAIDS and NCASC.

12

HIV/AIDS IN SRI LANKA: THE PROBLEM AND THE RESPONSE

Iyanthi Abeyewickreme

In South Asia, Sri Lanka is considered to be a country with a low prevalence of HIV. However, most of the risk behaviours that facilitate the spread of HIV exist within the country. A large sexually-active and potentially susceptible population aged between 15 and 49 years accounts for almost 55 per cent of the total population of 19 million. The 23-year-old conflict in the northern and eastern parts of the country resulted in an increasing number of military personnel and displaced persons. Further, the recent Memorandum of Understanding between the government of Sri Lanka and the Liberation Tigers of Tamil Eelam, a separatist Tamil group, in the north and east of the country has caused an influx of large numbers of displaced persons who had sought refuge in southern India, a high HIV prevalence area, posing an additional threat. External economic migration among large numbers of unskilled and semi-skilled workers, especially women, progressive urbanisation, and the increasing pace of economic development and change could all potentially promote the spread of HIV in Sri Lanka. In addition, close proximity to India, which has high HIV prevalence, leads to frequent travel between the inhabitants of the two countries, opening a yet another route for HIV to gain a foothold in Sri Lanka.

On the other hand, Sri Lanka is a small island whose population has a high literacy rate, a well-established health infrastructure and health indicators that are comparable with those observed in a developed nation.

Epidemiology

Sri Lanka, with a population of 19 million, has an estimated 7,200 adults and children living with HIV infection as of December 2001. According to the UNAIDS classification (UNAIDS/WHO 2000), Sri Lanka has a 'low-level HIV epidemic' as prevalence of HIV has not consistently exceeded 5 per cent in any defined sub-population.

The first case of HIV infection in Sri Lanka was reported in 1986 in a foreign national. By the end of December 2002, a cumulative total of 455 HIV infections had been reported to the National STD/AIDS Control Programme (NSACP) of the Ministry of Health. Of these, 139 have been diagnosed as AIDS and 108 have died. In addition, a further 43 foreigners were also detected to be HIV positive.

New infections that have been reported annually since 1987 reached a peak in 1993, declined over the next few years, and peaked again in 1998. In 2002, 50 new infections were reported (Table 12.1).

Table 12.1
Reported HIV and AIDS Cases in Sri Lanka: 1987–2002

Year	HIV			AIDS		
	Male	Female	Total	Male	Female	Total
1987	2	0	2	2	0	2
1988	3	0	3	2	0	2
1989	8	3	11	1	2	3
1990	6	1	7	2	0	2
1991	10	3	13	2	1	3
1992	19	8	27	8	2	10
1993	26	11	37	8	3	11
1994	15	8	23	13	1	14
1995	12	10	22	9	2	11
1996	20	10	30	9	2	11
1997	16	16	32	3	6	9
1998	29	26	55	11	4	15
1999	24	18	42	7	5	12
2000	34	20	54	9	5	14
2001	28	19	47	11	2	13
2002	26	24	50	6	1	7
Total	**278**	**177**	**455**	**103**	**36**	**139**

Source: National STD/AIDS Control Programme (NSACP).

Of the 414 HIV-infected persons with known age, 82 per cent were between 15 and 49 years, with the maximum number reported being in the age group 30 to 39 years. Since HIV affects the most productive age group in the society, it is estimated that the morbidity it causes will result in productivity loss of approximately US$ 30 million per year with 225,000 person years of productive life lost. The population in the productive age groups has increased. In addition, the unemployment rate is high in the 15 to 29 age group (Central Bank of Sri Lanka 2000). The age at marriage has increased for both sexes. It is 25.5 years for females and 27.7 years for males.

In the first five years of the epidemic (1987–91), the male to female ratio was 4:1, which decreased to 2:1 in the next five years. By the end of 2002 women made up 39 per cent of reported HIV cases, demonstrating the gradual increase in the number of women reported. By December 2001, 48 per cent of the reported HIV-infected women (cumulative) had been employed abroad. Most countries that employ these workers insist that they be subjected to compulsory HIV testing. Nearly 160,000 persons seek foreign employment annually and women account for around 70 per cent of them. The increased vulnerability of women to HIV transmission has implications for the vulnerability of children, who have a significant chance of becoming infected at birth from their mothers.

In the initial phase of the epidemic, HIV transmission was mainly due to homosexual or bisexual exposure, but subsequently it has become evident that in Sri Lanka heterosexual transmission is the predominant mode. In 103 (22 per cent) of the 455 HIV-infected persons, the mode of transmission is not known. Of the remainder, 302 (85.8 per cent) were heterosexual, 40 (11.4 per cent) homo- or bisexual, two (0.5 per cent) infected through blood and eight (2.3 per cent) infected through perinatal transmission (Figure 12.1).

HIV transmission via injecting drug use is yet to be reported. It is estimated that of the 40,000 heroin users in Sri Lanka, only approximately 2 per cent are injecting users.

The first case of indigenous transmission of HIV was detected in 1989. Since then the percentage of reported cases attributed to indigenous transmission has varied between 9 and 51 per cent. In 2002 indigenous transmission accounted for 44 per cent of the reported infections.

HIV has been reported from all nine provinces in Sri Lanka, with the maximum number of cases (63 per cent) from the Western Province.

Figure 12.1
Mode of Transmission of HIV in Sri Lanka

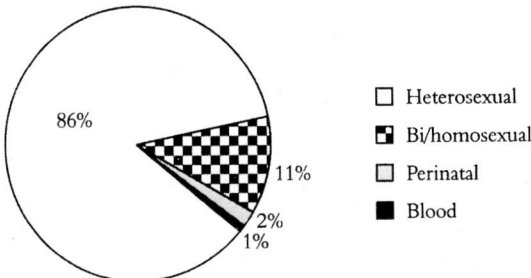

Source: NSACP.

Surveillance and Monitoring

To monitor the geographic, temporal and demographic spread of HIV infection among the population, sero-surveillance surveys have been conducted in sentinel sites since 1993. Such seroprevalence surveys are unlinked and anonymous. By 2002 eight sites were in operation covering eight of the nine provinces. Female sex workers, STD clinic attendees and patients with tuberculosis are screened at these sites annually. A few HIV positives were detected at some sites in 1993, 1995, 1998, 1999, 2000, 2001 and 2002. More HIV positives among STD clinic attendees were detected since the 2000 survey, but the numbers were too few to detect any significant trend. Ad hoc surveys among military and police recruits and remand prisoners using unlinked anonymous testing in 1998 did not reveal any HIV-positive cases. Screening of antenatal clinic attendees (17,601 samples) using unlinked anonymous testing during the year 2002 did not detect any HIV positives.

In Sri Lanka behaviour surveillance for HIV has been included as a component of knowledge and attitude surveys in the past. Behaviour surveillance systems (BSS) are yet to be established on a national scale. Sero-surveillance in combination with behavioural surveillance is recommended as combined data will generate a more complete picture of the national epidemic and response.

STIs and HIV/AIDS are not notifiable in Sri Lanka. However, the epidemiological patterns of these diseases could be inferred from data reported by the clinics of the National STD/AIDS Control Programme.

It has been estimated that around 200,000 new episodes of STIs occur annually of which only about 10 to 15 per cent are seen in government STD clinics. Most persons with STIs seek treatment in the private sector where no statistics are reported to the NSACP.

Non-gonococcal infections, genital herpes, syphilis, gonorrhoea, genital warts and trichomonal infections are the most frequently reported STIs. It is significant that a rising incidence of genital herpes has been noted in the last seven years (MOH 2000). Genital herpes has replaced syphilis as the leading cause of genital ulceration in Sri Lanka. However, syphilis still remains a major cause of morbidity due to STI.

Most males attending STD clinics admit to having had sexual exposures with female sex workers at least once. Despite the prohibition by law of soliciting clients for sex, there are an estimated 30,000 commercial sex workers active on the streets and in unlicensed 'massage parlours' (undercover commercial sex establishments) and brothels in many of the major commercial and industrial cities. Sex work is nourished as a consequence of the 23-year-old conflict in parts of the country, which has given rise to a greater military presence, displacement of citizens, increased numbers of widows and orphans, and women and children having to exchange sex sometimes for safety and security.

During the past 10 to 12 years 6,000 to 8,500 new cases of TB have been reported annually. The highest incidence rates are in the 45 to 74 year age group (MOH 2000). Patients newly diagnosed with TB have been screened for HIV during sentinel surveillance since 1993 and only two patients were found to be HIV positive. Tuberculosis is a common opportunistic infection diagnosed amongst reported AIDS patients in Sri Lanka.

Sri Lanka's Response

The government of Sri Lanka (GOSL), realising the importance of a concerted response to HIV/AIDS, formed the National AIDS Task Force in 1986. This was later expanded to form the multi-disciplinary, multi-sectoral National AIDS Committee (NAC) chaired by the secretary of health. The NAC advises the GOSL on policy related to the prevention and control of HIV/AIDS. Subcommittees on blood safety, laboratory services and surveillance, legal and ethical issues, care of the HIV infected including counselling, and information, education and communication (IEC) strategies related to HIV/AIDS function under the NAC. There is also a subcommittee on NGOs. Through the NAC, other ministries have been sensitised to the issue of HIV/AIDS and the importance of conducting activities related to AIDS in the workplace. With the devolution of health administration to the provinces, the provincial director of health services is responsible for the implementation of STD/HIV/AIDS prevention activities with the assistance of the Provincial AIDS Committee.

The formulation and implementation of the first Medium-term Plan (MTP) and the formation of the NAC, the formulation and implementation of the Medium-term Plan 11 (MTP11) in 1994, the formation of the UN Theme Group on HIV/AIDS in 1996 and the formulation and execution of the National Integrated Work Plan in 1998 are some of the progressive actions that have been undertaken. External reviews of the National AIDS Programme were held in 1994 and 2000. The National Strategic Plan (NSP) for the Prevention and Control of STD/HIV/AIDS 2002–6 has been developed in collaboration with all stakeholders and support from the WHO and UNAIDS.

Prevention and control of HIV/AIDS was integrated into the existing STD Control Programme in 1985. The NSACP is a public health programme of the Ministry of Health (MOH). There is close collaboration between the NSACP and other relevant health programmes of the MOH, particularly the National Blood Transfusion Service (NBTS), The Respiratory Diseases Control Programme, the Health Education Bureau (HEB), the Family Health Bureau, the Medical Research Institute and the Epidemiology Unit.

Information, Education and Communication on Prevention

Preventive education aimed at persons at increased risk as well as the public in general commenced in the mid-1980s and continue to be implemented both through the government and NGOs. Attempts to modify sexual behaviour through information and education have been one of the major prevention strategies adopted by the MOH. IEC activities aim to combat ignorance and prevent stigmatisation and discrimination, and emphasise the need for prevention of HIV transmission especially by practising safe sex. The HEB and its network of health education officers in the provinces are responsible for implementing health promotion and health education activities. The National Institute of Education and the National Youth Services Council in collaboration with the HEB have focused on youth in schools as well as those out of school. Mass media, discussions, lectures, debates, posters and leaflets, and poetry and drama are some of the methods and approaches used to deliver preventive messages. The UNFPA, UNICEF, UNDP, WHO and World Bank havse provided financial assistance for these activities. The NSACP is responsible for providing technical assistance to all agencies involved in education and training activities.

Although it is difficult to measure reliably the impact of these efforts, studies carried out in 1988, 1992, 1997 and 2000 showed measurable improvement in general awareness of the risks of HIV. A population survey based on WHO protocol to measure prevention indicators for evaluation of HIV/AIDS programmes carried out by the NSACP in 1997 in a rural and urban district showed that 89 to 97 per cent of sexually active persons surveyed were aware of HIV/AIDS (NSACP/WHO 1997). However, only around half in either area were aware of the protective role of the condom. Given the fact that heterosexual transmission is the predominant mode of HIV transmission in Sri Lanka, the results of the prevention indicator survey has clearly indicated a need to more actively promote condoms. Condoms are currently provided free of charge through STD clinics. Phase I of the social marketing programme, which actively promote condoms for disease prevention (approved by the NAC), has been completed. Phase II was due to commence in 2003.

The Sri Lanka Demographic and Health Survey in 2000 surveyed 6,385 ever-married women (15 to 49 years), excluding those from the northern and eastern provinces. Awareness of AIDS was widespread among women in all age groups (90 per cent) in all sectors except in the estate sector where only 40 per cent were aware of AIDS and only 10 per cent had heard about STDs (Department of Census and Statistics 2000).

Provision of Care

Provision of comprehensive care in the management of STIs is another major strategy adopted for the prevention of HIV through sexual transmission. National guidelines on clinical management of STIs have been developed and distributed. Syndromic management of STIs has been introduced at primary health care level.

In keeping with government policy, all HIV-infected patients requiring institutional care are now admitted to general wards. Domiciliary care, however, is encouraged. The NSACP has developed guidelines on clinical management of HIV/AIDS to facilitate uniform and improved management of patients. Persons with HIV infection are also managed on an outpatient basis whenever possible. Counselling services to patients and their families are provided, and large numbers of medical and nursing staff have been trained in counselling. Facilities for HIV testing are available in every province. Very few NGOs assist the government in providing care for patients with HIV and AIDS.

In addition, the antiretroviral drug zidovudine (AZT) is also given as prophylactic therapy free of charge following accidental exposure to HIV in health care settings. Combination antiretroviral therapy is available on prescription, but patients have to pay for it themselves.

Protection of Blood Supply

Sri Lanka was one of the first South Asian countries to reform its blood banks to prevent HIV transmission within the health system. Screening of donor blood for HIV antibodies was started in 1987 by the NSACP in collaboration with the NBTS. The MOH made screening of all donor blood mandatory. The Central Blood Bank in Colombo and 56 regional blood banks distributed throughout the country screen donated blood on-site. All blood and blood products are screened for HIV, hepatitis B, syphilis and malaria before transfusion. For the period 1987 to December 2001 nearly 1.5 million blood units were screened of which 21 were HIV positive, giving a seropositivity rate of 1.4 per 100,000.

Currently around 70 per cent of NBTS supplies come from voluntary blood donations. The rest are replacement donations. Given this scenario, the possibility of paid donors entering the system has to be acknowledged. The NBTS aims to collect all its requirements through voluntary donations in future.

Guidelines on safer blood has been developed and circulated to all health care institutions in the public and private sector. A national blood policy has been approved by the cabinet and is due to be presented to Parliament.

Multi-sectoral Collaboration

The government, NGOs and community-based organisations as well as the private sector are responsible for the implementation of the National AIDS Programme. The NSACP provides technical assistance to all collaborating agencies in order to enable them to implement activities effectively. In Sri Lanka NGOs are already delivering HIV prevention services to key vulnerable and high-risk groups. However, their

208 Iyanthi Abeyewickreme

activities are not coordinated and not strategic, and their coverage remains very limited (estimated to be less than 10 per cent). Participation by the private sector has been minimal and needs to be actively promoted.

Future Directions

Effective action to control and prevent the spread of HIV/AIDS requires national leadership and political commitment. Continued and sustained advocacy is critical to convince policy makers and opinion leaders on the need for clearly stated policies and resources. This is particularly important in Sri Lanka because HIV prevalence is still low and the devastating effects of the epidemic are yet to be experienced.

With the exception of the recently formulated National Blood Policy, even after a decade of HIV/AIDS in Sri Lanka there is an absence of policies pertaining to AIDS in the workplace, human rights issues and legal policies. A National AIDS Policy has been drafted is to be presented to the stakeholders for comments and discussion. Formulation of policies will also facilitate the active enlisting and participation of other government sectors. This holistic approach is critical for a national thrust to the prevention and care of HIV/AIDS to be established. In consideration of the grave economic consequences of HIV/AIDS, private sector participation will be encouraged.

HIV/AIDS is not only a health problem. It is a development issue that raises economic and social causes and consequences. Experiences from other countries show that the epidemic cannot be tackled only through medical interventions. It requires a multi-sectoral approach, involving sectors other than health. In the National Strategic Plan (NSP) other *line* ministries, such as education, defence, labour, women's affairs and youth affairs are encouraged to formulate their own action plans for HIV prevention interventions. Such sectors would draw upon their own existing institutional arrangements, which are better positioned to reach and work with vulnerable populations such as soldiers, migrant workers and youth.

Although NGOs have long been active in the field of HIV/AIDS, with the exception of a few NGOs, their activities are limited to IEC/awareness programmes. The critical need of fostering behaviour change appears to be beyond the technical capacities of NGOs and there is a general reluctance to shoulder the emerging need of providing community and home-based care for those affected with HIV/AIDS.

Networking among NGOs and capacity building of NGOs to deliver targeted interventions for vulnerable populations have been identified in the NSP. According to UNAIDS/WHO, surveillance efforts in low-level epidemics should focus on tracking behaviour and other markers of risk in sub-populations where risk of HIV infection is concentrated. This recommendation has been taken into consideration in the NSP and steps have been taken to establish BSS as soon as possible. Experience from other low-level epidemic countries in the region such as Bangladesh will be taken into account when planning the surveys.

HIV can be transmitted from mother to child before birth, during labour and delivery, and after birth through breast milk. In the absence of any intervention, about 30 per cent of HIV-positive pregnant women who breastfeed would pass HIV infection to their children. In Sri Lanka this amounts to an estimated 100 HIV-positive children born to women living with HIV (cumulative figure up to 2001). Research has shown that a short course of the antiretroviral drug AZT during pregnancy and labour can reduce the probability of HIV transmission from mother to child among breastfeeding mothers by half (Shaffer et al. 1999).

To reduce the impact of the AIDS epidemic on children, Sri Lanka has implemented a policy of providing free HIV testing to pregnant women and, for those who are HIV positive, a short course of AZT. Currently, only those pregnant women who are considered to be at risk of HIV infection are tested. Because fertility is low and the number of children infected is small, this intervention is affordable in Sri Lanka.

For this intervention to be successful, all pregnant women should be screened and the cost would include counselling, training, supervision and consumables (for example, HIV test kits). A pilot project on prevention of mother-to-child transmission is due to be implemented in two districts in 2003 to work out an effective model that could be expanded nationally. In Sri Lanka 95 per cent of pregnant women attend antenatal clinics and 97 per cent deliver in hospitals (Department of Census and Statistics 2000).

Although there is no cure for AIDS at present, there are antiretroviral treatment options that can prolong and improve the quality of life of such patients. ART suppresses HIV, maintaining the integrity of the immune system and postponing development of life-threatening opportunistic infections. It must be taken indefinitely.

An effective response to HIV/AIDS must, however, include treatment for individuals who are already infected in addition to primary prevention for those who are not. The MOH has recognised and accepted the need to provide ART to HIV-infected persons and is currently reviewing the logistics involved. The cost of providing combination antiretroviral drugs indefinitely, laboratory equipment and reagents for monitoring the response to therapy, testing for adverse effects and resistance testing, and training of health care providers are issues that need careful consideration.

Sri Lanka, with its deep historical commitment to human development, a highly literate population, especially among women, and a well developed health infrastructure, is in a strong position to confront and control the spread of HIV infection in the country. The recently formulated National Strategic Plan draws on these strengths to address the priority areas in the prevention and control of HIV/AIDS.

REFERENCES

Central Bank of Sri Lanka (2000). *Report of the Central Bank of Sri Lanka*. Colombo: Central Bank of Sri Lanka.

Department of Census and Statistics (2000). *Sri Lanka demographic and health survey*. Colombo: Department of Census and Statistics.

Ministry of Health (MOH) (2000). *Annual health bulletin*. Colombo: MOH.

NSACP/WHO (1997). National STD/AIDS control programme and WHO Sri Lanka priority prevention indicator survey. Unpublished report, Colombo.

Shaffer, Nathan et al. on behalf of the Bangkok Collaborative Perinatal HIV Transmission Study Group (1999). Short-course zidovudine for perinatal HIV-1 transmission in Bangkok, Thailand: A randomised controlled trial. *Lancet*, 353(9155).

UNAIDS/WHO (2000). *Guidelines for second generation HIV surveillance*. Geneva: UNAIDS.

13

Response in a Post-conflict Setting: HIV and Vulnerability in Afghanistan

Anne Bergenström and Naqibullah Safi*

Afghanistan is evolving into a transitional country following over 25 years of war and civil strife. In post-conflict and humanitarian situations, HIV prevention is frequently overlooked because of other competing priorities. Yet it is exactly in such circumstances that HIV/AIDS thrives, as experienced by other war-affected countries such as Cambodia and Myanmar. Until reliable data on STIs and HIV become available, immediate interventions are required to avert possible HIV transmission among vulnerable populations, including drug users, refugees and mobile populations, men and women who exchange sex for money or drugs, and uniformed personnel and their families. In responding to the global HIV epidemic, all countries have faced a decision between early and late intervention to reduce the impact on society, communities and individuals. Delayed response is mostly associated with greater adverse impact at different levels, including higher HIV/AIDS prevention- and care-related costs, while early intervention has the potential to maintain HIV prevalence at low levels. Afghanistan still benefits from a window of opportunity for embarking on an early HIV prevention strategy for averting a rapid increase of HIV prevalence among vulnerable populations as experienced in neighbouring countries in Asia.

While beginning to rebuild following prolonged war and social instability, Afghanistan ranked at the bottom of the UNDP Human Development Index when it was last included in 1996. Between 6 and 10 per cent of the population suffers from acute malnutrition (Safi 2003), with economic activity in recent years having mostly been diverted to war. Literacy rate among women was 21 per cent in 2000 (UNICEF 2004). The low socio-economic status of women renders them particularly vulnerable. While no HIV or STI prevalence data has been available due to absence of surveillance (WHO/UNAIDS 2002), there is evidence of several HIV risks faced by the Afghan people. These should be considered as warning signs of a potential HIV epidemic.

Risk Factors for HIV

Blood Supply

Globally some 5 to 10 per cent of all HIV infections are acquired through unsafe blood transfusions and blood products (UNAIDS 1997a). The main factors that contribute to HIV transmission through blood or blood products include lack of 'safe' blood donors and presence of unsafe blood donations, absence or lack of universal screening, insufficient infection control measures, inappropriate testing, or unnecessary or incorrect use of blood.

During the 1980s a central blood bank (CBB) was established in Kabul (Dupire et al. 1999) with branches across the country. The report flow was hampered from provinces to the centre, and the surveillance system became non-functional after 1992 due to political conflict and lack of human and financial resources. HIV testing is now carried out as routine. Though Dupire et al. (ibid.) reported a low prevalence of 0.3 per cent of hepatitis B and C, the situation can change rapidly. The current coverage of blood screening by the CBB is limited to its own catchment area in Kabul and the majority of blood donations are derived from relatives when required. Only 11 out of 32 provincial blood banks are currently reporting to the CBB (Safi 2003). Over half of the transfused blood is believed not to have been tested for HIV currently, though no reliable estimates are available (GFATM 2002).

To maintain a supply of safe blood in the long term, it is crucial to ensure:

- support to the local authorities, including budget for supply of HIV, syphilis and hepatitis B and C test kits;
- ongoing training of health care staff in blood safety and infection control;

- recruitment and selection of blood donors on a voluntary and unpaid basis, including encouraging blood donations by relatives;
- screening of all donated blood and blood products for HIV; and
- appropriate and rational use of blood.

Availability of safe blood supply for blood transfusions is an essential component of any health care system and as such requires ongoing monitoring efforts.

Drug Production, Trafficking, Use and Needle Sharing

Afghanistan continues to be a major producer of opium globally. Opium production increased by 6 per cent from 3,400 tons in 2002 to 3,600 tons in 2003 (UNODC 2003b) and an estimated three-quarters of global opium supply was derived from Afghanistan in 2003 (UNODC 2003a). Although the Taliban authorities imposed a total ban on opium cultivation in 2001, lack of alternative income generation activities and severe droughts experienced in many areas make growing alternative crops difficult. Consequently, many individuals and communities depend on opium production for their livelihoods. The cultivation ban resulted in a 10-fold increase in the price of opium and in 2002 gross income form opium totaled $1.2 billion ($6,500 per family) (UNODC 2003a). Despite the ban on cultivation and subsequent ban on trading set by the Karzai administration in 2002, the opium economy is thriving. Dismantling this complex economy poses a major challenge for Afghanistan and the international community.

Evidence suggests that opium and heroin abuse appear to be more severe in areas where these drugs are produced (Poschyachinda 1993). All countries in Central Asia have reported increasing levels of injecting drug use and, therefore, increasing risk of blood-borne diseases, including HIV (UNODC 2003a). Already some 105,000 persons in neighbouring countries have been reported with HIV (UNAIDS 2002). The majority of these HIV infections were among injecting drug users in Pakistan and Iran. Uzbekistan and Tajikistan as well as China have each reported outbreaks of HIV among injecting drug users, with reported HIV prevalence rates among IDUs ranging from 50 to 70 per cent in China (Zhang and Ma 2002). In Iran between 710,000 and 1.2 million people are reported to use opiates (UNODC 2003a). In Pakistan there are an estimated of 500,000 heroin-dependent persons (UNODC, 2002) of whom some 15 per cent inject. A prevalence of 89 per cent of hepatitis C, an indicator of HIV risk, among IDUs has been reported in Pakistan (UNDCP and UNAIDS 1999). Recently, one study reported significant increase in needle sharing among IDUs in Lahore (Strathdee et al. 2003). The change in injecting behaviour may have been indirectly or directly affected by the war in Afghanistan in 2001 (ibid.). As in neighbouring countries, it is clear that injecting drug use is a major risk factor for HIV transmission in Afghanistan.

Data on injecting drug use and HIV in Pakistan is of particular relevance as Pakistan has hosted a large Afghan refugee population, which is currently undergoing voluntary repatriation to Afghanistan. For several years Pakistan reported very low prevalence of HIV among IDUs despite high prevalence of hepatitis C. Recently, in a survey of 100 IDUs who were imprisoned and tested for HIV in Sindh province in southern Pakistan, 17 showed HIV (UNOCHA 2003). Though the survey raised questions about ethical and sampling issues, it is a reminder of the rapidly deteriorating HIV situation in the IDU population in Pakistan. Previously, Thailand, Myanmar, Manipur state in India, and more recently Nepal and Indonesia have each experienced how fast HIV prevalence can rise among IDUs (Sarkar et al. 2003; WHO/UNAIDS 2002).

The impact of long-term civil strife, combined with political, social and economic problems, has been associated with an increase in drug use in both rural and urban areas, as well as in refugee settings (Reid and Costigan 2002). Use of heroin, opium and hashish appears to be on the rise, but reliable data on the actual extent of the drug use problem is scarce (ibid.). In 2002 a five-district study reported 50 per cent of households to have a hashish user, almost 10 per cent to have someone with a problem of pharmaceutical use and 2 per cent an opium user (ibid.). Misuse of pharmaceuticals is frequent due to wide availability of over-the-counter medicines. An estimated 0.64 per cent of the households surveyed reported heroin use (ibid.).

According to a recent community-based assessment, some 10,774 individuals in Kabul are addicted to opium, 7,000 to heroin and 14,300 to pharmaceuticals (UNODC 2003a). An estimated 7 per cent use the injecting route of administering heroin and sharing of injecting equipment has been reported (ibid.). The low cost of heroin has been reported to be associated with an increase in the number of heroin users, while another reason is linked to the large populations of returning refugees from the neighbouring countries, many of whom became addicted while abroad (ibid.). Data on actual injecting practices are scarce, although there are reports of heroin injecting among Afghan refugees living outside the country as well as returning refugees (ibid.). One study had found needle sharing between four to six other users in Quetta, Pakistan (UNDCP 2000). A recent study of Pakistani and Afghani drug users in Quetta reported extremely low HIV knowledge and high HIV risk behaviours, such as low level of condom use (Zafar et al. 2003). Available data indicates an increase of hepatitis C over time, from a reported 82 cases in 2002 to 148 cases in 2003 (Safi 2003). Data on HIV prevalence or hepatitis C among IDUs, a surrogate marker for HIV, are currently unavailable in Afghanistan.

The reported number of HIV infections in Afghanistan is 22, while the National AIDS Control Programme of the Ministry of Health estimate there are between 200 to 300 persons living with HIV/AIDS (Ministry of Health 2003, personal communication). In view of the findings from one study that reported an estimated of 40 per cent of Afghan drug users having initiated drug use in neighbouring Pakistan or Iran (UNDCP 2001) and the reports of a high percentage of new HIV infections attributable to injecting drug use in Iran (MAP 2001), there is much cause for concern about the potential introduction of HIV through returning refugees. Nevertheless, every effort should be made to prevent compulsory HIV testing and to avoid stigmatisation of returning Afghan nationals on these grounds. Previous research on HIV VCT among IDUs has demonstrated that HIV testing or knowledge of HIV status alone does not result in behaviour change by IDUs (Sarkar et al. 1995).

Experience from other countries suggests that when opium becomes unavailable, for example, due to successful eradication programmes, drug dependent persons frequently shift to injecting, thus increasing their vulnerability to HIV (Panda et al. 1997). Fluctuations in the market price of opium may also have an impact on the number of users (McCarthy 2001). Such a decrease may result in an increased number of drug users. Injecting may also become the preferred option due to lower cost of a 'fix' (Reid and Costigan 2002). At the same time, should the interim government successfully destroy existing opium crops, resulting in a decrease in smokable opium, there is a fear that many current drug users may switch to injecting.

In the light of the vulnerability of IDUs to HIV, prevention interventions are paramount to avert new infections among drug dependent persons. Furthermore, evidence suggests that low level of condom use among IDUs in mainstream relationships is associated with STDs and HIV among sexual partners of IDUs (Panda et al. 2000). Female sexual partners of drug users, whether drug users themselves or not, are at high risk of STIs and HIV (WHO International Collaborative Group 1994). In Pakistan the number of Afghan drug users has been estimated to account for some 15 to 20 per cent of all drug users (Zafar Syed 2002). Condom use has been reported to be almost non-existent among drug users (ibid.), thus rendering female Afghan refugees and sexual partners highly vulnerable to HIV.

Although there is currently no HIV prevalence or incidence data among IDUs in Afghanistan, the prevalence is thought to be low, a situation that could change rapidly given the efficiency of HIV transmission through sharing of injecting equipment. Drug and HIV awareness programmes are on a limited scale and there is a need to conduct a mapping of the scale of injecting drug use, including in refugee settings in Pakistan and Iran, followed by scaling up of outreach programmes for IDUs, including distribution of injecting equipment and drug treatment services. HIV interventions, including treatment options, focused at IDUs are limited, with the main focus having been on eradication of drug supply. It is crucial that drug supply control measures form a part of a comprehensive intervention programme, which includes drug treatment with methadone or buprenorphine, syringe and needle exchange programmes, condom distribution, outreach, peer education and access to HIV VCT, care and support (Sarkar et al. 2003; United Nations 2000). Active participation of drug users at all stages of the response and a comprehensive coverage of the IDU population and their partners is essential to achieving an impact.

Essential components of interventions aimed at averting HIV transmission among drug dependent persons include:

- access to information about modes of HIV transmission through outreach and peer education;
- universal coverage to provide access to clean syringes and needles, including in refugee settings in neighbouring countries;
- access to drug treatment programmes;
- access to STI treatment services and STI prevention programmes; and
- protection from discrimination and stigmatisation.

Sexual Risk Behaviour

In most countries the HIV epidemic is driven by one or more established risk factors and behaviours, some of which are related to sexual behaviour, including unprotected sex in non-regular sexual partnerships, men who have sex with men (MSM), and sex in exchange for money, food, protection, drugs, etc. In addition, low rate of condom use is also an established indicator of unsafe sexual behaviour. Information on the trends of sexual behaviour is crucial for identification of populations most at risk for acquiring HIV and for planning focused interventions to reduce HIV vulnerability among these groups. In case of Afghanistan scientifically sound behavioural data, including the size of the high-risk populations, are yet to be collected. However, sex between men has been reported across Asia (Aggleton et al. 1999) and the Middle East (Jenkins and Robalino 2003), in both Islamic and non-Islamic societies, and it is unlikely that Afghanistan would be an exception. Similarly, exchange of sex for money, protection or other reasons is well documented in conflict and post-conflict countries in the Asia region (Beyrer 2001). Others are simply forced into sex work and many are sold into the trade (Ohshige et al. 2000).

In Afghanistan as well as in other parts of South Asia a large proportion of women experience poverty and struggle for a daily survival for themselves and their children. Such a low socio-economic status, combined with lack of economic opportunities, may result in an increase in the numbers of women, and possibly men, turning to sex work to meet their basic needs. In Peshawar a consistent increase in the number of Afghan women turning to sex work was reported in 2002 (McGee, personal communication). Presence of Afghan commercial sex workers has also been reported in Kabul (Baldauf 2003). However, without scientific behavioural surveys no conclusions can be drawn on the actual numbers of female and male sex workers inside or outside the country.

Also vulnerable to HIV are the highly mobile populations, including long-distance truck drivers and their assistants. Border crossing areas between countries have been identified as places that foster risk-taking behaviour (Haour-Knipe et al. 1999). Truckers and their assistants frequently spend long time away from home and their communities. Self-reported sexual encounters within other members of the trucker community as well as along the route are well documented in India (UNAIDS 2001), Bangladesh (Dunston et al. 1993; Gibney et al. 2001). Several cities in Pakistan, including Peshawar, Lahore and Karachi, serve as major stopping points for truckers in the region. Similarly, Afghan truckers transport large quantities of goods to and from Central Asian republics as well as Pakistan and Iran. Consequently, mobile populations, including truckers and their assistants in and outside Afghanistan are also likely to be vulnerable to STIs and HIV.

In order to identify the extent and range of HIV risk factors related to sexual behaviour, and to design HIV prevention interventions focused at the most vulnerable groups, there is an urgent need to:

- conduct a rapid assessment of sexual behaviour in specific population groups and geographic locations;
- assess the extent and range of risk behaviours, including size of the populations and level of condom use among different populations; and
- utilise the data to design and implement HIV prevention interventions focused on vulnerable groups, including marginalised groups such as IDUs and sex workers, and to provide appropriate services.

Vulnerability Factors for HIV

HIV/AIDS in Post-conflict and Humanitarian Settings

Evidence from other countries has shown that HIV/AIDS thrives in conflict areas, post-conflict situations, and areas with high numbers of internally displaced populations and refugees (Khaw et al. 2000; UNAIDS 1997b, 1997c, 1998). The HIV epidemic has been particularly widespread in countries with long-term civil war, political instability and human rights violations (Beyrer 1998). War can have an indirect or direct impact on established HIV risk behaviours such as drug use and injecting practices (Strathdee et al. 2003).

Refugee Settings

Of over 3.5 million Afghans who became refugees due to war, nearly 2 million have voluntarily repatriated from Pakistan and Iran by January 2003. Some 665,000 Afghans continued to be internally displaced as of January 2003 (UNHCR 2003). Refugees and internally displaced persons are especially vulnerable to HIV for various reasons, such as involuntary displacement to a higher HIV prevalence area, potential exposure to sexual abuse, violence, commercial sex work, trafficking, lack of access to information, education, services and safe injecting equipment, as well as potential exposure to contaminated blood used in transfusion (UNAIDS 1997b). Many Afghan refugees, including women and young people, crossed the border to neighbouring countries in search of safety or better economic prospects. Although there are currently no published scientific data on the exposure of these refugees and migrants to other potential HIV risks, such as trafficking and sexual exploitation (Salama and Dondero 2001), resulting in a greater risk of STIs (Carballo et al. 1996), these cannot be ruled out. Interviews of 70 Afghan refugees residing in Islamabad found low knowledge of STIs and HIV, combined with self-reported HIV risk factors including unprotected sexual behaviour, multiple partners and history of STIs. Yet reported condom use was low and knowledge of and access to health services was poor (Nazir 2002). According to the Ministry of Health, new HIV infections have been diagnosed among returning refugees (UNHCR OCM Afghanistan 2004).

The basic minimum HIV/AIDS response in refugee settings should consist of the following interventions:

- access to STI and TB treatment and reproductive health care;
- availability of condoms and clean injecting equipment for drug using populations;
- access to information and skills on how to protect themselves and their children from HIV/AIDS;
- ensuring a safe physical environment, in particular for women and girls;
- universal HIV screening of all blood to be used for transfusion; and
- availability of required supplies for universal precautions.

HIV and Uniformed Personnel and Prisoners

Peacekeeping forces, uniformed personnel and the families of both are especially vulnerable to HIV/AIDS (O'Grady and Miller 2001). Evidence from other countries frequently indicates higher HIV seroprevalence levels among military personnel and the police force compared with the general population (ibid.). It is well known that presence of STIs, in particular, ulcerative ones, increase the probability of HIV transmission (Dallabetta et al. 1999). Among armed forces, STI rates have been reported to be two to five times higher compared with the civilian population during peacetime, and this difference may be greater during conflict (UNAIDS 1998). Similarly, several studies have shown HIV prevalence to be higher among military personnel compared with civilians (ibid.). For example, in Cambodia a seroprevalence of 6 per cent has been reported among the military and the police force (Phalla et al. 1998).

Concern about the potential impact of HIV/AIDS on peacekeeping forces has been stated in the UN Security Council Resolution in July 2001, which calls for international collaboration between member states and highlights the need for HIV/AIDS education, prevention, access to voluntary counselling and HIV testing, as well as treatment, care and support. The essential services in complex emergency settings should include:

- access to the means to prevent HIV, in particular condoms and clean injecting equipment, combined with HIV/AIDS information and education;
- access to STI and TB treatment and reproductive health care for uniformed personnel and their families;
- measures to prevent nosocomial transmission of HIV, in particular prevention of transmission through blood transfusion through adherence to a policy of universal precautions and access to materials and equipment;
- training of health care staff; and
- ensuring the human rights of vulnerable individuals, such as prisoners and people living with HIV/AIDS.

Other operational measures to be considered include pre-deployment HIV prevention education, access to voluntary counselling and HIV testing, and ongoing condom distribution and promotion. Finally, prisoners are also at an increased risk of HIV due to their vulnerability to possible sexual abuse. They should have equal access to STI and HIV prevention measures, treatment and care.

Limited Health and Education Infrastructure

Other HIV vulnerability factors faced by the Afghans include low levels of HIV awareness, lack of access to education and information for girls and women, limited access to good-quality general health services, such as STI treatment, lack of trained health care workers, unsafe blood supply and poor medical practices. For example, one syringe is frequently used up to five to ten persons for injections and one lancet for up to 50 persons in the laboratory. Rebuilding the infrastructure for education and health services is a long-term challenge as much of the infrastructure collapsed during the last decade. In the short term, there is an urgent need to ensure access to quality STI treatment, safe blood transfusion, condoms, reproductive health care, and voluntary counselling and testing for HIV. In the long term, challenges involved in management of opportunistic infections and delivery of antiretroviral treatment will need to be addressed.

Low Socio-economic Status of Women and Lack of Access to Employment Opportunities

During the 1970s Afghan women enjoyed relatively high levels of education and freedom. In the last decade women were systematically excluded from public and professional life. However, their empowerment is key to rebuilding the society as evidence from other development projects has shown that women's empowerment is critical for improving key health and social indicators. Currently, Afghan women and girls are facing severe malnutrition, maternal and infant mortality is staggering, and their education and health care needs have been neglected. Fertility per woman is high at 6.9 children (UNFPA 2002) and maternal mortality, at approximately 1,600 per 100,000, is among the leading causes of mortality in Afghanistan (UNICEF/CDC 2002). Lack of access to information and education renders women especially vulnerable to STIs and HIV. Reports from other countries that have experienced conflicts have shown that lack of employment opportunities for women may force some into sex work as a means of survival for themselves and their children.

In the neighbouring South Asian countries gender inequality has resulted in low social status of girls and women, high level of illiteracy, sexual abuse as well as a high risk of HIV (UNICEF 2001). In India one study showed that 90 per cent of women diagnosed as HIV positive had only had one sexual partner, their husband (Gangakhedkar et al. 1997). In Bangladesh 90 per cent of girls could not name one method to prevent HIV (UNICEF 2001). In Afghanistan literacy rates among girls and women has plummeted and are now among the lowest in the world. Some 78 per cent women and 48 per cent men are illiterate

(UNICEF 2000). Lack of empowerment and poor access to information, education and employment opportunities is likely to make many girls and women highly vulnerable to STIs and HIV. While there is an immediate short-term need to provide for the essential nutritional requirements, primary health care and educational needs for women and girls, long-term reconstruction efforts must focus on capacity building, income generating activities and empowerment of women.

Surveillance for HIV and Risk Behaviours

An activity with special importance attached to it in a low HIV prevalence setting is the HIV and STI surveillance system. Experience has shown that HIV surveillance efforts need to be tailored according to the state of the epidemic (FHI and UNAIDS 2001). Many countries have experienced sub-epidemics among certain groups of people, such as sex workers, IDUs and MSM. Once HIV prevalence reaches a critical threshold among such a group, the epidemic becomes sustainable and is likely to spread to the general population through the 'bridge population', which includes current and ex-partners of drug users and clients of sex workers. In low-prevalence countries such as Afghanistan, prevalence monitoring alone is likely to show low rates of HIV. In the absence of HIV prevalence data, second-generation behavioural surveillance data is the primary source of an early warning for a possible 'hidden' HIV epidemic. For example, in Bangladesh the behavioural surveillance system was implemented when HIV prevalence rates according to sentinel surveillance were comparable to those in Afghanistan. Yet presence of other HIV risk factors, such as high level of STIs, was evident (Tarantola et al. 1999). An essential component of HIV surveillance in low-prevalence countries such as Bangladesh and Afghanistan is to collect both STI and behavioural data to allow planning and implementation of HIV interventions for especially vulnerable populations early in the epidemic. Community involvement in the planning and implementation of successful behavioural surveillance is an essential element.

The National and International HIV/AIDS Response

Despite presence of multiple HIV risk indicators, Afghanistan currently benefits from an exceptional window of opportunity to avert an HIV epidemic experienced globally by many nations. Relative absence of data on HIV/AIDS (WHO/UNAIDS 2002) and other STIs in Afghanistan should no longer be a reason for limited priority given by the leaders and the international community for addressing a potentially silent HIV epidemic. While a preliminary assessment was completed in 2003, there is a scope for a detailed quantitative approach with systemic collection of size, range of different risk populations and risk behaviours, study on biologic markers and surrogate indicators. Timely readjustment of the National Strategic Plan (2003–7) developed in 2003 according to the detailed situation and response analysis remain crucial in order to seize the current window of opportunity of low prevalence but high HIV vulnerability. The potential impact of failure to seize this chance for a country already struggling to rebuild its general and health infrastructure could be devastating. Capacity and resources need to be ensured and political barriers, if any, need to be minimised. In long-term reconstruction efforts the possibility of a hidden HIV epidemic must be taken seriously, while there is an immediate need for addressing the reproductive and other health care needs of women and girls, in particular high maternal and infant mortality. Though the current burden of HIV-related disease may not be very high, the weak health infrastructure, unless significantly strengthened, is likely to pose a major challenge in future efforts to provide services such as HIV VCT, prevention of mother-to-child transmission, treatment of opportunistic infections, and treatment and monitoring for antiretroviral therapy.

In terms of planning for and implementing HIV/AIDS interventions, local government, communities and opinion leaders play a key role as they have in-depth knowledge of and insight into cultural and social norms, know the local languages and other such factors. In fact, experience from other countries has shown that, with the support of the national government, community-based HIV interventions can successfully reach their communities with effective HIV prevention projects (Granich and Mermin 2001). For example, the experience of the community-based SHAKTI (Stopping HIV and AIDS through Knowledge and Training Initiative) project in another Muslim country, Bangladesh, has shown reduced rates of STIs, HIV and injecting drug use among community members (Abdul-Quader 1997). Afghanistan could benefit by learning from successful HIV responses by the communities and governments from other predominantly Muslim countries. Religious leaders in Afghanistan have been quick to respond to the challenge of HIV/AIDS, and after participating in an inter-faith consultation on HIV/AIDS in Nepal in 2003, follow-up plans involve development of training materials and information tools. Up to now, some 500 *mullahs* have received training on HIV/AIDS.

In low-prevalence settings, such as Afghanistan, 'targeted' HIV interventions focused at sub-populations at higher risk of HIV transmission, such as IDUs, and their injecting and sexual partners, are essential. The earlier such community-led interventions are planned and implemented, the greater the opportunity to avert an HIV epidemic among subpopulations and the general population. As an effective HIV prevention response takes time, an early strategic and coordinated response by the communities, government and the international community is necessary to avert an impending HIV epidemic in Afghanistan. The establishment of an HIV Technical Working Group in 2002 demonstrates the commitment of international agencies in supporting the government in planning a multi-sectoral strategic response to HIV/AIDS. The Ministry of Health has expressed concern about the spread of HIV, in particular transmission related to unsafe blood, and the current HIV/AIDS response focuses on increasing blood safety, awareness raising, media training and formative research. In addition, two NGOs engage in condom social marketing. However, the HIV response needs to expand fast to include behavioural interventions in order to avert potential sub-epidemics among individuals at high risk of HIV transmission, particularly IDUs and their partners.

Short-term and Long-term Intervention Strategies

In terms of planning for a strategic response to HIV /AIDS, there is an urgent need to conduct a rapid situation analysis to understand the current behavioural risk factors for HIV, if any, and to obtain a prevalence of HIV or its surrogates (STI, hepatitis B/C) in blood transfusion settings and vulnerable groups such as IDUs, sex workers, MSM, migrant and mobile populations, and uniformed personnel. These studies could be conducted by rapid assessment methods developed in recent years and frequently used by HIV researchers (Fitch et al. 2000). Recommendations emerging from these surveys should guide the strategic planning process for short-term and long-term activities. An evidence-based national strategic plan that forms the basis for development of a national plan for action needs to be developed. A national plan needs to be costed and supported by specific targets. A recently conducted analysis of regional resources revealed a significant resource gap in Afghanistan, consisting of $53,000 government funds and an allocation of the Global

Fund to Fight AIDS, Tuberculosis and Malaria (GFATM) funding (GFATM 2002; UNAIDS 2003). The resource gap, coupled with a late release of earmarked GFATM funds and poor absorptive capacity, can pose significant barriers to scaling up a comprehensive HIV response. While capacity building in planning and management are required to manage donor funding issues, rapid interventions for populations at highest risk, such as IDUs and sex workers, can significantly slow the progress of the epidemic. Immediate capacity building to enable surveillance and focused interventions must be prioritised.

Therefore, the recommendations should consist of the following:

1. Ensuring implementation of the proposed detailed situation assessment for HIV and STIs, and introduction of second-generation surveillance that includes both behavioural and serological surveys, and size estimation of the at-risk population.
2. Readjustment of the strategic plan and implementation plan based on the results of situation assessment, including prioritisation of target populations, and estimation of financial and human resources required to implement the plan.
3. Rapid saturation of interventions for refugees, uniformed personnel and populations most at risk.
4. Fostering a coordinated multi-sectoral response with clear objectives, targets and output indicators.
5. Strengthening the capacity, both technical and managerial, of the Ministry of Health, combined with advocacy with political and religious leaders.
6. Ensuring strategic use and smooth flow of external donor funds that have been mobilised so far from GFATM and other sources with continued resource mobilisation efforts.
7. Establishment of monitoring and evaluation for tracking the progress of the response and course correction.

In the final analysis, the extent of the success would largely depend on the commitment of the national leadership and capacity to launch a multi-sectoral response. It remains to be seen how Afghanistan will respond in the post-conflict era. Response to HIV/AIDS should be viewed as part of the reconstruction and rebuilding process.

N OTE

* The authors are grateful to Dr. Swarup Sarkar, Dr. Olavi Elo, Dr. Yon Heerackers, Dr. Phillipe Calain, Dr. Hasan Orooj and Dr. Andrew McGhee. The views expressed are those of the individual authors.

R EFERENCES

Abdul-Quader, A. (1997). Women in need: Street-based female sex workers in Dhaka city. SHAKTI project report, CARE, Dhaka, July.

Aggleton, P., S. Khan and **R. Parker** (1999). Interventions for men who have sex with men. In L. Gibney, R.J. Diclemente and S.H. Vermund (eds.), *Preventing HIV in developing countries: Biomedical and behavioral approaches* (pp. 313–28). New York: Plenum Press.

Baldauf, S. (2003). AIDS follows Afghanistan's miniglobalisation. *Christian Science Monitor*, 17 October.

Beyrer, C. (1998). Burma and Cambodia: Human rights, social disruption, and the spread of HIV/AIDS. *Health Human Rights*, 2(4), 84–97.

——— (2001). Shan women and girls and the sex industry in Southeast Asia: Political causes and human rights violations. *Social Science Medicine*, 53(4), 543–50.

Carballo, M., M. Grocutt and **A. Hadzihasanovic** (1996). Women and migration: A public health issue. *World Health Statistics Quarterly*, 49(2), 158–64.

Dallabetta, G., D. Serwadda and **D. Mugrditchian** (1999). Controlling other sexually transmitted diseases. In L. Gibney, R.J. Diclemente and S.H. Vermund (eds.), *Preventing HIV in developing countries: Biomedical and behavioral approaches* (pp. 109–33). New York: Plenum Press.

Dunston, A., Sattar Gale and **A. Naila** (1993). A literature review of factors related to the spread of STDs and HIV/AIDS in Bangladesh. UNICEF, Dhanmondi, Dhaka, November.

Dupire, B., A.K. Abawi, C. Ganteaume, T. Lam, P. Truze and **G. Martet** (1999). Establishment of a blood transfusion center at Kabul, Afghanistan. *Sante*, 9(1), 18–22.

FHI and **UNAIDS** (2001). *Effective prevention strategies in low prevalence settings*. Geneva: UNAIDS.

Fitch, C., T. Rhodes and **G.V. Stimson** (2000). Origins of an epidemic: The methodological and political emergence of rapid assessment. *International Journal of Drug Policy*, 11(1–2), 63–82.

Gangakhedkar, R.R., M.E. Bentley, A.D. Divekar, D. Gadkari, S.M. Mehendale, M.E. Shepherd, R.C. Bollinger and **T.C. Quinn** (1997). Spread of HIV infection in married monogamous women in India. *Journal of American Medical Association*, 278(23), 2090–92.

Gibney, L., N. Saquib, J. Metzger, P. Choudhuri, M. Siddiqui and M. Hassan (2001). Human immunodeficiency virus, hepatitis B, C and D in Bangladesh's trucking industry: Prevalence and risk factors. *International Journal of Epidemiology*, 30(4), 878–84.

Global Fund to Fight AIDS, Tuberculosis and Malaria (GFATM) (2002). Proposal by the Global Fund Commission in Afghanistan (GFCA). Geneva, July, http://www.theglobalfund.org/en/.

Granich, R. and J. Mermin (2001). *HIV, health & your community: A guide for action*. Berkeley: The Hesperian Foundation.

Haour-Knipe, M., M. Leshabari and G. Lwihula (1999). Interventions for workers away from their families. In L. Gibney, R.J. Diclemente and S.H. Vermund (eds.), *Preventing HIV in developing countries: Biomedical and behavioral approaches* (pp. 257–79). New York: Plenum Press.

Jenkins, C. and D.A. Robalino (2003). *HIV/AIDS in the Middle East and North Africa: The costs of inaction*. Washington, DC: World Bank.

Khaw, A.J., P. Salama, B. Burkholder and T.J. Dondero (2000). HIV risk and prevention in emergency-affected populations: A review. *Disasters*, 24(3), 181–97.

McCarthy, R. (2001). Opium growing doubles in Northern Alliance zones. *The Age*, 23 October, p. 11.

Monitoring the AIDS Pandemic (MAP) (2001). The status and trends of HIV/AIDS/STI epidemics in Asia and the Pacific. MAP, Melbourne, 4 October.

Nazir, M. (2002). Factors contributing to risks and vulnerabilities for contracting STDs/HIV/AIDS in Afghan refugees. M.Sc. thesis, Fatima Jinnah Women University, Rawalpindi, Pakistan.

O'Grady, M. and N.N. Miller (2001). The civil–military project on HIV/AIDS: An international joint venture for HIV/AIDS prevention. In Bunmi Makinwa and Mary O'Grady (eds.), *FHI/UNAIDS best practices in HIV/AIDS prevention collection*. Geneva and Arlington: UNAIDS and Family Health International.

Ohshige, K., S. Morio, S. Mizushima, K. Kitamura, K. Tajima, A. Suyama, S. Usuku, P. Tia, L.B. Hor, S. Heng, V. Saphonn, O. Tochikubo and K. Soda (2000). Behavioural and serological human immunodeficiency virus risk factors among female commercial sex workers in Cambodia. *International Journal of Epidemiology*, 29(2), 344–54.

Panda, S. et al. (1997). Injection drug use in Calcutta: A potential for an explosive HIV epidemic. *Drug and Alcohol Review*, 16(1), 17–23.

Panda, S., A. Chatterjee, S.K. Bhattacharya, B. Manna, P.N. Singh, S. Sarkar, T.N. Naik, S. Chakrabarti and R. Detels (2000). Transmission of HIV from injecting drug users to their wives in India. *International Journal of STD and AIDS*, 11(7), 468–73.

Phalla, T., L. Hor Bun, S. Mills, A. Bennett, P. Wienrawee, P. Gorback and J. Chin (1998). HIV and STD epidemiology, risk behaviours, and prevention and care response in Cambodia. *AIDS*, 12(Supplement B), S11–18.

Poschyachinda, V. (1993). Drug injecting and HIV infection among the population of drug abusers in Asia. *Bulletin of Narcotics*, 45(1), 77–90.

Reid, G. and G. Costigan (2002). *Revisiting 'the hidden epidemic': A situation assessment of drug use in Asia in the context of HIV/AIDS*. Melbourne: Centre for Harm Reduction and Burnet Institute.

Safi, N. (2003). Background paper on health and nutrition, National Development Report, Afghanistan.

Salama, P. and T.J. Dondero (2001). HIV surveillance in complex emergencies. *AIDS*, 15(Supplement 3), 4–12.

Sarkar, S., A. Chatterjee and A. Bergenstrom (2003). Drug-related HIV in South and South-East Asia. *Journal of Health Management*, 5(2), 277–95.

Sarkar, S., S. Panda, K. Sarkar, C.Z. Hangzo, L. Bijaya, N.Y. Singh, N. Das, A. Agarwal, A. Chatterjee, B.C. Deb and R. Detels (1995). A cross-sectional study on factors including HIV testing and counselling determining unsafe injecting practices among injecting drug users of Manipur. *Indian Journal of Public Health*, 39(3), 86–92.

Strathdee, S.A., T. Zafar, H. Brahmbhatt, A. Baksh and S. ul Hassan (2003). Rise in needle sharing among injection drug users in Pakistan during the Afghanistan war. *Drug Alcohol Dependency*, 71(1), 17–24.

Tarantola, D., P.R. Lamptey and R. Moodie (1999). The global HIV/AIDS pandemic: Trends and patterns. In L. Gibney, R.J. Diclemente and S. H. Vermund (eds.), *Preventing HIV in developing countries: Biomedical and behavioral approaches* (pp. 9–38). New York: Plenum Press.

UNAIDS (1997a). *UNAIDS technical update: Blood safety and HIV*. October.

———— (1997b). *UNAIDS technical update: Refugees and AIDS*. September.

———— (1997c). *UNAIDS point of view: Refugees and AIDS*. April.

———— (1998). *Point of view: AIDS and the military*. May.

———— (2001). *An HIV/STD intervention in the transport sector: A case study*. New Delhi: UNAIDS.

———— (2002). *Report on the global HIV/AIDS epidemic*. Geneva: UNAIDS.

———— (2003). Estimated resource need for Asia Pacific countries. Unpublished data, draft report of a regional workshop, New Delhi, September.

UNDCP and UNAIDS (1999). Baseline study of the relationship between injecting drug use, HIV and hepatitis C among male injecting drug users in Lahore. UNDCP and UNAIDS, Islamabad.

UNDCP (2000). *Community drug profile # 3: A comparative study of Afghan street heroin addicts in Peshawar and Quetta, Pakistan*. Islamabad: UNDCP.

———— (2001). *Community drug Profile # 4: An assessment of drug problem in rural Afghanistan—The GAI target districts, Afghanistan*. Islamabad: UNDCP.

UNFPA (2002). Information note, http://www.unfpa.org/news/2002/pressroom/afghanistan_rept.htm.

UNHCR (2003). *Refugees by numbers*. January.

UNHCR OCM Afghanistan (2004). *Return information update*. Issue 49, 1–15 January.

UNICEF (2000). ACO: Multi indicators cluster survey (MICS). UNICEF.

———— (2001). *The state of world's children 2001*. Geneva: UNICEF.

———— (2004). *The state of world's children 2004*. Geneva: UNICEF.

UNICEF/CDC (2002). CDC/UNICEF preliminary findings for maternal mortality survey.

UN Office for Coordination of Humanitarian Affairs (UNOCHA) Pakistan (2003). New cases of HIV among drug users. *IRIN News*, 23 July, http://www.irinnews.org/default.asp.

United Nations (2000). Preventing the transmission of HIV among drug abusers. Position paper of the United Nations System.

UNODC (2002). *Drug abuse in Pakistan: Results from the year 2000 national assessment.* New York: UNODC.

—— (2003a). *The opium economy in Afghanistan: An international problem.* New York: United Nations.

—— (2003b). *Afghanistan opium survey 2003.* Islamabad: UNDCP and UNAIDS.

WHO International Collaborative Group (1994). Multi-city study on drug injecting and risk of HIV infection. Document WHO/PSA/(4.4), WHO, Geneva.

WHO/UNAIDS (2002). *Epidemiological Fact Sheet, Afghanistan.* Geneva: WHO/ UNAIDS.

Zafar Syed, T. (2002). War on terrorism: Triggering injecting drug use and HIV/ AIDS in Pakistan—Strategies and programs to minimize damage. 13th International Conference on the Reduction of Drug Related Harm, Ljubljana, Slovenia, 3–7 March (abstract A633).

Zafar, T., H. Brahmbhatt, G. Imam, S. ul Hassan and S.A. Strathdee (2003). HIV knowledge and risk behaviors among Pakistani and Afghani drug users in Quetta, Pakistan. *Journal of Acquired Immunodeficiency Syndromes,* 1(32), 394–98.

Zhang, K.L. and S.J. Ma (2002). Epidemiology of HIV in China. *British Medical Journal,* 325(7362), 803–4.

PREVENTION OF TRANSFUSION-
TRANSMISSIBLE HIV IN MYANMAR | 14

Myint Zaw

HIV infection in Myanmar started among injecting drug users and then the higher-risk commercial sex workers were infected (Myo Thet Htoon 1994). From CSWs the infection moved on to clients, who acted as a bridge population to transfer HIV infection to their wives and regular partners. The last population to be affected were infants and children from their infected mothers (National AIDS Programme 2000).

The National Blood Safety Programme in Myanmar started in 1985. Since then blood donors and other sub-population groups are tested for HIV antibodies in many major cities by the Department of Medical Research. Starting from 1987, the National Health Laboratory took the responsibility of testing blood donors. The Central National Blood Bank and other blood banks then tested for HIV among blood donors, which expanded to other states and divisions, districts and townships. By 1996 about 70 per cent of the blood drawn was tested and by the end of 1998 all blood donated up to the township level was screened (Figure 14.1).

The administrative setup of the National Blood Safety Programme by the Ministry of Health has brought in many collaborations within and outside the health sector. It works in line with guidelines laid down by National Health Committee and detailed framework of the National AIDS Committee. The National AIDS Programme coordinates with many departments to ensure adequate HIV test equipment, training of health personnel and recruitment, and retaining voluntary and safe blood donors. NGOs like the Myanmar Red Cross Society and the Myanmar Maternal and Child Welfare Association play major roles in the recruitment of safe blood and healthy blood donors.

Figure 14.1
Proportion of Blood Screened for HIV Antibodies per Year: 1989-98

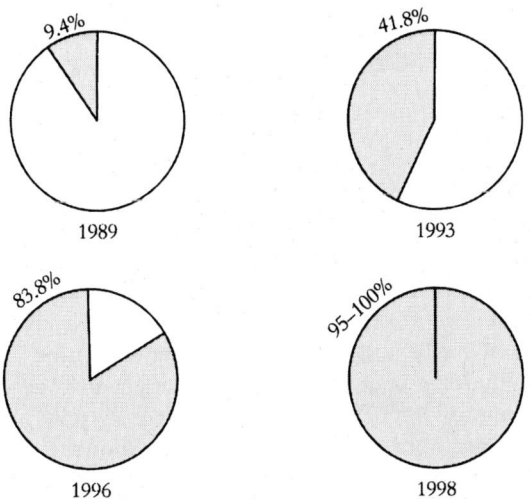

Source: National AIDS Programme, Yangon.

About half of the total blood units collected all over the country is from Yangon and Mandalay. Of the rest, 20 per cent is drawn from state/division general hospitals and the remaining 30 per cent is from districts, townships and peripheral hospitals.

The expansion of the blood safety programme has been rapid in Myanmar. The central laboratory in Myanmar, the National Health Laboratory, started to test donated blood since 1987. This was followed by the Public Health Laboratory from Mandalay and the Central National Blood Bank of Yangon, catering to their respective hospitals and catchment areas. Blood safety then quickly expanded in its scope and geographical coverage, and by 1996 most hospitals and blood banks were covered.

Three main types of HIV antibody testing systems are used for the blood safety programme in Myanmar. An ELISA test, which is the cornerstone of all blood donor testing programmes, is used in five major areas. The HIV Spot test, a rapid qualitative test with 100 per cent specificity, is mainly used in smaller hospitals and in testing for emergency operative procedures. District and township hospitals use the Passive

Particle Agglutination test, which is both high in sensitivity and specificity.

The blood testing strategy adopted in Myanmar adheres to WHO/UNAIDS guidelines. Different test systems are used to screen blood donors. Apart from HIV testing, recruitment and retention of voluntary non-remunerative blood donors are other useful strategies used to ensure safe blood.

The total amount of blood screened for HIV in 1989 was only 9.4 per cent. But with guidance from the National Health Committee, and advocacy and commitment from the Ministry of Health it expanded to 83.8 per cent coverage in 1996. By 1998 all blood donated and transfused in the public sector was screened before every donation.

The marked improvement in the expansion of an HIV-safe blood supply system in Myanmar within a short period of time is noticeable. What was only 70 per cent coverage in 1996 reached 100 per cent coverage by the end of 1998 due to keen interest from policy makers and specific guidance from the National Health Committee. The Ministry of Health contributed US$ 100,000 worth of HIV test kits every year.

A cross-sectional blood use and HIV screening study was carried out across the country by the National AIDS Programme between 1996 and 1998. Due to the policy of rational use of blood in all public sector hospitals under the Ministry of Health guidelines, blood use decreased while the blood tested for HIV increased (Figure 14.2).

The five main strategies adopted by the Ministry of Health for safe blood transfusion system in the country were: replenishment of HIV test kits, recruitment and retainment of blood donors, referral to blood banks, reporting and returns, and research of best practice methods.

In big urban hospitals like state and division hospitals, general and specialist hospitals and in major blood banks the importance of proper donor education and systematic deferral are in the forefront of activities. Then donors are tested for HIV. Here, the role of blood donor groups, which are many in Myanmar, ensures voluntary donation and safer blood products. There are medical officers, social workers and counsellers in continuous attendance giving education and counselling to potential donors.

A different model called 'walking blood banks' is used in township hospitals and station hospitals in remote settings where voluntary donors are recruited from Red Cross, Myanmar Maternal and Child Welfare Association (MMCWA), Union Solidarity and Development Association (USDA), youth organisations, religious organisations and from the

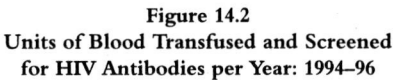

Figure 14.2
Units of Blood Transfused and Screened
for HIV Antibodies per Year: 1994–96

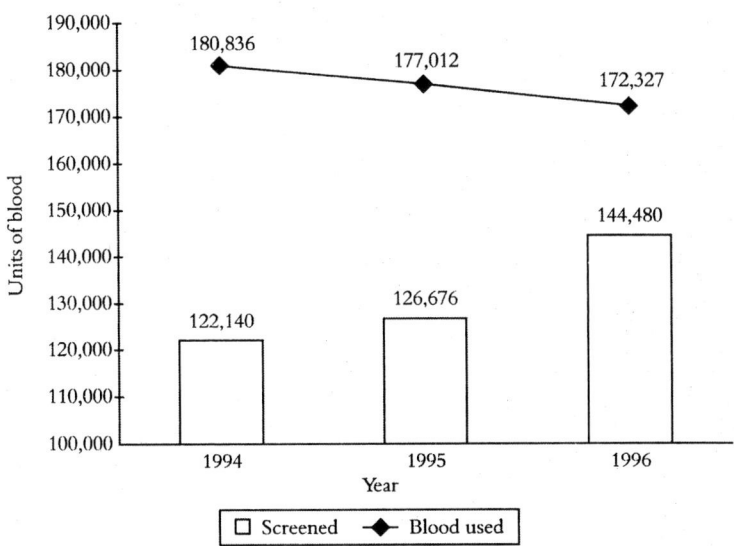

Source: National AIDS Programme, Central Blood Bank, National Health Laboratory, Public Health Laboratory, Hospital Reports, 1996 survey results.

community. Here, the blood is tested voluntarily after pre-test counselling and the list of eligible donors is kept with the respective township medical officer confidentially. These 'walking blood banks' are continually assessed with education and retesting if necessary. When a hospital needs blood these safe donors are ready for donation at any time. There are a very few paid donors in Myanmar. Now, with rapid HIV test kits available to test these volunteers, the blood donation system in rural areas is made doubly safe.

The blood programme research carried out in Myanmar since 1993 up to the present includes seroprevalence studies, risk behaviour studies, field evaluation of test kits (both hospital based and laboratory based), donor deferral best practice studies and the ever-expanding HIV/AIDS/STD-related behavioural studies among blood donors.

This experience shows Myanmar's commitment and technical preparations for a safe and reliable blood supply system. While there is much progress in the public sector, the private sector blood transfusion system still needs to be tightened up and tidied to some extent. But there are now blood laws, laboratory accreditation laws and drug laws, which need to be strictly followed to have a healthy and efficient blood supply system in Myanmar.

REFERENCES

Myo Thet Htoon (1994). HIV/AIDS in Myanmar. *AIDS*, 8(Supplement 2), S105–9.

National AIDS Programme (2000). *Report of HIV/AIDS surveillance*. Yangon: National AIDS Control Programme, Ministry of Health.

OCCURRENCE AND MANAGEMENT
OF OPPORTUNISTIC INFECTIONS
ASSOCIATED WITH HIV/AIDS IN ASIA

15

Subhash K. Hira

Introduction

Systemic symptoms among HIV-seropositive individuals occur progressively and are correlated with the degree of immune suppression along the continuum (Legg 1994). These symptoms and diseases are categorised into the following three groups: (*a*) when CD4 counts are above 500 cells per microlitre, causes of systemic symptoms are less likely to be related to HIV infection; (*b*) when CD4 counts are between 200 and 500 cells per microlitre, frequent infections such as bacterial pneumonia and sinusitis occur, which sometimes are debilitating, but these are not considered opportunistic infections (OI); and (*c*) when CD4 counts fall below 200 cells per microlitre, a host of OI such as *Cryptococcus neoformans*, cytomegalovirus, *Strongyloides stercoralis*, *Candida* spp. and *Cryptosporidium parvum* occur (Figure 15.1). Also, common infections occur with uncommon clinical presentations during this late stage of HIV disease.

A study in Australia defined the correlation between CD4 cell count and occurrence of OI (Crowe et al. 1991). These were broadly categorised into the following five groups: asymptomatic infection, CD4 greater than 500/cmm; oral candidiasis and tuberculosis, range 250–500/cmm; Kaposi's sarcoma, lymphoma and *Cryptosporidium*, range 150–200/cmm; *Pneumocystis carinii* pneumonia, disseminated *Mycobacterium avium* complex, *Herpes simplex*, toxoplasmosis, cryptococcosis and oesophageal candidiasis, range 75–125/cmm; and cytomegalovirus retinitis, CD4 less than 50/cmm (Table 15.1).

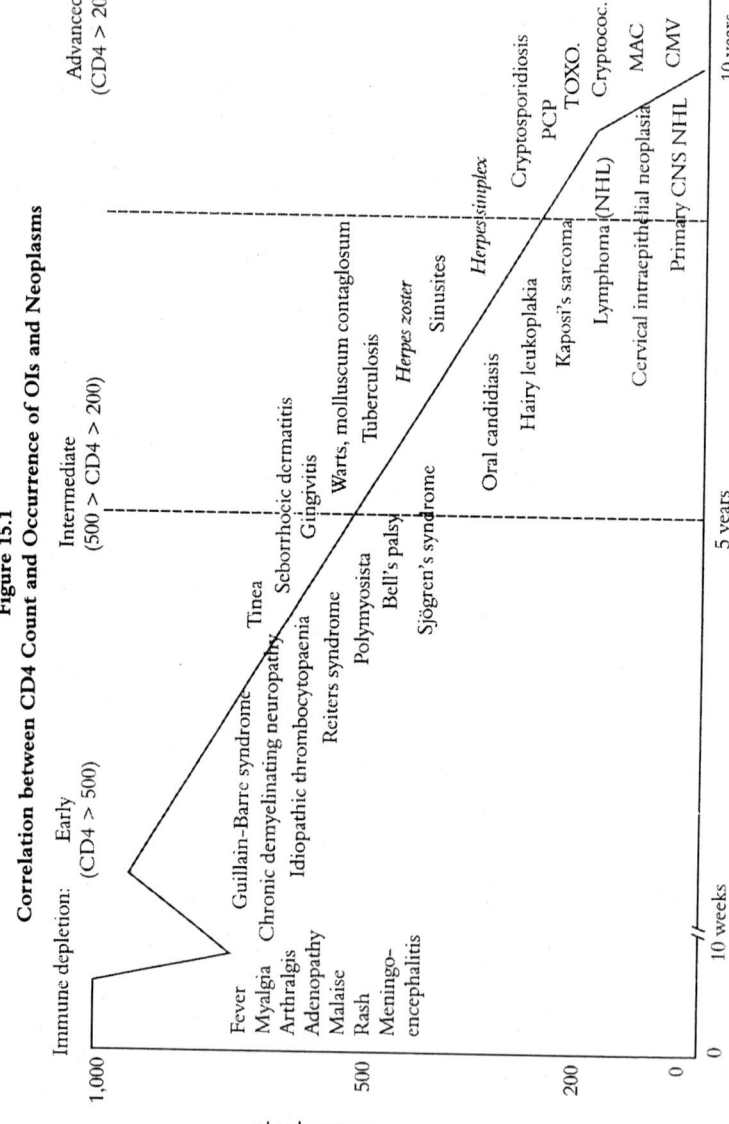

Figure 15.1
Correlation between CD4 Count and Occurrence of OIs and Neoplasms

Table 15.1
**Mean and Median CD4 Numbers per Cubic Millimetre
for Each Category of Opportunistic Infection**

Illness	Number of events	Mean	Median
Asymptomatic	20	692.0	575.0
Tuberculosis	7	340.0	159.0
Oral candidiasis	22	275.6	170.0
Cryptosporidium	11	213.0	134.0
Herpes simplex	9	117.6	110.0
Pneumocystosis	70	111.9	70.5
M. avium complex	46	98.4	50.0
Toxoplasmosis	16	93.1	57.5
Cryptococcosis	11	73.2	46.0
Esophageal candidiasis	15	66.5	45.0
Cytomegalovirus retinitis	31	29.0	17.0
Kaposi's sarcoma	43	169.5	110.0
Lymphoma	6	166.5	81.5

Source: Crowe et al. (1991).

Definition of Opportunistic Infections

OIs are defined as infections that otherwise may be present as latent infections in an immune competent host without producing systemic symptoms of diseases/malignancies. However, in the presence of profound immune suppression, such as that occurring with AIDS, there is activation of latent infections and production of serious life-threatening symptoms and diseases. For example, *Pneumocystis carinii* pneumonia (PCP) is the most common AIDS-defining OI in the United States and Europe (CDC 1992).

Immune Mechanisms that Precipitate OIs and non-OIs

OIs are precipitated by severe qualitative and quantitative defects of T-helper (CD4) cells that have been described in patients with HIV-related disease and AIDS (Bowen et al. 1985; Lane et al. 1985). There is incomplete knowledge as to how the presence of the HIV genome in a minority of CD4+ T-cells leads to the destruction of immune system. In-vitro observations suggest that HIV's envelope glycoprotein gp120 interacts with the receptor CD4 and this may impair the functions of CD4+

cells, both infected and non-infected T-cells (Moore and Blanc 1991). The latter action is possibly mediated through cytokine cascade. The qualitative defects of the CD4 cells weaken the helper role of these cells, both in relation to the monocyte–macrophage system and B-cell immunoglobulin production (Lane et al. 1985). The phagocytic function of monocytes and macrophages remains intact, but their chemotaxis and intracellular killing capacity is hampered (Nottet et al. 1993). A recent study indicated that there was virologic cross-talk between B-cells and CD4 T-cells, within the micro-environment of lymphoid tissue and to a lesser extent between cells in the lymph nodes and peripheral blood. Thus, most of the virus in the plasma originates from cells other than the CD4 T-cells in the peripheral blood and lymph nodes (Malaspina et al. 2002).

The common non-OIs that occur in individuals with HIV infection and AIDS are:

1. Bacterial:

   - *Salmonella* spp.
   - *Streptococcus pneumoniae*
   - *Hemophilus influenzae*
   - *Mycobacterium tuberculosis*
   - *Staphylococcus aureus* (most common cutaneous bacterial infection)
   - *Pseudomonas aeruginosa* (chronic leg ulcer)
   - Sexually-transmitted infections such as *Treponema pallidum, Chlamydia trachomatis, Haemophilus ducreyi* and *C.granulomatis.*

2. Fungal:

   - *Histoplasma* spp.
   - *Aspergillus fumigatus*
   - *Nocardia* spp.
   - *Tinea* spp.

3. Viral:

   - *Molluscum contagiosum*

4. Parasitic:

   - *Giardia lamblia*
   - *Sarcoptes scabei*

Non-OIs may occur due to the following mechanisms:

1. Quantitative defect such as granulocytopaenia is reportedly associated with hampered chemotaxis, phagocytosis and impaired bacterial killing capacity (Murphy et al. 1988; Pitrak et al. 1993). This defect, for example, predisposes an HIV-infected individual to *Staphylococcus aureus, Pseudomonas aeroginosa* and gram-negative enteric bacteria.

2. B-cell abnormality may present as an increase in the spontaneous secretion of immunoglobulins or as impaired response to a variety of antigens (Pahwa et al. 1984). This defect, for example, predisposes an individual to infection with encapsulated bacteria such as *Streptococcus pneumoniae* and *Haemophilus influenzae.* Both occur as non-opportunistic infections with increased frequency among HIV-infected persons. The lack of antibody response to new infections can be devastating in patients who had no opportunity to develop antibody to the infecting pathogen before developing B-cell dysfunction. Such a situation frequently occurs in children with perinatally acquired HIV infection. Thus, these children do not have recall antibodies with which to protect themselves from new infections.

Pattern of Opportunistic Infections in Asia

The occurrence and frequency of opportunistic infections correlate with the prevalence of microbes in geographic regions of the world. Few OIs are region specific. For the purpose of simplicity, their salient features are presented here.

Bacterial Opportunistic Infections

Mycobacterium tuberculosis

The disseminated and miliary forms of tuberculosis occur frequently as OIs in severely immuno-compromised individuals in Asia. It is the most common OI reported from the region. It is associated with severe weight loss, fever, cough, raised ESR and anergic tuberculin test. High prevalence of HIV among individuals with abdominal tuberculosis is reported from India (Rathi et al. 1997). The prevalence of HIV among patients with tuberculosis in Chiang Rai in Thailand increased from

1.5 per cent in 1990 to 45.5 per cent in 1994. The HIV-seropositive tuberculosis group showed annual mortality rate of 68 per cent despite adequate tuberculosis treatment (Yanai et al. 1996). Mixed infection with *M. tuberculosis*, and *Pneumocystis carinii* and *C. neoformans* in 10 per cent of cases with respiratory involvement among patients with AIDS in Thailand suggests that poly-aetiology is a frequent phenomenon in severely immuno-compromised individuals (Mootsikapun et al. 1996). Several autopsy studies have established tuberculosis as the most frequently identified infection (Bhoopat et al. 1994; Lanjewar et al. 1996b). The radiographic presentation in pulmonary disease resembles primary tuberculosis of immuno-competent hosts (prominent hilar and mediastinal adenopathy, non-cavitatory infiltrates and no upper lobe predominance) or miliary infiltrates (Lee et al. 1993). An Australian study showed that despite lack of cavitatory lung lesions in a patient with advanced HIV disease, nosocomial transmission of tuberculosis occurred among HIV-infected patients exposed to the index case in an HIV outpatient facility (Couldwell et al. 1996). This was also demonstrated in 1998 in the Chiang Rai province of Thailand where cases of tuberculosis attributable to immunosuppression caused by HIV proportionately rose to 72 per cent in male patients and 65.8 per cent in females (Siriarayapon et al. 2002).

The most difficult form of tuberculosis that has presented a greater challenge to public health is drug-resistant tuberculosis (MDR-TB). Resistance to multiple drugs emerges due to: (*a*) inadequate treatment doses; (*b*) irregular intake of drugs; (*c*) incorrect prescriptions; and (*d*) improper monitoring and supervision. The WHO defines MDR-TB as resistance to two or more drugs. Chiang Rai province of Thailand reported rising prevalence of primary resistance in an HIV endemic area, namely, 13.2 per cent to INH, 10.8 per cent to rifampicin, 15.6 per cent to streptomycin and 5.8 per cent to ethambutol. It reported MDR-TB at 6.3 per cent (Yoshiyama et al. 2001). Even worse, a study conducted among HIV–TB dually-infected patients in Mumbai revealed a high level (72 per cent) of patients who were resistant to four of the five first-line anti-TB drugs and more than 60 per cent were resistant to four of the five second-line drugs. The individual drug resistance was high, ranging from 62 to 100 per cent (Birdi et al. 2003).

The natural history of HIV-1 among adults in Mumbai reveals that HIV-infected persons with tuberculosis were three times at risk of early death (Hira et al. 2003). The study established the annual incidence of tuberculosis at 4.8 per 100 person-years and a lifetime risk of developing tuberculosis as 60 per cent with a consistent correlation between mortality and occurrence of tuberculosis (Hira and Dholakia 2002; Hira et al. 1998). Another study in Mumbai based on post-mortem examinations established tuberculosis as the predominant cause of death in 74 per cent of dually-infected cases (Lanjewar et al. 1998a).

With the advent of antiretroviral therapy, there is an increasing evidence that the occurrence of OIs can be significantly reduced, including that of tuberculosis. A recent study in South Africa demonstrated that after initiation of ART, the incidence of HIV-1-associated tuberculosis was reduced by over 80 per cent in an area that was endemic for both TB and HIV (Badri et al. 2002).

Mycobacterium avium Complex

Mycobacterium avium and *Mycobacterium intracellulare* are collectively known as the *Mycobacterium avium* complex (MAC) because the distinction between the two is rather difficult even with modern diagnostics. It simulates classical tuberculosis such that differentiation can become difficult. Pulmonic involvement is common. It may also involve the skin and the musculoskeletal system, and its coexistence with HIV causes dissemination with anaemia, fever, leukocytocis, lymphadenopathy, hepatosplenomegaly and hypergammaglobulinaemia. Occasional reports of identification of *M. avium-intracellulare* from patients with advanced HIV disease have appeared from Australia (Choo and McCormack 1995; Jackson et al. 1992) and Thailand (Manatsathit et al. 1996). Recognition of atypical mycobacteria is important in the treatment of infections in these patients and in the understanding of epidemiology of atypical mycobacterial infections. It is suggested that a liquid culture medium such as BACTEC be employed for primary isolation of mycobacteria from AIDS patients (Choo and McCormack 1995). Due to non-availability of diagnostic facilities in the developing countries of Asia, it is likely that MAC is under-reported.

Fungal Opportunistic Infections

Candidia spp.

Candida usually presents as oral thrush where there is a presence of grey-white or brown plaques in the oral mucosa, located on the buccal or palatal mucosa. Scraping these plaques reveals a bleeding surface underneath. The other sites it may affect are the upper GI tract, skin and the respiratory tract. Upper GI *Candida* may present as odynophagia or severe oesophagitis. Extensive, recurrent candidial infection of the GI tract, lungs and skin is observed among severely immunosuppressed individuals (Chacko et al. 1995; George et al. 1996; Giri et al. 1995; Kumarasamy et al. 1995). A study conducted in Mumbai, India, reported 54 per cent of oral candidiasis among individuals with HIV disease caused by *Candida tropicalis* (Medak et al. 1996). An Australian study identified that 5 per cent of oral lesions were caused by genetically atypical *C. albicans* strains. These atypical strains produced greater amounts of extracellular proteinase, adhered to a greater degree to buccal epithelial cells and were less susceptible to the anti-fungal drug 5-flucytosine. The results of this study indicated that these genetically atypical *C. albicans* strains possessed increased virulence in comparison with typical *C. albicans* strains (McCullough et al. 1995).

Cryptococcus neoformans

This is the second most common opportunistic infection reported in patients with AIDS in Asia (George et al. 1996; Giri et al. 1995; Manatsathit et al. 1996; Mootsikapun et al. 1996). In Victoria, Australia, the incidence of 3.0 cases of cryptococcosis per 1 million population per year increased to 5.0 cases per 1 million population per year over the decade as a result of the AIDS epidemic. A distinct association was observed between immune status and *C. neoformans variety*: all *C. neoformans variety gattii* infections occurred in healthy hosts and 90 per cent of *C. neoformans variety neoformans* infections occurred in immunosuppressed hosts. The mortality among patients with *C. neoformans variety neoformans* infection was high, while none of those patients with *C. neoformans variety gattii* died, but often had neurological sequelae that required surgery and prolonged therapy (Speed and Dunt 1995). Similarly, 133 out of 139 isolates of *Cryptococcus* obtained from patients with AIDS in different parts of Thailand were identified as *C. neoformans variety gattii*. Anti-fungal susceptibility tests using five anti-fungal agents including amphotericin B, fluconazole, flucytosine, itraconazole and micronazole against 50 selected strains of *C. neoformans* showed that they were sensitive to all of the anti-fungal agents (Poonwan et al. 1997). While secondary prophylaxis was recommended in the pre-ART era, a recent study in Taiwan showed that discontinuation of fluconazole prophylaxis in patients on ART when their CD4 counts rose to above 300 cells/µl. and sustained for three months was safe (Sheng et al. 2002).

Penicillium marneffei

It was first reported as a frequent opportunistic infection from Thailand (Chariyalertsak et al. 1996). Very little was known about the epidemiology and natural reservoir of *P. marneffei* except that its occurrence increased during the rainy season (ibid. 1996, 1997). Skin lesions, usually papules with central necrotic umbilication, provide the most significant clue to the diagnosis. Early diagnosis based on finding *P. marneffei* in the skin smear or lymph node provides the basis for prompt administration of anti-fungal therapy (Sirisanthana and Sirisanthana 1995). Disseminated infection presents clinically with generalised lymphadenopathy (90 per cent), hepatomegaly (90 per cent), fever over 38.5 degrees Celsius (81 per cent), papular skin lesions with central umbilication (67 per cent), splenomegaly (67 per cent), failure to thrive in children (52 per cent), severe anaemia (43 per cent) and thrombocytopaenia (21 per cent) (ibid.). The response rate in patients who are treated with appropriate anti-fungal therapy (amphotericin B, fluconazole or ketoconazole) is good. There are few other reports of penicillosis among travellers in the South Asian region (Heath et al. 1995).

Viral Opportunistic Infections

Herpes simplex

Herpes simplex causes both primary and secondary or recurrent lesions, intra-orally and extra-orally, at any age. In individuals with severe immune-suppression, recurrent herpes episodes are frequent, likely to be painful and healing is slow. When lesions are persistent for a duration of over one month, it is taken as an AIDS-defining illness (Luo et al. 1995). It is associated with a relatively better prognosis than Kaposi's sarcoma. A cross-sectional study of 41 Thai patients with AIDS did not report oral herpes simplex, possibly due to low occurrence of this opportunistic infection in some countries of Asia or due to difficulty in establishing diagnosis (Nittayananta et al. 1997). Dissemination of infection may lead to herpes simplex encephalitis. The latter condition is reported to be fatal unless treated vigorously (Satishchandra et al. 1993).

Varicella zoster

The *Varicella zoster* virus causes herpes zoster (shingles). It is frequently reported as a muco-cutaneous marker of HIV infection (Chacko et al. 1995; Panda et al. 1994). It is characterised by clustered vesicles along a dermatome on the skin or mucosae. A recurrent episode of herpes zoster is an AIDS-defining illness associated with a relatively better prognosis (Luo et al. 1995). A longitudinal study of herpes zoster among HIV-seropositive individuals showed that their clinical presentation was more likely to be multi-dermatomal, recurrent, thoracic (below T6), and had a longer post-herpetic neuralgia as compared with HIV-negative individuals (Dandvate et al. 1998).

Cytomegalovirus

Disseminated cytomegalovirus (CMV) infection is an AIDS-defining illness. It causes encephalitis, pneumonitis (Giri et al. 1995), gastro-enteritis (Lanjewar et al. 1996a; Manatsathit et al. 1996), pancreatitis, retinitis (Biswas et al. 1995) and interstitial renal disease. Mucosal ulcers appearing as superficial ulcers mimicking aphthous ulcers have been reported (Heinic et al. 1993). A recent study from Madrid showed that CMV does not play any significant pathologic role in most of the cutaneous lesions appearing due to other infections and conditions (Dauden et al. 2001). Atypical presentation as cerebral mass has been reported from Australia (Dyer et al. 1995). Despite therapy, prognosis for long-term survival is poor (Maschke et al. 2002).

Oral Hairy Leukoplakia (OHL) and Epstein-Barr Virus

OHL presents as striated white lesions on the lateral margins of the tongue, and less frequently on buccal and genital mucosa. It occurs in about 20 per cent of those with asymptomatic HIV infection and becomes more common as the CD4 count falls (Feigal et al. 1991). Diagnosis of OHL is a clinical indicator of rapid disease progression. A recent study at the University of California showed that 26 per cent of individuals developed oral candidiasis and 42 per cent developed OHL within five years after sero-conversion (Lifson et al. 1994). Another longitudinal study in the US showed that 47 per cent and 67 per cent of individuals developed AIDS within two and four years of occurrence of OHL respectively (Katz et al. 1992). Aetiology of OHL has been attributed to a herpes virus, namely the Epstein-Barr virus (De Souza et al. 1989). Several studies in Asia have reported occurrence of OHL (Chacko et al. 1995; Nittayananta et al. 1997).

Non-Hodgkin's Lymphoma: Malignancy with Viral Aetiology

High-grade B-cell non-Hodgkin's lymphoma (NHL) is an increasingly important condition in individuals infected with HIV (Chacko et al.

1995; Nittayananta et al. 1997). It is associated with relatively poor prognosis for survival (Luo et al. 1995). Central nervous system NHL occurs more frequently when CD4 counts fall below 50 cells/µl. NHL is possibly due to viral antigenic–mitogenic stimulation leading to cytokine-mediated B-cell overproliferation, and/or emergence of Epstein-Barr virus (EBV)-infected and immortalised B-cells. Fifty per cent of these tumours harbour the EBV with a reported equal frequency of EBV A and B sub-types in the tumours (Boyle et al. 1993). An international collaboration on HIV and cancer pooled results of 20 published studies on AIDS-related lymphoma. The adjusted incidence rates showed a decline from 1992–96 to 1997–99 with a relative risk ratio of 0.58. This decline, attributed to the widespread introduction of ART, was most marked for primary cerebral lymphoma, but was also significant for systemic NHL (Beral et al. 2000; Bower and Fife 2001).

Kaposi's Sarcoma: Neoplasia with Viral Aetiology

Kaposi's sarcoma (KS) is a frequent occurrence in the early stages of HIV disease among homosexual men in the US and Europe. With progression of HIV disease, KS tends to become extensive and disseminated when CD4 cell count falls below 50 cells/µl. It may be the first manifestation of late-stage HIV disease. In Asia, where HIV is predominantly transmitted heterosexually, fewer cases of KS have been reported. In decreasing order of frequency, KS is reported most commonly in men (Bhoopat et al. 1996; Dore et al. 1996; Grulich et al. 1997; Luo et al. 1995), women (Rubsamen-Waigmann et al. 1993) and children (Bhoopat et al. 1996; Pruksachatkunakorn et al. 1995). Lymph node, oral, gastrointestinal, respiratory, hepatic and cerebral involvement are reported from the region. The introduction of ART since 1995 has reduced the incidence of Kaposi's sarcoma and NHL precipitously.

Protozoan and Parasitic Opportunistic Infections

Pneumocystis carinii

Pneumocystis carinii pneumonia (PCP) is an AIDS-defining illness. Its presenting features include dyspnoea, fever, weight loss, fatigue and dry cough. Chest radiographs showing interstitial markings should be investigated with specific laboratory tests to demonstrate *P. carinii* cysts. Dissemination to several other systems of the body has been reported (Telzak et al. 1990). PCP is being reported with increasing frequency among the severely immunosuppressed in India (Arora et al. 1996; Bijur et al. 1996; George et al. 1996; Giri et al. 1995), Thailand (Yanai et al. 1996) and Australia (Blackmore et al. 1994; Mallal et al. 1994). PCP may mimick pulmonary tuberculosis (Arora et al. 1996) or present as thick-walled pulmonary cavities (Blackmore et al. 1994). A study conducted in Spain suggested that primary and secondary prophylaxis against PCP could be safely discontinued after the CD4 cell count increased to above 200 cells/μl and were sustained for more than three months (Lopez Bernaldo de Quiros et al. 2001).

Toxoplasma gondii

Toxoplasma gondii is recognised as a major cause of neurologic morbidity and mortality among severely immunosuppressed individuals. Primary route of infection is from animal faeces, such as that of cat or pig, and also associated with eating poorly cooked meat. This latent infection gets activated in immunosuppressed hosts. In the US 22 to 45 per cent of patients with advanced HIV disease have IgG antibodies against *T. Gondii* (Grant et al. 1990). Clinical toxoplasmosis may present as encephalitis, focal neural deficits, lymphadenopathy, hepatosplenomegaly or chorioretinitis. Contrary to therapy for most other opportunistic infections, anti-toxoplasmosis therapy produces good response. Toxoplasmosis of the CNS (Birdi et al. 2003; Handa et al. 1996), respiratory system (Handa et al. 1996) and eye (Wongkamchai et al. 1995) is reported from Asia. Acute encephalitis caused by *Toxoplasma gondii* was diagnosed at autopsy in 20 per cent of patients at Sir J.J. Hospital in Mumbai, suggesting that toxoplasmosis should be considered as an important cause of CNS infections in patients with AIDS (Lanjewar et al. 1998b).

Cryptosporidium parvum

Cryptosporidial diarrhoea is one of the AIDS-defining illnesses in Asia (Chacko et al. 1995; George et al. 1996; Giri et al. 1995; Lanjewar et al. 1996b; Manatsathit et al. 1996). In individuals with AIDS, it produces chronic watery diarrhoea, which then leads to malabsorption, malnutrition, dehydration and weight loss. It has limited treatment options. The probability that diarrhoea will resolve or remit decreases with HIV disease progression. An Australian study found temporal clustering in cryptosporidial detection, but no association with the season, rainfall or environmental temperature (Stuart et al. 1997). Chronic diarrhoea due to *C. parvum* is reported in 20 to 25 per cent of patients with AIDS in India (Ananthasubramanian et al. 1997; Lanjewar et al. 1996b; Panda et al. 1994) and in 19 per cent adults and 8 per cent children with AIDS in Thailand (Moolasart et al. 1995).

Microsporidium

Microsporidium is recognised as a diarrhoeal pathogen in a substantial percentage of cases previously attributed to non-specific AIDS enteropathy (Greenson et al. 1991). Its occurrence correlates with severe immune-suppression (Eeftinck-Schattenkerk et al. 1991). A case of pulmonary microsporidial infection in an HIV-seronegative female patient with chronic myeloid leukaemia undergoing allogeneic bone marrow transplant has been reported in Mumbai, India (Kelkar et al. 1997). A case each of intestinal microsporidiosis has been reported among individuals with AIDS in Thailand and Australia (Lumb et al. 1993; Pitisuttithum et al. 1995).

Strongyloides stercoralis

Studies of non-specific AIDS enteropathy have identified *S. stercoralis* as an opportunistic infection in severely immunosuppressed individuals (Lanjewar et al. 1996b; Manatsathit et al. 1996). Such patients present with abdominal pain and diarrhoea. The infection responds well to broad-spectrum anti-helminthic drugs, and therapy is then followed up with secondary prophylaxis.

Clinical Syndromes and Their Management

In Asia few clinicians are willing to provide care and support to persons living with HIV/AIDS. The laboratory infrastructure required for identification of opportunistic infections is grossly inadequate. Hence, most published reports present frequency of syndromes such as chronic diarrhoea, weight loss greater than 10 per cent of body weight, recurrent fever, chronic cough, persistent headache and cutaneous manifestations caused by a host of opportunistic infections (Chacko et al. 1995; George et al. 1996; Hira et al. 1990, 1996, 1998). Management of clinical syndromes is recommended in accordance with guidelines published by the WHO (WHO 1998) and the national AIDS control programmes. An indicative list based on individual opportunistic infection is presented in Table 15.2.

Management comprises regular monitoring of seropositive individual at two- to three-month intervals. Regular visits include clinical

Table 15.2
Site of Occurrence and Treatment of Opportunistic Infections

Pathogen/infection	Site of infection	Treatment
Aspergillus	Lungs, sinuses or disseminated	IV amphotericin B, itraconazole
Bacterial	Lungs, sinuses or disseminated	Standard antibiotics, IV immunoglobulins
Candidiasis	Mucous membranes, skin, lungs	Ketoconazole, fluconazole
Cytomegalovirus	Retina, GIT, lungs, brain, heart, kidneys, adrenals	IV ganciclovir, IV foscarnet
Coccidioidomycosis	Lungs, lymph nodes, spleen	IV amphotericin B
Cryptococcus	Brain, lungs or disseminated	Fluconazole, IV amphotericin
Cryptosporidium	GIT, lungs	Paromomycin, azithromycin
Leukoplakia	Hairy tongue, buccal mucosa	Topical podophyllin, acyclovir
Herpes simplex	Mouth, lips, genitals	Acyclovir
Herpes zoster	Trunk, face, extremities	Acyclovir, foscarnet
Histoplasmosis	Lungs, skin, GIT	IV amphotericin B, itraconazole
HPV	Genitalia, anus	Cryotherapy, intralesional alpha interferone, topical 5-FU
Isospora belli	Intestines	Cotrimoxazole
Kaposi's sarcoma	Skin, lymph nodes, GIT, lungs	IV vincristine, IV amphotericin B, IV doxorubicin
MAC	Lungs, disseminated	Rifampin, ethambutol, ciprofloxacin, clofazimine Clarithromycin
Microsporidium	GIT	Metronidazole, albendazole
Molluscum	Skin	Cryotherapy
PCP	Lungs, lymph nodes, spleen, liver	Cotrimoxazole, IV pentamidine
Salmonellosis	GIT, disseminated	Ciprofloxacin, cotrimoxazole, ampicillin
Neurosyphilis	CNS	IV crystalline penicillin
Toxoplasmosis	Brain, lungs, lymph glands	Sulfadiazine + pyrimethamine or clindamycin + pyrimethamine or azithromycin + pyrimethamine
Tuberculosis	Lungs, lymphatic system, CNS	INH + rifampin + pyrazinamide + ethambutol for 2 mo then, rifampin + INH for 7 mo

examination along with minimal laboratory investigations comprising: FBC-ESR, montaux test, urine, stool and radiology for the chest and other organs. But these may not always be possible in resource-limited settings. Hence, clinical judgement may have to be used to initiate treatment.

Lymphadenopathy is common with HIV/AIDS and presents as the enlargement of a single or multiple lymph nodes. The causes may range from local or focal infections, tuberculosis, lymphoma or HIV itself. Initially, the dictum is to treat with tetracycline 500 mg four times daily or erythromycin 500 mg four times daily for 15 days. Alternatively, a long-acting penicillin may be used. Tuberculosis should be ruled out for matted lymph nodes associated with fever, anorexia and weight loss, and treated accordingly. The presence of a genital ulcer along with lymph nodes is presumptive of syphilis and benzathine penicillin 2.4 million IU intramuscularly is recommended. Persistent generalised lymphadenopathy due to HIV is common and is defined as enlarged lymph nodes at two or more extra-inguinal sites, more than 1.5 cm in diameter, for more than one month, with no contiguous infections to explain their existence. If the individual is asymptomatic, he/she should be closely monitored. Alternatively, rapidly growing lymph nodes or those not responding to empiric treatment should be appropriately investigated to rule out lymphomas, Kaposi's sarcoma or systemic fungal infection, and treated accordingly (WHO 1998).

Diarrhoea is treated with TMP-SMX, two tablets twice daily for five days to manage bacterial infections. Metronidazole 400 mg, one tablet three times a day for seven days is useful if there is no response to the earlier drug. Fever and bloody stools are indicative of bacterial rather than parasitic infections. After every unformed stool, an anti-secretory agent like loperamide is started; initially 2 mg, followed by 4 mg after every unformed stool (maximum 16 mg a day). Anti-helminthic agents like albendazole (400 mg stat) or mebendazole (100 mg, two times a day for three days) can be given prior to constipating agents. Patients with bloody diarrhoea should not be given constipating agents to prevent the risk of megacolon. A relapse of diarrhoea may occur usually due to inadequate treatment and a prolonged course of therapy may be justified in that case. Disabling diarrhoea needs to be referred to an in-patient facility with better care and support.

Oral thrush and/or odynophagia or severe oesophagitis may present together and candida is the common causative OI. However, in case of oesophagitis there is need to rule out CMV and *Herpes simplex* virus. The usual treatment for mild oral candida includes oral application of gentian violet 1 per cent aqueous solution twice a day for seven days or nystatin washes (100,000 every four hours for seven days) or tablets to be sucked (500,000 IU every six hours). Alternatively, miconazole gel may be used as local application. In case of severe oral candida with oesophagitis or pharyngeal lesions or lesions not responding to the first line of treatment, oral fluconazole 200 mg twice daily may be given up to two to three weeks. Recurrent infections are quite likely and are indicative of a high risk of other OIs. Acyclovir can be given 800 mg five times a day if herpes simplex oesophagitis is suspected or ganciclovir IV if CMV is the causative organism that is identified.

Respiratory conditions present as persistent or worsening cough, dyspnoea, with or without fever, anorexia and weight loss. Most of the times, the X-ray of chest may show bilateral basal interstitial infiltrates that are suggestive of PCP. When diagnostics are not available the condition may be treated symptomatically with broad-spectrum antibiotics for three days. Thereafter, if improvement is noticed, the treatment should be continued for five to seven days. If there is no improvement, shift to penicillin V 250 mg four times daily. In case of no response, a trail of another antibiotic such as TMP-SMX may be given for seven to ten days. There is need to assess the benefit regularly. Initially the pneumonia may worsen; hence, the treatment should be continued for at least 14 days. In case the patient cannot tolerate the full course of penicillin V, change to pentamidine—isothionate 3 mg/kg body weight is recommended. Corticosteroids, for example, prednisone, 20 mg twice daily, may be considered in severely ill patients (WHO 1998).

Headache is a common occurrence and needs to be evaluated if it is persistent and not responding to common analgesics, or if it is accompanied with neurological or focal signs such as change in mental state, dementia, paresis, cerebral palsies, seizures and/or fever. With resurgence of malaria in several parts of Asia, this should be considered as a differential diagnosis and treated with chloroquine. Alternative treatment with other antibiotics like benzyl penicillin 12 to 24 million IU given intravenously four hourly or chloramphenicol 2 to 4 g intravenously four hourly may be considered. A lumbar puncture with CSF examination may be required to rule out tuberculous meningitis, toxoplasmosis or cryptococcal meningitis. Toxoplasmosis usually responds well to sulfadiazine (4 to 6 g daily) and pyremethamine (loading dose 75 and 100 mg, then 25 to 30 mg) daily in four doses. Later, a maintenance dose can be continued lifelong with pyremethamine 25 mg and sulfadiazine 2 to 4 g daily. Cryptococcal infection may be treated with amphotrecin B 0.5 to 0.7 mg/kg intravenously for six weeks or fluconazole 200 to 400 mg daily for 12 weeks. A maintenance dose may be continued with amphoterecin B 1 mg/kg given intravenously weekly or fluconazole oral 200 mg daily (WHO 1998).

Dermatoses are common with HIV/AIDS. Palliative care may be given for itching using oral administration of cetrizine or chlorphenaramine, and local application of soothing agents like calamine. This may or may not be accompanied with antibiotics depending on the type of lesions. Candidiasis may be treated with local application of miconazole and in case of persistent lesions, oral fluconazole may be given. Severe forms of herpes zoster are treated with oral acyclovir 800 mg five times a day for seven days. Post-herpetic neuralgia is common and should be treated with phenytoin or carbamezapine. The recurrence rate of *Molluscum contagiosum* is high if treated with local pricking of lesions with a needle dipped in phenol or trichloroacetic acid. Alternatively, cryotherapy or glacial acetic acid may be used locally. Condylomata acuminata may be treated with glacial trichloroacetic acid. Dermatophytosis may be treated with topical anti-fungals like clotrimezole 1 per cent and oral ketoconazole or griseofulvin 500 mg twice daily. Other allergic conditions may need local glucocorticoids applications (WHO 1998).

Management of HIV/TB Co-infections

So far this paper has dealt with and revealed that immune-suppression due to HIV is the most potent inducer of tuberculosis. It is also documented that co-infection with tuberculosis leads to early progression of disease by stimulating the HIV-infected macrophages and CD4 lymphocytes to produce more viruses. But tuberculosis is different from other OIs because it is treatable, curable and preventable. The treatment of tuberculous co-infection in HIV-infected patients is similar to that given to seronegative individuals. But the focus should be on early diagnosis. Regular monitoring with clinical examination for fever, anorexia, weight loss, lymphadenopathy, diarrhoea, along with investigations such as FBC, ESR, mantoux, chest X-ray, sputum AFB, sputum culture, CT scan for CNS or abdominal TB and lymph-node biopsy (FNAC) to rule out other pathogens and PCR can be useful for early diagnosis of tuberculosis. DOTS (Directly Observed Therapy Short Course) is the preferred form of therapy to prevent relapse and defaulters, and thus prevent the occurrence of MDR TB.

The prophylaxis of opportunistic infections has been one of the major factors responsible for improved patient survival. Primary prophylaxis of opportunistic infections is an attractive concept, as the majority of opportunistic infections are reactivations of latent infections. Primary prophylaxis against PCP and MAC is both effective and necessary, but the role for primary prophylaxis against other infections is as yet unclear. Secondary prophylaxis of most opportunistic infections is warranted, although in most cases the optimal regimens that are least toxic and affordable remain to be determined (Carr et al. 1993; Centres for Disease Control and Prevention 1999; USPHS/IDSA 2000).

There is always a need for repeated sessions of counselling and comfort for patients with HIV/AIDS. Counselling should cover areas of adherence to treatments, especially with chronic infections such as tuberculosis or toxoplasmosis. Additional nutritional counselling may be required for all patients. Other areas of specialised counselling are sexuality, bereavement and inheritance.

Impact of ART

The increased availability of antiretroviral therapy has significantly reduced the incidence of opportunistic infections. The most striking benefit of ART is the reduction in the incidence of HIV-1-associated tuberculosis by more than 80 per cent (95 per cent CI 62–91) (Badri et al. 2002).

Studies from Spain (Soriano et al. 2000), Brazil (Guimaraes 2000) and Chile (Wolff et al. 2000) showed the declining annual trends for the occurrence of OIs after widespread introduction of ART and safe discontinuation of OI prophylaxis. Italian ART studies reported significantly fewer infections and consequent shorter hospital stay (Arici et al. 2001) and modification of the natural history of cryptosporidiosis and microsporidiosis (Maggi et al. 2000). Other studies have reported prolonged survival and decreased risk of death (McNaghten et al. 1999, 2000; Oka 2002), increased survival of patients with progressive multifocal leukoencephalopathy (Geschwind et al. 2001) and NHL (Dore et al. 2002), fewer episodes of oral candidiasis (Munro and Hube 2002), marked improvement in psychosocial depression (Brechtl et al. 2001) and AIDS-associated Kaposi's sarcoma (Dupont et al. 2000).

ART is shown to bring about immune reconstitution and to do away with prophylaxis of major OIs. Several studies have shown that following ART, primary and secondary prophylaxis against PCP can be safely discontinued after the CD4 cell counts increase to 200 cells/μl for more than three months (Grant et al. 1990). Similarly, azithromycin prophylaxis for MAC when the CD4 cell counts rise above 100 cells/μl (El-Sadr et al. 2000), and cessation of secondary prophylaxis for cryptococcal meningitis after CD4 counts increase above 200 cell/μl (Nwokolo et al. 2002) can be discontinued. In a way, the improved access to ART has ushered in a new era in the management of OIs.

R EFERENCES

Ananthasubramanian, M., S. Ananthan, R. Vennila and **S. Bhanu** (1997). *Cryptosporidium* in AIDS patients in south India: A laboratory investigation. *Journal of Communicable Diseases*, 29(1), 29–33.

Arici, C. et al. (2001). Long term clinical benefit after highly active antiretroviral therapy in advanced HIV-1 infection, even in patients without immune reconstitution. *International Journal of STD and AIDS*, 12(9), 573–81.

Arora, V.K., A. Tumbanatham, S.V. Kumar and **C. Ratnakar** (1996). *Pneumocystis carinii* pneumonia simulating as pulmonary tuberculosis in AIDS. *Indian Journal of Chest Diseases and Allied Sciences*, 38, 253–57.

Badri, M., D. Wilson and **R. Wood** (2002). Effect of highly active antiretroviral therapy on incidence of tuberculosis in South Africa: A cohort study. *Lancet*, 359(9323), 2059–64.

Beral, V. et al. (2000). Changes in AIDS related lymphoma (ARL) in the era of HAART. *Proc ASCO*, 19 (abstract 17a).

Bhoopat, L. et al. (1994). Histopathologic spectrum of AIDS-associated lesions in Maharaj Nakorn Chiang Mai Hospital. *Asian Pacific Journal of Allergy and Immunology*, 12(2), 95–104.

Bhoopat, S.K., P. Vithayasai and **C. Pruksachatkunakorn** (1996). AIDS-associated Kaposi's sarcoma: A rare entity at Maharaj Nakorn Chiang Mai Hospital. *Asian Pacific Journal of Allergy and Immunology*, 14(2), 115–20.

Bijur, S. et al. (1996). *Pneumocystis carinii* pneumonia in human immunodeficiency virus infected patients in Bombay: Diagnosed by bronchoalveolar lavage cytology and transbronchial lung biopsy. *Indian Journal of Chest Diseases and Allied Sciences*, 38, 227–33.

Birdi, T., Y.N. Dholakia, D.T. D'souza, B. Oza, S.K. Hira and **N.H. Antia** (2003). A preliminary report on initial mycobacterium drug resistance in HIV-TB dual infection in Mumbai. *Indian Journal of Tuberculosis*, 51(2), 212–16.

Biswas, J., N. Madhavan and **S.S. Badrinath** (1995). Ocular lesions in AIDS: A report of first two cases in India. *Indian Journal of Ophthalmology*, 43(2), 69–72.

Blackmore, T.K., J.P. Slavotinek and **D.L. Gordon** (1994). Cystic pulmonary lesions in *Pneumocystis carinii* infection. *Australian Radiology*, 38(2), 138–40.

Bowen, E.J., H.C. Lane and **A.S. Fauci** (1985). Immunopathogenesis of the acquired immunodeficiency syndrome. *Annals of Internal Medicine*, 103(5), 704–8.

Bower, M. and **K. Fife** (2001). Current issues in the biology of AIDS-related Lymphoma. *HIV Medicine*, 2(3), 141–45.

Boyle, M.J. et al. (1993). The role of Epstein-Barr virus subtypes in human immunodeficiency virus-associated lymphoma. *Leukemia and Lymphoma*, 10(1–2), 17–23.

Brechtl, J.R., W. Breitbart, M. Galietta, S. Krivo and **B. Rosenfeld** (2001). The use of highly active antiretroviral therapy (HAART) in patients with advanced HIV infection: Impact on medical, palliative care, and quality of life outcomes. *Journal of Pain and Symptom Management*, 21(1), 41–51.

Carr, A., R. Penny and **D.A. Cooper** (1993). Prophylaxis of opportunistic infections in patients with HIV infection. *Journal of AIDS*, 6(Supplement 1), S56–60.

Centres for Disease Control (CDC) (1992). HIV/AIDS surveillance report. Atlanta, CDC, 1–22.

Centres for Disease Control and Prevention (1999). 1999 USPHS/IDSA guidelines for the prevention of opportunistic infections in persons infected with the human immunodeficiency virus. *Morbidity and Mortality Weekly Reports*, 48(RR–10), 1–66.

Chacko, S., T.J. John, P.G. Babu, M. Jacob, A. Kaur and **D.J. Mathai** (1995). Clinical profile of AIDS in India: A review of 61 cases. *Journal of the Association of Physicians in India*, 43(8), 535–38.

Chariyalertsak, S., T. Sirisanthana, K. Supparatpinyo and **K.E. Nelson** (1996). Seasonal variation of disseminated *Penicillium marneffei* infections in northern Thailand: A clue to the reservoir? *Journal of Infectious Diseases*, 173(6), 1490–93.

Chariyalertsak, S., T. Sirisanthana, K. Supparatpinyo, J. Praparattanapan and **K.E. Nelson** (1997). Case-control study of risk factors for *Penicillium marneffei* infection in human immunodeficiency virus-infected patients in northern Thailand. *Clinical Infectious Diseases*, 24(6), 1080–86.

Choo, P.S. and **J.G. McCormack** (1995). *Mycobacterium avium*: A potentially treatable cause of pericardial effusions. *Journal of Infection*, 30(1), 55–58.

Couldwell, D.L. et al. (1996). Nosocomial outbreak of tuberculosis in an outpatient HIV treatment room. *AIDS*, 10(5), 521–25.

Crowe, S.M. et al. (1991). Predictive value of CD4 lymphocyte numbers for the development of opportunistic infections and malignancies in HIV-infected persons. *Journal of AIDS*, 4(8), 770–76.

Dandvate, V., S.K. Hira and **C. Oberai** (1998). The natural history of *Herpes zoster* in the era of AIDS. *Indian Journal of Dermatology*, 43, 169–72.

Dauden, E., Fernandez-Beuzo, J. Fraga, L. Cardenoso and **A. Garcia-deiz** (2001). Mucocutaneous presence of CMV associated with human immunodeficiency virus infection: Discussion regarding its pathogenic role. *Archives of Dermatology*, 137(4), 443–48.

De Souza, Y.G. et al. (1989). Localisation of Epstein-Barr virus in the epithelial cells of oral hairy leukoplakia using in situ hybridisation of tissue sections. *New England Journal of Medicine*, 320(23), 1559–60.

Dore, G.J. et al. (1996). Declining incidence and later occurrence of Kaposi's sarcoma among persons with AIDS in Australia: The Australian AIDS cohort. *AIDS*, 10(12), 1401–6.

Dore, G.J., Y. Li, A. McDonald, H. Ree and **J.M. Kaldor** (2002). National HIV surveillance committee: Impact of highly active antiretroviral therapy on individual AIDS-defining illness incidence and survival in Australia. *Journal of AIDS*, 29(4), 388–95.

Dupont, C. et al. (2000). Long term efficacy of Kaposi's sarcoma with highly active anti-retroviral therapy in a cohort of HIV-positive patients: Centre d'information et de soins de l'immunodeficience humaine. *AIDS*, 14(8), 987–93.

Dyer, J.R., M.A. French and **S.A. Mallal** (1995). Cerebral mass lesions due to Cytomegalovirus in patients with AIDS: Report of two cases. *Journal of Infection*, 30(2), 147–51.

Eeftinck-Schattenkerk, J.K. et al. (1991). Clinical significance of small intestinal microsporidiosis in HIV-1 infected individuals. *Lancet*, 337(8746), 895–98.

El-Sadr, W.M. et al. (2000). Discontinuation of prophylaxis for MAC disease in HIV-infected patients who have a response to antiretroviral therapy. *New England Journal of Medicine*, 342(15), 1085–92.

Feigal, D.W. et al. (1991). The prevalence of oral lesions in HIV-infected homosexual and bisexual men: Three San Francisco epidemiological cohorts. *AIDS*, 5(5), 519–25.

George, J., A. Hamide, A.K. Das, S.K. Amarnath and **R.S. Rao** (1996). Clinical and laboratory profile of sixty patients with AIDS: A South Indian study. *Southeast Asian Journal of Tropical Medicine and Public Health*, 27(4), 686–91.

Geschwind, M.D., R.I. Skolasky, W.S. Royal and **J.C. McArthur** (2001). The relative contributions of HAART and alpha-interferon for therapy of progressive multifocal leukoencephalopathy in AIDS. *Journal of Neurovirology*, 7(4), 353–57.

Giri, T.K., I. Pande, N.M. Mishra, S. Kailash, S.S. Uppal and **A. Kumar** (1995). Spectrum of clinical and laboratory characteristics of HIV infection in northern India. *Journal of Communicable Diseases*, 27(3), 131–41.

Grant I.H. et al. (1990). Toxoplasma gondii serology in HIV-infected patients: The development of central nervous system toxoplasmosis in AIDS. *AIDS*, 4(6), 519–21.

Greenson, J.K. et al. (1991). AIDS enteropathy: Occult enteric infections and duodenal mucosal alterations in chronic diarrhoea. *Annals of Internal Medicine*, 114(5), 366–72.

Grulich, A.E., J.M. Kaldor, O. Hendry, K. Luo, N.J. Bodsworth and **D.A. Cooper** (1997). Risk of Kaposi's sarcoma and oroanal sexual contact. *American Journal of Epidemiology*, 145(8), 673–79.

Guimaraes, M.D. (2000). Temporal study in AIDS-associated diseases in Brazil, 1980–1999. *Cadernos de Saude Publica*, 16(Supplement 1), 21–36.

Handa, R. et al. (1996). Toxoplasma encephalitis in AIDS. *Journal of the Association of Physicians in India*, 44, 838.

Heath, T.C., A. Patel, D. Fisher, F.J. Bowden and **B. Currie** (1995). Disseminated *Penicillium marneffei*: Presenting illness of advanced HIV infection; a clinico-pathological review, illustrated by a case report. *Pathology*, 27(1), 101–5.

Heinic, G.S., D. Greenspan and **J.S. Greenspan** (1993). Oral CMV lesions and the HIV infected: Early recognition can help prevent morbidity. *Journal of American Dental Association*, 124(2), 99–105.

Hira, S.K. et al. (1990). Clinical and Epidemiologic features of HIV infection at a referral clinic in Zambia. *Journal of AIDS*, 3(1), 87–91.

Hira, S.K. and **Y.N. Dholakia** (2002). *HIV-TB interface: Round Table Conference series*. New Delhi: Ranbaxy Foundation.

Hira, S.K., H.L. Dupont, D.N. Lanjewar and **Y.N. Dholakia** (1998). Severe weight loss: The predominant clinical presentation of TB in patients with HIV infection in India. *National Medical Journal of India*, 11(6), 256–58.

Hira, S.K., C. Oberoi and **H. Gharpure** (1996). Clinical profile of persons with single and dual HIV-1/2 infections in Bombay, India. Paper presented at the 10th International Conference on AIDS, Vancouver.

Hira, S.K., H.J. Shroff, D.N. Lanjewar, Y.N. Dholakia, V.P. Bhatia and **H.L. Dupont** (2003). The natural history of adult patients infected with Human Immunodeficiency Virus in Mumbai. *National Medical Journal of India*, 16(3), 126–30.

Jackson, K., A. Sievers, B.C. Ross and **B. Dwyer** (1992). Isolation of a fastidious *Mycobacterium* species from two AIDS patients. *Journal of Clinical Microbiology*, 30(11), 2934–37.

Katz, M.H. et al. (1992). Progression to AIDS in HIV-infected homosexual and bisexual men with hairy leukoplakia and oral candidiasis. *AIDS*, 6(1), 95–100.

Kelkar, R., P.S. Sastry, S.S. Kulkarni, T.K. Saikia, P.M. Parikh and **S.H. Advani** (1997). Pulmonary microsporidial infection in a patient with CML undergoing allogeneic marrow transplant. *Bone Marrow Transplant*, 19(2), 179–82.

Kumarasamy, N., S. Solomon, S.A. Jayaker Paul, R. Venilla and **R.E. Amalraj** (1995). Spectrum of opportunistic infections among AIDS patients in Tamil Nadu, India. *International Journal of STD and AIDS*, 6(6), 447–49.

Lane, H.C. et al. (1985). Qualitative analysis of immune function in patients with the acquired immunodeficiency syndrome: Evidence for a defect in soluble antigen detection. *New England Journal of Medicine*, 313(2), 79–84.

Lanjewar, D.N., B.S. Anand, R. Genta, M.B. Maheshwari, M.A. Ansari, S.K. Hira and **H.L. DuPont** (1996a). Major differences in the spectrum of gastrointestinal infections associated with AIDS in India versus the West: An autopsy study. *Clinical Infectious Diseases*, 23(3), 482–85.

Lanjewar, D.N., C. Rodrigues, D.G. Saple, S.K. Hira and **H.L. DuPont** (1996b). *Cryptosporidium, Isospora* and *Strongyloides* in AIDS. *National Medical Journal of India*, 9(1), 17–19.

Lanjewar, D.N., C.R. Shetty and **G. Katdare** (1998a). Profile of AIDS pathology in India: An autopsy study. In U.L. Wagholikar and K.P. Deodhar (eds.), *Recent advances in pathology* (pp. 83–98). New Delhi: Jaypee Brothers.

Lanjewar, D.N., K.B.V. Surve, M.B. Maheshwari, M.V. Shenghe and **S.K. Hira** (1998b). Toxoplasmosis of the central nervous system in the Acquired Immunodeficiency Syndrome. *Indian Journal of Pathology and Microbiology*, 41, 147–51.

Lee, K.S. et al. (1993). Adult onset pulmonary tuberculosis: Findings on chest radiographs and CT scans. *American Journal of Roentgenology*, 160(4), 753–58.

Legg, J.J. (1994). Systemic symptoms of HIV infection: Evaluation and management. In P.T. Kohen, M.A. Sande and P.A. Volberding (eds.), *The AIDS knowledge base* (pp. 1–10). Boston: Little Brown.

Lifson, A.R. et al. (1994). Time from HIV sero-conversion to oral candidiasis or hairy leukoplakia among homosexual and bisexual males enrolled in three prospective cohorts. *AIDS*, 8(1), 73–79.

Lopez Bernaldo de Quiros, J.C. et al. (2001). A randomised trial of the discontinuation of primary and secondary prophylaxis against PCP after HAART in patients with HIV infection. *New England Journal of Medicine*, 344(3), 159–67.

Lumb, R., J. Swift, C. James, K. Papanaoum and **T. Mukherjee** (1993). Identification of the microsporidian parasite, *Enterocytozoon bieneusi* in faecal samples and intestinal biopsies from an AIDS patient. *International Journal of Parasitology*, 23(6), 793–801.

Luo, K., M. Law, J.M. Kaldor, A.M. McDonald and **D.A. Cooper** (1995). The role of initial AIDS-defining illness in survival following AIDS. *Journal of AIDS*, 9(1), 57–63.

Maggi, P. et al. (2000). Effect of antiretroviral therapy on cryptosporidiosis and microsporidiosis in patients infected with human deficiency virus type-1. *European Journal of Clinical Microbiology and Infectious Diseases*, 19(3), 213–17.

Malaspina, A. et al. (2002). Human immunodeficiency virus type 1 bound to B cells: Relationship to virus replicating in CD4+ T cells and circula in plasma. *Journal of Virology*, 76(17), 8855–63.

Mallal, S.A., O.P. Martinez, M.A. French, I.R. James and **R.L. Dawkins** (1994). Severity and outcome of *Pneumocystis carinii* pneumonia (PCP) in patients of known and unknown HIV status. *Journal of AIDS*, 7(2), 148–53.

Manatsathit, S. et al. (1996). Causes of chronic diarrhoea in patients with AIDS in Thailand: A prospective clinical and microbiological study. *Journal of Gastroenterology*, 31(4), 533–37.

Maschke, M., O. Kastrup and **H.C. Diener** (2002). CNS manifestations of CMV infections: Diagnosis and treatment. *CNS Drugs*, 16(5), 303–15.

McCullough, M., B. Ross and **P. Reade** (1995). Characterisation of genetically distinct subgroup of *Candida albicans* strains isolated from oral cavities of patients infected with human immunodeficiency virus. *Journal of Clinical Microbiology*, 33(3), 696–700.

McNaghten, A.D., D.L. Hanson, J.L. Jones, M.S. Dworkin and **J.W. Ward** (1999). Effects of antiretroviral therapy and opportunistic illness primary chemoprophylaxis on survival after AIDS diagnosis: Adult/adolescent spectrum of disease group. *AIDS*, 13(13), 1687–95.

———— (2000). Erratum in *AIDS*, 14(12), 18–77.

Medak, S., S.K. Hira and **C. Oberai** (1996). *Candida tropicalis* is the predominant strain isolated from oral candidiasis with AIDS. Paper presented at the 11th International Conference on AIDS, Vancouver, July.

Moolasart, P., B. Eampokalap, M. Ratanasrithong, P. Kanthasing, S. Tansupaswaskul and **C. Tanchanpong** (1995). Cryptosporidiosis in HIV infected patients in Thailand. *Southeast Asian Journal of Tropical Medicine and Public Health*, 26(2), 335–38.

Moore, J.P. and **D.F. Blanc** (1991). Immunological incompetence in AIDS. *AIDS*, 5(4), 455–56.

Mootsikapun, P., P. Chetchotisakd and **B. Intarapoka** (1996). Pulmonary infections in HIV infected patients. *Journal of Medical Association of Thailand*, 79(8), 477–85.

Munro, C.A. and **B. Hube** (2002). Anti-fungal therapy at the HAART of viral therapy. *Trends in Microbiology*, 10(4), 173–77.

Murphy, P.M. et al. (1988). Impairment of neutrophil bactericidal capacity in patients with AIDS. *Journal of Infectious Diseases*, 158(3), 627–32.

Nittayananta, W., S. Jealae and **S. Chungpanich** (1997). Oral lesions in Thai heterosexual AIDS patients: A preliminary study. *British Dental Journal*, 182(6), 219–21.

Nottet, H.S.L.M. et al. (1993). Phagocytic function of monocytes-derived macrophages is not affected by human immunodeficiency virus type 1 infection. *Journal of Infectious Diseases*, 168(1), 84–90.

Nwokolo, N.C., M. Fisher, B.G. Gazzard and **M.R. Nelson** (2002). Cessation of secondary prophylaxis in patients with cryptococcosis. *AIDS*, 15(11), 1438–39.

Oka, S. (2002). Pulmonary complications in patients with AIDS. *Kekkaku*, 77(1), 37–40.

Pahwa, S.G. et al. (1984). Defective B-lymphocyte function in homosexual men in relation to the acquired immunodeficiency syndrome. *Annals of Internal Medicine*, 101(6), 757–62.

Panda, S. et al. (1994). Clinical features of HIV infection in drug users of Manipur. *National Medical Journal of India*, 7(6), 267–69.

Pitisuttithum, P., B. Phiboonnakit, D. Chindanond, B. Punpoonwong, S. Leelasuphasri and **S. Vanijanond** (1995). Intestinal microsporidiosis: First reported case in Thailand. *Southeast Asian Journal of Tropical Medicine and Public Health*, 26(2), 378–80.

Pitrak, D.L. et al. (1993). Depressed neutrophil superoxide production in human immunodeficiency virus infection. *Journal of Infectious Diseases*, 167(6), 1406–12.

Poonwan, N. et al. (1997). Serotyping of *Cryptococcus neoformans* strains isolated from clinical specimens in Thailand and their susceptibility to various antifungal agents. *European Journal of Epidemiology*, 13(3), 335–40.

Pruksachatkunakorn, C., K. Uruwannakul and **L. Bhoopat** (1995). Kaposi sarcoma in a Thai boy with acquired immunodeficiency syndrome. *Pediatric Dermatology*, 12(3), 252–55.

Rathi, P.M. et al. (1997). Impact of human immunodeficiency virus infection on abdominal tuberculosis in western India. *Journal of Clinical Gastroenterology*, 24(1), 43–48.

Rubsamen-Waigmann, H. et al. (1993). Kaposi's sarcoma in an Indian woman infected with HIV-1 and HIV-2. *AIDS Research and Human Retroviruses*, 9(6), 573–77.

Satishchandra, P. et al. (1993). *Herpes simplex* encephalitis: A diagnostic and therapeutic reappraisal. *Journal of Association of Physicians in India*, 41(5), 277–78.

Sheng, W.H., C.C. Hung, M.Y. Chen, S.M. Hsieh and **S.C. Chang** (2002). Successful discontinuation of fluconazole as secondary prophylaxis for cryptococcosis in AIDS patients responding to HAART. *International Journal of STD and AIDS*, 13(10), 702–5.

Siriarayapon, P., H. Yanai, J.R. Glynn, S. Yanpaisarn and **W. Uthaivoravit** (2002). The evolving epidemiology of HIV infection and tuberculosis in northern Thailand. *Journal of AIDS*, 31(1), 80–89.

Sirisanthana, V. and **T. Sirisanthana** (1995). Disseminated *Penicillium marneffei* infection in human immunodeficiency virus-infected children. *Pediatric infectious Diseases Journal*, 14(11), 935–40.

Soriano, V., C. Dona, R. Rodriguez-Rosado, P. Barreiro and **J. Gonzalez-Laahoz** (2000). Discontinuation of secondary prophylaxis for OI in HIV-infected patients receiving ART. *AIDS*, 14(4), 383–86.

Speed, B. and **D. Dunt** (1995). Clinical and host differences between infections with the two varieties of *Cryptococcus neoformans*. *Clinical Infectious Diseases*, 21(1), 28–34.

Stuart, R.L. et al. (1997). Cryptosporidiosis in patients with AIDS. *International Journal of STD and AIDS*, 8(5), 339–41.

Telzak, E.E. et al. (1990). Extrapulmonary *Pneumocystis carinii* infection. *Review of Infectious Diseases*, 12(3), 380–86.

USPHS/IDSA (2000). Prevention of opportunistic infections working group: 1999 USPHS/IDSA guidelines for the prevention of opportunistic infections in persons infected with human immunodeficiency virus. *Clinical Infectious Diseases*, 30(Supplement 1), S29–65.

Wolff, M., C. Bustamante, T. Bidart, J. Dabanch, A. Diomedi and R. Northland (2000). Impact of antiretroviral therapy in mortality of Chilean HIV (+) patients: A case control study. *Revista Medica de Chile*, 128(8), 839–45.

Wongkamchai, S., B. Rungpitaransi, S. Wongbunnate and C. Sittapairochana (1995). Toxoplasma infection in healthy persons and in-patients with HIV or ocular disease. *Southeast Asian Journal of Tropical Medicine and Public Health*, 26(4), 655–58.

WHO (1998). *Clinical management of HIV and AIDS at the district level*. New Delhi: WHO Regional Office for South-East Asia.

Yanai, H. et al. (1996). Rapid increase in HIV-related tuberculosis, Chiang Rai, Thailand, 1990–1994. *AIDS*, 10(5), 527–31.

Yoshiyama, T. et al. (2001). Prevalence of drug resistant TB in HIV endemic area in northern Thailand. *International Journal of Tuberculosis and Lung Diseases*, 5(1), 32–39.

16

THE CHALLENGE OF HIV/TB IN ASIA

Jai P. Narain

Asia and the Pacific region accounts for nearly 60 per cent (37 per cent in South-East Asia [SEA] and 22 per cent in the Western Pacific regions) of the global burden of tuberculosis, with 2.2 million new cases occurring each year (WHO 2003) (Figure 16.1). Most of these cases are reported from six countries, namely, India, China, Indonesia, Bangladesh, Nigeria and Pakistan, which together contributes 55 per cent of all reported cases. Affecting the most productive age groups, TB levies enormous social and economic cost on individuals and nations—it has been estimated that 20 to 30 per cent of household incomes, and 4 to 7 per cent of national GDPs are lost on account of the morbidity and mortality due to TB, and that on the whole TB costs the SEA region alone around US$ 4 billion every year (ibid.).

Figure 16.1
Tuberculosis in Asia

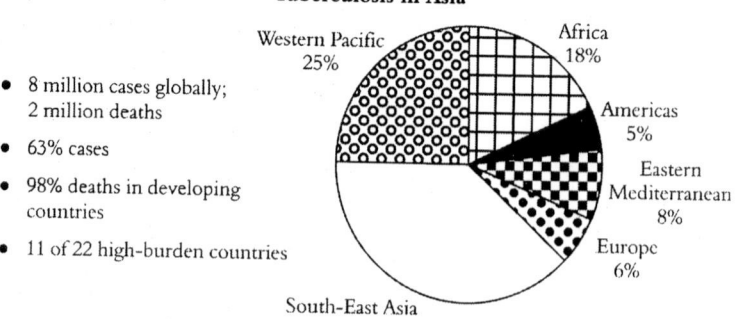

- 8 million cases globally; 2 million deaths
- 63% cases
- 98% deaths in developing countries
- 11 of 22 high-burden countries

Western Pacific 25%
Africa 18%
Americas 5%
Eastern Mediterranean 8%
Europe 6%
South-East Asia 38%

Source: WHO (2003).

The worldwide epidemic of HIV in the latter decades of the last century has fuelled the resurgence of tuberculosis in some regions of the world, notably Africa and including parts of Asia. TB and HIV are inextricably linked; HIV progressively weakens the immune system, making people vulnerable to a host of opportunistic infections such as tuberculosis. Moreover, the large majority of people with HIV/AIDS live in countries where the prevalence of tuberculosis is high. Actually, TB is the earliest manifestation of AIDS in over half of all cases, and accounts for about a third of AIDS deaths. It is, therefore, the leading killer of people living with HIV. Last but not the least, TB and HIV are both driven by poverty, homelessness, poor nutritional status and crowded living conditions. So to confront the twin challenges of TB and HIV is to confront issues fundamental to both health and human rights.

There is emerging evidence that the HIV epidemic can facilitate the emergence of multi-drug-resistant (MDR) strains of *Mycobacterium tuberculosis* (Fatkenheuer et al. 1999; Punnotok et al. 2000; Sacks et al. 1999). These findings have serious implications for TB control since the present armoury of anti-TB drugs may not be adequate to combat epidemics of MDR TB.

Unlike HIV, we have an effective weapon against TB. Known as DOTS, it ensures that people suffering from TB are fully treated with a powerful combination of drugs under the regular supervision of health workers or community volunteers. The treatment costs $10 or less for six months of drugs and uses primary care services. Over the past few years DOTS has turned the TB tide in several countries and more will follow suit.

Since 1993 10 million TB patients have been treated successfully worldwide, more than 90 per cent of them in developing countries. A total of 155 countries have now adopted the DOTS strategy, which is vital to ensuring high cure rates and preventing the spread of infection.

India, China and several other countries in Asia have shown remarkable progress in expanding population coverage while maintaining high cure rates (WHO 2003). India has the most rapid expansion unprecedented in the history of DOTS, which is now driving the global progress in TB control. Some 50,000 new TB patients are put on effective therapy each month in India. In China active TB cases fell by 35 per cent in areas applying DOTS over the last decade. Other countries, such as Nepal, DPR Korea, Maldives and Vietnam, have already surpassed 2005 targets for TB detection and treatment. However, the emerging spectre of interaction between HIV and TB may have grave implications for both TB and HIV programmes. Unless effectively tackled, this may undermine the progress being made in TB control, particularly in countries where HIV is spreading rapidly.

Interaction between HIV and TB: The Evidence

The close association between HIV and TB has been documented before (Narain et al. 1992, 2002). Of the 7 million adults with HIV in Asia and the Pacific region, about 2.8 million are likely to be infected with TB (Figure 16.2). Given that the annual risk of symptomatic tuberculosis is between 5 and 10 per cent among individuals who are dually infected (that is, with both HIV and latent tuberculosis), increases in new cases of tuberculosis seem inevitable (Figure 16.3). The increase in cases is likely to lead to further spread of the disease among the general non-HIV-infected population.

Figure 16.2
Distribution of TB and HIV in the World

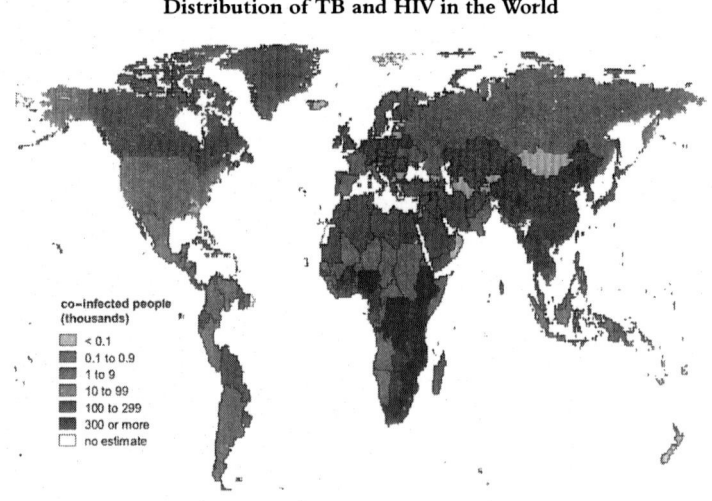

co-infected people
(thousands)

< 0.1
0.1 to 0.9
1 to 9
10 to 99
100 to 299
300 or more
no estimate

Source: WHO.

Sentinel surveillance in many countries shows that HIV rates are increasing rapidly among TB patients. In Chiang Mai 1,030 patients with tuberculosis were tested for HIV in 1989, 6.8 per cent of whom were found HIV positive. By 1995 this rate had increased to 40 per cent. Similarly, HIV rates among TB patients have gone up in Bangkok and

Figure 16.3
TB and AIDS

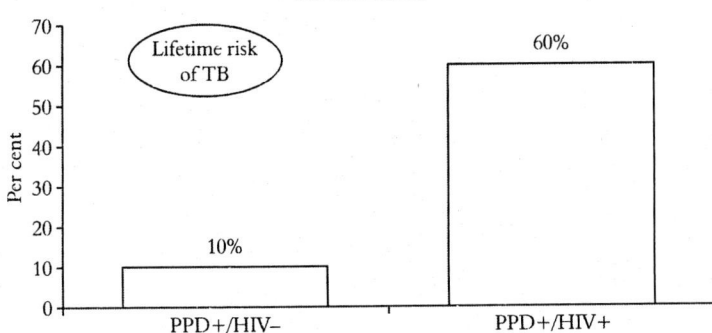

Source: WHO/SEARO.

Mumbai, and many other Asian cities (Mohanty and Basheer 1995; Paranjape et al. 1997; Rajasekaran et al. 2000; Supawitkul et al. 1998; Solomon et al. 1995; Tripathy et al. 1996). A review of data from 18 African countries shows a linear relationship between HIV prevalence and TB notification rates—the countries with high HIV prevalence rates are also those that are likely to have high incidence of tuberculosis (Figure 16.4).

Figure 16.4
Relationship between Estimated Incidence of TB (All Forms) and
HIV Prevalence in Adults for 18 African Countries: 1999

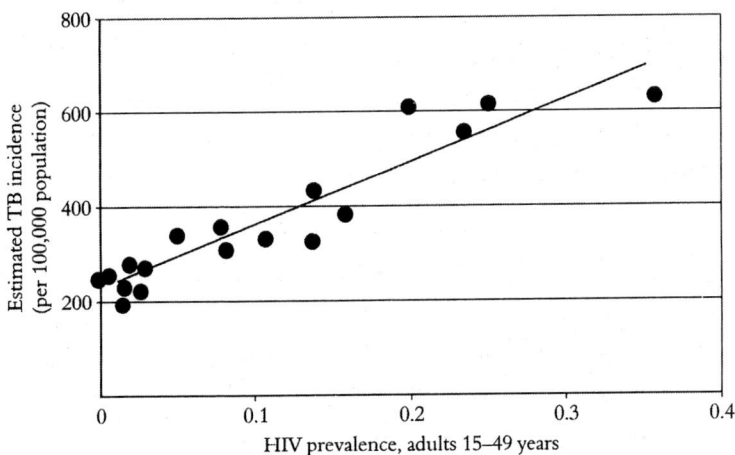

Source: WHO (2001).

Tuberculosis is now the most important life-threatening opportunistic infection associated with HIV in many parts of the world (Agarwal et al. 1998; Kumarasamy et al. 1995; Sunderam et al. 1986). In Thailand 60 per cent of AIDS patients have had pulmonary tuberculosis, Myanmar 80 per cent, India 56 per cent and Nepal 75 per cent (Figure 16.5). Across Asia TB has emerged as the biggest killer of AIDS patients, although it is a preventable and curable condition.

Figure 16.5
Tuberculosis among AIDS Patients (%)

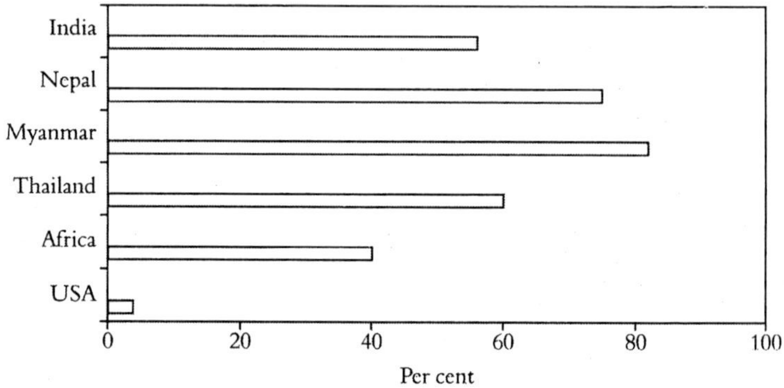

Source: WHO/SEARO HIV/TB Programme, 2003.

Emergence of drug-resistant tuberculosis worldwide, due in part to HIV, is also a serious concern, although the extent of the problem is presently unclear. However, recent data show that contrary to general belief, drug resistance is common in developing countries, albeit at a low level, and that drug resistance is more common among patients with HIV (Narain et al. 2002; Punnotok et al. 2000; Supawitkul et al. 1998). In a study in Thailand MDR prevalence among HIV-positive patients was 5.2 per cent compared to 0.4 per cent among HIV-negative patients ($p < 0.001$) (Punnotok et al. 2000). Other studies also show that drug-resistant tuberculosis organisms are spreading in the community (Supawitkul et al. 1998). Therefore, an advanced HIV epidemic contributes to the emergence of drug-resistant strains of TB, which often do not respond to treatment.

Large increases in TB notifications over the past decade in many countries in Sub-Saharan Africa, including Zimbabwe, Malawi, Kenya, Tanzania and Zambia, are largely attributable to the HIV epidemic. Since the mid-1980s in many African countries, including those with well-organised programmes, annual TB cases notification rates have risen by up to four-fold, reaching peaks of more than 400 cases per 100,000 population. Up to 70 per cent of patients with sputum-smear-positive pulmonary TB are HIV positive in some countries. The countries most badly affected by TB/HIV are those where HIV prevalence is the highest. In these countries TB is becoming manageable and the achievement of 85 per cent cure rate and 70 per cent case detection is becoming difficult.

In the SEA region the impact of HIV on TB has so far been observed in areas where HIV prevalence is high. For example, in one of the provinces in northern Thailand (Chiang Rai) the rate of HIV seropositive TB patients increased from about one in 100,000 in 1990 to over 50 per 100,000 in 2000. Simultaneously, TB notification rates increased from about 50 per 100,000 in 1991 to about 130 in 2000 (Figure 16.6). The increase was seen in all categories of TB—smear-positive pulmonary TB, smear-negative pulmonary TB and extra-pulmonary TB. A number of reports indicate that the proportion of TB patients with HIV infection increased sharply after 1991. TB registry data from Chiang Rai Provincial

Figure 16.6
New TB Rate by HIV Status per 100,000
in Chiang Rai, Thailand: 1987–2000

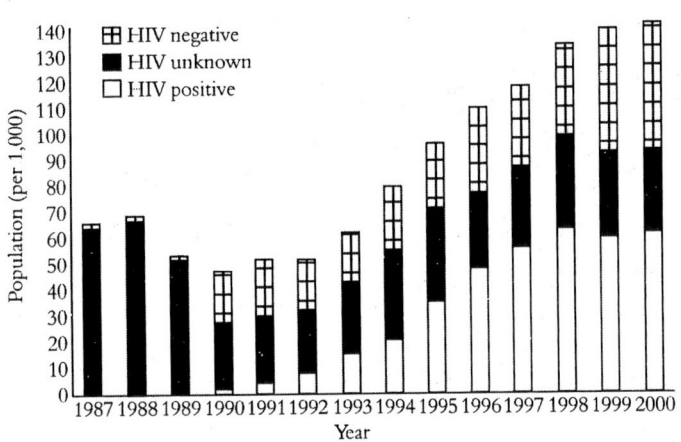

Source: TB/HIV Research Project, RIT-JATA, Provincial Health Office Chiang Rai, Ministry of Public Health, Thailand.

Hospital, which started confidential HIV testing in October 1989, indicated a steady and rapid increase in the number and proportion of HIV-seropositive TB patients from 1.5 per cent in 1990 to 45.5 per cent in 1994, and 72 per cent in male patients and 65.8 per cent in female patients by 1998 (Siriarayapon et al. 2002; Yanai et al. 1996). The HIV/TB epidemic exerts a negative impact on existing TB and AIDS programmes in several ways. HIV infection is now considered the most potent risk factor for tuberculosis; it not only increases the risk of reactivating latent MTB infections but also increases rapid progression of clinical TB soon after natural infection. The increased risk of active TB among HIV-infected persons compared with those not HIV-infected has been shown in both cohort as well as case control studies with the magnitude of the relative risk varying from 5 to 20 per cent. While part of this variation is explained by differences in study design, the strength of association between HIV and TB is likely to increase with increasing number of HIV-infected persons being immuno-compromised. In much of Africa, therefore, spread of HIV is primarily responsible for driving the parallel epidemic of TB, often at a rate of 6 per cent per year. HIV-infected TB patients are considered less infectious because they have fewer cavitations and are less likely to be smear positive. Nevertheless, increase in TB is expected to enhance TB transmission in the community. However, in many countries it has been noted that while TB incidence continues to increase due to reactivation by HIV, the annual risk of TB infection in children shows no increase; there is even a decline in areas where DOTS is being expanded. This has important implications for TB control programmes.

Impact on the TB and HIV Programmes

The HIV/TB epidemic exerts a negative impact on existing TB and AIDS programmes in several ways.

On TB

Tuberculosis is already a huge problem overstretching the fragile health infrastructure in much of Asia and the Pacific. With the increasing TB caseload attributable to HIV, there will be greater demand to diagnose and treat TB cases, which otherwise would not have occurred. In Chiang

Rai, Thailand, the TB notifications increased from 40 per 100,000 population to 144 per 100,000 between 1990 and 2002, a three-fold increase in TB mostly attributable to HIV.

HIV-associated TB poses difficult clinical challenges. Patients are relatively more likely to be sputum negative, posing difficulty in diagnosis since sputum smear examination is the mainstay of diagnosing the disease. Moreover, the pathogenesis of both tuberculosis infection and the disease relates directly to cell-mediated immunity (CMI), especially CD4+ T-lymphocytes. Not surprisingly, HIV infection that induces CD4+ T-lymphocyte depletion, also leads to defective immunological response to *M. tuberculosis*. The pathogenesis of TB can be altered by HIV either through reactivation of latent tuberculosis infection to active disease (more common) or by causing rapid progression from recent infection with *M. tuberculosis* to tuberculosis disease. As HIV infection progresses, CD4+ lymphocytes decline in number and function. The immune system is, therefore, less able to prevent the growth and local spread of *M. tuberculosis*. As a result, disseminated and extra-pulmonary disease is more commonly seen. Nevertheless, pulmonary TB is still the most common form of TB even in HIV-infected patients. Pulmonary involvement can occur in 70 to 90 per cent of all patients with TB.

The presentation of pulmonary TB depends on the degree of immunosuppression. In advanced HIV infection the presence of many opportunistic infections affecting the lungs may cause difficulties in the diagnosis of TB. The occurrence of hilar and/or mediastinal adenopathy seen in a chest X-ray can also suggest the diagnosis of TB in an HIV-infected patient. The most common forms of extra-pulmonary involvement include lymphadenopathies, pleural effusion, pericardial disease, miliary disease and meningitis. Cervical, supraclavicular and auxillary lymphnodes are the most common sites of peripheral lymphadenitis. Examination of the percutanous needle aspiration of the lymph nodes can be useful in establishing the diagnosis.

In most cases, particularly at early stages of HIV infection, the presentation of tuberculosis among such patients with HIV is indistinguishable from other cases. However, some may show a bizarre pattern with a higher proportion of cases tending to have a negative sputum smear. In spite of that, sputum smear examination remains an essential component in the diagnosis of tuberculosis in countries where HIV infection is common, because of its ability to identify infectious cases.

The diagnosis of TB in HIV-positive patients is difficult for three main reasons:

1. The sensitivity of the direct sputum smear examination is reduced in HIV-positive patients. Compared to HIV-negative patients with pulmonary TB, a lesser proportion of HIV-positive patients with pulmonary TB will have positive sputum smears.
2. X-ray abnormalities, which are not specific for TB in HIV-negative patients, are even more non-specific in the HIV-infected, with only minor abnormalities seen on chest X-ray or with abnormalities that do not look like classical TB.
3. Patients infected with HIV have frequent illnesses with pulmonary involvement caused by agents other than *M. tuberculosis*.

The response to anti-TB therapy is similar among for HIV-positive and HIV-negative TB patients. HIV-related immunosuppression does not interfere with the effectiveness of therapy for TB. Since the management of TB and the response to standard short-course regimen is similar in patients with or without HIV, there is no rationale for HIV tests in clinical settings from the patient management point of view.

Adverse reactions are generally more common in HIV-positive than in HIV-negative TB patients. Most reactions occur in the first two months of treatment. Skin rash and hepatitis are more common and most often attributed to rifampicin. The usual drug responsible for fatal skin reactions such as exfoliative dermatitis, Steven-Johnson syndrome and toxic epidermal necrolysis is thiacetazone. Therefore, thiacetazone should never be given to HIV-positive TB patients. From a programmatic point of view, thiacetazone should not be prescribed in areas where HIV prevalence is shown to be high.

Rifampicin is a potent inducer of the hepatic cytochrome P450 enzyme system and can reduce the activity of several medications commonly used in HIV-infected patients. These include ketoconazole, fluconazole, methadone and several antiretroviral compounds such as the non-nucleoside reverse transcriptase inhibitors and protease inhibitors. Although the combination of anti-TB medications and zidovudine is well tolerated, pharmacokinetic data suggest that rifampicin may increase hepatic clearance of zidovudine and decrease zidovudine plasma levels. There are also reports of decreased rifampicin absorption attributed to simultaneous administration of ketoconazole. On the other hand some protease inhibitors decrease the metabolism of rifampicin and increase the rifampicin blood level, thereby resulting in increased frequency of side effects. In such a situation the appropriate dosage of the above-mentioned drugs should be closely monitored and adjusted as needed in order to minimise the side effects from rifampicin and to maximise the effectiveness of other medications being given simultaneously. If possible, treatment for TB should be completed before starting protease inhibitors.

On HIV

HIV and *M. tuberculosis* are both intracellular pathogens and act on the cell-mediated immunity. Patients with HIV infection are uniquely susceptible to TB and TB on the other hand accelerates the course of infection. Besides contributing to progression from HIV infection to AIDS, contribution of TB to AIDS deaths is substantial: up to 40 per cent of AIDS deaths are due to TB. The mortality rate for HIV-infected persons with TB is approximately four times greater than the rate for TB patients not infected with HIV. The high mortality rate amongst patients with TB appears to be due mainly to progressive HIV infection and caused by other infections such as septicaemia, salmonella, etc. The degree of immunosuppression is the most important predictor of survival of HIV-infected patients with TB, and low CD4 counts are associated with increased mortality. These data indicate that the relationship is one of deadly symbiosis; each potentiating the effect of the other.

The evidence that TB may accelerate HIV-induced immunological deterioration is as follows:

1. active TB is associated with transient CD4+ T-lymphocyte depletion;
2. TB causes immune stimulation and increased production of cytokines, such as the tumour necrosis factor (TNF), which increases HIV replication in vitro; and
3. HIV-infected persons with TB appear to have a higher risk of opportunistic infections and death than do HIV-infected patients with similar CD4+ T-lymphocyte counts but without TB.

The shorter survival among patients with HIV partly attributable to death from TB has been observed both in developing and developed countries. The fact that TB accelerates the progression of HIV is observed by a six- to seven-fold increase in the HIV viral load as compared to the load in those without TB and by the decline in CD4 counts among people with HIV. Effective treatment of TB using DOTS has been shown to prolong the survival of patients living with AIDS.

Thanks to major reduction in prices of antiretrovirals, these drugs are now available in many countries. Due to the high prevalence of tuberculosis among HIV-infected individuals living in Asia and the Pacific, many patients who are candidates for ART will have active TB (Narain et al. 2002). In addition, patients already receiving ART may develop clinical TB. Effective treatment and control of TB is a central priority when developing treatment strategies for co-infected patients. The management of HIV and TB co-infection is complicated because some antiretroviral agents produce unacceptable drug interactions with anti-tubercular agents and/or can increase toxicity of TB treatment (Kumarasamy et al. 1995, 1998). Tuberculosis treatment following the DOTS strategy should be initiated promptly in diagnosed cases of TB.

Combating HIV/TB: The Progress So Far

Global Level

Combating HIV/TB is accorded a high priority by the WHO. In order to decrease the burden of TB/HIV, the WHO has established a Global TB/HIV Working Group, which met in Geneva, Switzerland, in 2001 and Durban, South Africa, in 2002. It is one of the working groups instituted under the Global Stop TB partnership, launched by the director-general of the WHO in November 1998. During the first meeting the working group reviewed and endorsed the WHO Strategic Framework to Decrease the Burden of TB/HIV. At the second meeting the Draft Guidelines Implementing Collaborative TB and HIV Programme Activities were endorsed. The group is committed to providing stronger country-level support to TB and HIV programmes to enable collaborative planning and implementation of TB/HIV activities, and to advocate for increased resources with which to fight the dual epidemic.

In Asia

In 2001 the first SEA Regional Office (SEARO) National TB and National AIDS Programme managers meeting held in Chiang Mai, Thailand, recommended the development of a TB/HIV regional framework, promoting greater collaboration and interaction between existing

TB and AIDS control programmes, and capitalising on the strengths of each programme to implement TB/HIV interventions delivered through existing health care systems. Several countries in Asia have responded positively. For example, in India a national policy of coordination of common activities for HIV/AIDS and TB is being formulated by the National AIDS Control Organisation (NACO) and the Central TB Division. TB and HIV/AIDS are reciprocally included in the national policies of the two programmes. The following tools were developed: (*a*) treatment guidelines for TB in HIV-infected individuals; (*b*) TB/HIV guide for health workers; and (*c*) HIV/TB training manual for medical officers. Voluntary counselling and testing (VCT) services at the sub-district level will incorporate screening for TB symptoms and referral to diagnosis and treatment of TB and AIDS care. National HIV/TB consultants are expected to facilitate the local coordination of service delivery, referral, NGO involvement, cross-training and infection control in the six high HIV prevalence states.

In Myanmar HIV/AIDS is a priority and increasing HIV prevalence in defined sub-populations for sentinel surveillance has been reported since 1995. An estimated 70 per cent of AIDS patients develop active TB. Collaborative HIV/TB activities include counselling of TB patients on HIV and vice versa, training of health care providers in TB and HIV services, HIV prevalence surveys among TB patients, evaluating treatment outcome of TB among co-infected patients, and developing a model for cross-border disease control for TB/HIV in 15 border townships in collaboration with the Thai government. Future plans include scaling up cross-border collaboration on control of TB, HIV/AIDS and malaria with Thailand.

In Nepal a planned collaboration between the national AIDS and TB programmes includes the following components: joint policy and strategy on HIV/TB; joint planning, evaluation and logistics management; information sharing and dissemination; training of health workers; and advocacy and operational research. The national TB programmes (NTP) have carried out HIV prevalence surveys in TB patients in selected TB centres since 1993–94. A HIV/TB centre has been established.

Thailand is more advanced in containing the HIV epidemic and in the response to TB/HIV. A national TB/HIV working group has been established as an interface between national AIDS programme (NAP) and NTP, providing guidance to collaborative HIV/TB activities. The working group developed a national policy for integrated HIV/TB strategies for the prevention and control of TB. A technical advisory group on INH preventive therapy has also been established. In northern Thailand where HIV prevalence in active TB is the highest compared to the country average, the concerned ministry conducted an assessment of INH preventive therapy services and drafted technical and operational guidelines on it for people living with HIV/AIDS. Currently INH preventive therapy is being used in 22 sites in northern Thailand since 2001 using the aforementioned guidelines and is being expanded to more sites countrywide. In October 2002 the restructuring of the Ministry of Public Health lead to the formation of a Department of Disease Control with a structural integration of the TB, AIDS and STD divisions under one umbrella.

At the regional level the WHO is promoting the concept of joint planning and coordination of both TB and AIDS programmes for generating evidence for advocacy, mobilising partnership and resources, education of communities and for managing HIV-related TB. The principles that guide the regional strategy include establishing a functional collaboration between two programmes, not integration, so that both programmes will benefit. The idea is to assess the capacities of both programmes and strengthen where needed, then establish collaboration by identifying responsibilities of each programme and including areas where both would work together. This idea is presently being tested in pilot districts in some countries. Based on these experiences, the collaborative initiatives are likely to be scaled up in coverage.

Conceptual Framework for HIV/TB Interventions

The control of TB/HIV and mitigating its impact requires an understanding of its natural history and pathogenesis. In most cases tuberculosis infection comes first and HIV is contracted subsequently when the person achieves adolescence or adulthood (Figure 16.7). Once co-infected, the progression to active TB occurs quite rapidly, which could be prevented through the use of isoniazid prevention therapy (IPT). Those who progress to active TB could be managed with DOTS and through provision of care and support, including the use of anti-retroviral therapy. Therefore, at each point in the scheme, interventions can be planned and implemented to try and interrupt TB and HIV infection from progressing to active TB and/or AIDS. Management of

HIV-associated TB through DOTS can prevent community transmission of tuberculosis, as has been demonstrated in many studies.

Figure 16.7
Combating TB/HIV: The Conceptual Framework and Intervention Points

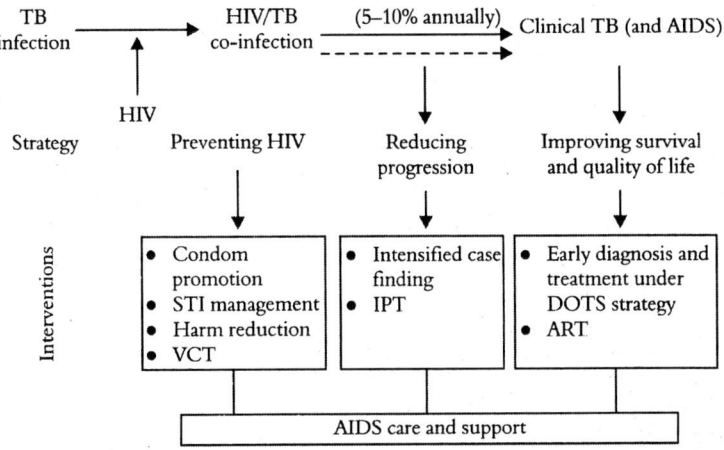

The above figure presents the strategic framework with points where the effects of TB and HIV can be either prevented or reduced through specific interventions.

Major Interventions

Preventing HIV Infection

Prevention of HIV infection, the most potent risk factor, is essential to prevent the devastating impact on tuberculosis. The strategy calls for support and care of those who have been infected with HIV, whether they are still healthy or have developed illnesses associated with their infection, including AIDS. The support and care of HIV-infected persons is not only humane, it is vital for the success of prevention. The majority, up to 85 to 90 per cent of the infections result through sexual transmission of HIV and additional 5 per cent by injecting drug use. Changing sexual and injecting behaviour are thus the prime foci of action for interrupting transmission. Action for prevention of HIV transmission must include: (*a*) information and education aimed at all men and women, particularly those at high risk of infection, includingsex workers and injecting drug users; (b) health and social services, especially for the purpose of providing condoms, clean needles and syringes to reduce harm, and the early diagnosis and treatment of sexually-transmitted infections using syndromic approach; and (c) creating an enabling environment to reduce the stigma and discrim-ination directed against people living with HIV/AIDS or those at risk. These should be linked with strategies aimed for the social and economic empowerment of women, and reducing the vulnerability of young people by providing accurate information about HIV transmission to pre-adolescent and adolescent girls and boys, and enabling them to learn and practise the related prevention skills.

Reducing Progression to Active TB

Preventing the occurrence of clinical TB among co-infected persons requires that people with HIV be diagnosed in the first place. The primary intervention required for it is expansion and wide availability of VCT services. Those found infected both with TB and HIV can use TB preventive therapy with isoniazid (INH) to prevent progression to TB. Co-infected persons must be screened for active TB through intensified case finding. Screening patients for clinical or active TB is important since they may require short-course chemotherapy over a period of six months instead of preventive therapy, as recommended by national TB programmes. VCT, therefore, provides an entry point not only identifying HIV-infected persons, but also of co-infected individuals who could benefit from TB preventive therapy as well as for diagnosing patients with active TB who could require TB treatment.

IPT with isoniazid may play a role in limiting a possible increase in the number of cases of symptomatic tuberculosis that is expected from the pool of HIV/TB co-infected individuals. This approach is supported by the knowledge that TB in HIV-infected people is predominantly caused by the endogenous reactivation of dormant foci, that it can happen with a higher frequency among co-infected individuals than in the general population, and that the disease can, therefore, be prevented by chemotherapy. The efficacy of INH in preventing TB in HIV-positive people has been proven. However, it must be administered to the patient for a long period, for at least six months, a factor that may challenge patient compliance. A two-month course of rifampicin and pyrazinamide daily is an alternative regimen.

In many countries in Asia and the Pacific facilities for VCT are yet to become widely available and tuberculin testing to identify TB infection is operationally difficult to implement in the field situation. There is also problem of energy, since many with advanced HIV infection may not be able to mount immune response. Moreover, persons who live far away from TB service sites are unlikely to complete the course of preventive therapy. The WHO, therefore, recommends TB preventive chemotherapy on an individual basis, as part of an HIV/AIDS care package wherever suitable, for those infected with both TB and HIV.

Preventing Death and Improving Quality of Life

Experiences in the region show that early diagnosis and treatment of HIV-associated TB is critical for improving survival and enhancing quality of life of patients. Intensive case finding of such patients should be followed by referral to a DOTS centre for further investigation and treatment for active TB, and for prophylaxis for other opportunistic infections.

Short-course chemotherapy under the DOTS strategy is as effective among HIV-positive TB patients as in HIV-negative patients in curing patients of TB and thereby rendering them non-infectious. Thus, besides lowering individual suffering, implementing DOTS through effective TB control programmes can reduce the transmission of TB infection, even in the context of increased HIV prevalence.

During the course of HIV infection, the immune system becomes less efficient in preventing the growth and spread of *M. tuberculosis*. As a result, disseminated and extra-pulmonary TB is more commonly seen in HIV-positive than in HIV-negative patients. Nevertheless, pulmonary TB is still the most common form of TB seen even in HIV-infected patients, with or without concomitant extra-pulmonary TB.

Strengthening the capacity of health services to be able to diagnose patients with TB, both pulmonary and extra-pulmonary, contributes to greater case finding and for putting them on the DOTS strategy. The quality of diagnostic infrastructure and of a responsive health service will improve the situation. The DOTS strategy depends primarily on passive case finding. However, in view of the close association between TB and HIV, actively looking for TB cases may be a helpful approach, particularly in high HIV prevalence areas. Clinical presentation, and radiological and laboratory findings depend greatly on the stage of HIV infection and on the degree of suppression of host defences. For example, in the advanced stages of HIV, the mycobacterial load in patients are high pulmonary lesions, mostly infiltrative, sputum smears are often negative and frequently the lesions are extra-pulmonary. The common forms of extra-pulmonary involvement of tuberculosis include lymph-adenopathy, pleural effusion, pericardial disease, miliary disease and meningitis.

In most cases the clinical presentation of tuberculosis in patients particularly at an early stage of HIV infection is indistinguishable from those patients who do not have HIV infection. Nonetheless, sputum smear examination remains an essential component in TB diagnosis, even in countries where HIV infection is common because of its ability to identify infectious cases.

Common problems with treating HIV-infected TB patients include non-adherence to therapy, increased adverse reactions to anti-TB drugs and concomitant occurrence of other opportunistic diseases. The clinical and bacteriological response of HIV-positive TB patients to treatment should, therefore, be closely monitored. Therapy may be prolonged only for patients with slow or sub-optimal responses. The clinical, radio-logical and microbiological responses to short-course chemotherapy in HIV-positive and HIV-negative TB patients are similar in the two groups, barring HIV-positive patients who may die due to other causes. The bactericidal activity of anti-TB drugs on the tubercle bacilli is similar in HIV-positive and HIV-negative patients. Hence, the same drug regi-mens are employed in the two populations.

Antiretroviral Therapy in People with TB and HIV Co-infection

ART can significantly decrease viral replication in the organism and restore immune function. This leads even under programme conditions to decreased morbidity and mortality, including incidence of HIV-associated opportunistic infections such as tuberculosis.

The WHO recommends that ART be provided to HIV-infected individuals with symptomatic HIV disease (stage III and IV) and CD4 counts of less than 350. Given the toxicity associated with taking three anti-TB and three ARV drugs concomitally, it may be better to treat the TB first and then add ARV drugs once the initial intensive phase of TB treatment has stabilised the patient. After the first two months of treatment, patients are generally switched to a continuation phase of only two drugs (often INH–RIF) for the remaining four months. It is at this stage that ARV treatment can be considered if the patient warrants it based on their CD4 count and underlying clinical condition.

WHO recommendations issued in December 2003 (WHO 2003) state that people with TB/HIV co-infection complete their TB therapy prior to beginning ARV treatment unless there is a high risk of HIV disease progression and death during the period of TB treatment (that is, a CD4 cell count of less than 200/mm^3 or disseminated TB is present). In cases where a person needs TB and HIV treatment concurrently, the first line treatment option is (ZDV or d4T) + 3TC + EFZ (the dose of EFZ should be increased to 800 mg/day when administered with rifampicin if the patient can tolerate it) (Table 16.1). While NVP should be avoided when used in combination with rifampicin because of the potential for

Table 16.1
Antiretroviral Therapy for Individuals with Tuberculosis Co-infection

Situation	Recommendations
Pulmonary TB and CD4 cell count <50/mm^3 or extra-pulmonary TB	Start TB therapy; start the following ARV regimen simultaneously: (d4T or ZDV) + 3TC + EFZ[*][†]
Pulmonary TB and CD4 cell count 50–200/mm^3 or total lymphocyte count <1200/mm^3 or signs of clinically advanced HIV infections	Start TB therapy; start the following ARV regimen after completing two months of TB therapy: (d4T or ZDV) + 3TC + EFZ[*][†]
Pulmonary TB and CD4 cell count >200/mm^3 or total lymphocyte count >1200/mm^3 or signs of clinically advanced HIV infections	Treat TB; monitor CD4 cell counts if available; start ART after completion of TB treatment

Notes: [*] If clinically feasible EFZ should be increased to 800 mg/day in adults when co-administered with rifampicin.
[†] Alternatives to EFZ include SQV/r or ABC. The use of ZDV/3TC/ABC must be considered in the context of the ACTG A5095 results. However, it is a reasonable consideration when HIV and TB must be co-treated, particularly if EFZ is not an option.

additive hepatotoxicity and a major drug interaction that can lead to sub-optimal levels of NVP; this should be used with caution in case no other ARV combination is available. There are concerns regarding the risk of NVP resistance and treatment failure. Although viable alternatives for ARV therapy in conjunction with RIF exist (for example, EFZ, ABC, SQV), these are not always available in some countries due to high costs.

Mobilising National and International Support

The worsening co-epidemics of TB and HIV in Asia and the Pacific require urgent and effective attention. The two epidemics need a joint effort employing different but complementary strategies. The best approach to curb the HIV epidemic is—so far—based on an integrated prevention and care interventions. Prevention interventions should target all the possible ways of transmission, but especially the ones most frequently involved in the ongoing transmission in a given country. Unlike HIV, TB can be cured, even in people with HIV infection. The DOTS strategy has been demonstrated to achieve TB cure rates of over 85 per cent. This is the most successful approach to stop further spread of the disease. A strategic framework is necessary to integrate the different interventions needed to combat the dual TB/HIV epidemic and to avoid wasting the already scarce resources available.

Analysis of HIV/TB surveillance and research data is crucial for generating evidence and for promoting collaborative action between the HIV and TB control programmes. This will also be helpful for developing the strategic framework to address the HIV/TB co-epidemic in a given country. Multiple sources of data can be evaluated to generate the evidence of the association between HIV and TB and to quantify the extent of the problem. In a few countries these data are already available since HIV surveillance activities include TB patients as part of the sentinel population. Other sources of data include TB notifications; HIV prevalence surveys among TB patients and the general population; cohort and case control studies evaluating risk of TB by HIV status; clinical and autopsy data indicating the proportion of AIDS patients having TB; and finally obtaining the population attributable fraction that indicates the proportion of all TB cases that would be attributable to HIV. Epidemiological data are extremely useful to obtain the baseline, monitor trends that can be helpful evidence to be used for advocacy, programme planning and for mobilising resources (human and financial). The basis for good advocacy lies especially in skilful communication and articulation of available data and facts.

Partnerships at country level between the government, NGOs, private health sector, corporate bodies, foundations, universities and committed individuals are needed, and these are fortunately being forged to stop TB and HIV. A new initiative in the form of the Global Fund to Fight AIDS, TB and Malaria (GFATM) is a major contributor to this work and is bringing unprecedented opportunities to mobilise substantial additional financial resources to fight AIDS, TB and malaria. Through support from the GFATM and other partners, hundreds of millions of more dollars are available now than in previous years for DOTS expansion, for innovative response to HIV-associated TB and drug-resistant TB, and for research and development for new diagnostics, drugs and vaccines. Many experiences in countries, particularly in Myanmar and Thailand, show that joint collaboration between national TB and HIV/ AIDS programmes is feasible. Among activities, development of a national policy and strategic framework, a joint TB and AIDS programme team, and coordination at central level have been identified as the most crucial.

Implementing HIV/TB Interventions:
A Step-by-Step Approach

In order to combat HIV/TB, a clear strategic framework is needed based on epidemiological and public health rationale. The strategy should promote a coordinated and integrated approach and build on the existing activities to prevent and control both HIV and TB. This mandates clearly defining the interventions and activities that must be planned for and implemented, including the roles that can be played by various stakeholders. A coordination mechanism, both at policy as well as at implementation levels, is needed as a matter of urgency.

At the regional level the WHO is promoting the concept of joint planning and coordination of both TB and AIDS programmes for generating evidence for advocacy, mobilising partnership and resources, for educating communities and for managing HIV-related TB. The principles that guide regional strategy include establishing a functional collaboration between the two programmes, not integration, so that both programmes will benefit from the collaboration. The idea is to first assess the capacities of both programmes and strengthen them where needed, then establish collaboration by identifying responsibilities of each programme and including areas where both programmes would work together.

The HIV and TB programmes have traditionally functioned separately along different perspectives. HIV programmes have focused on prevention and care under a broad multi-sectoral approach with emphasis on the involvement of the community and civil society. TB programmes on the other hand have more of a medical or clinical approach, where TB prevention and control is carried out primarily through a case management approach. Communication and involvement of the civil society are only now beginning to get attention as an important part of the programme. More recently, however, the two programmes are adopting approaches that are becoming more complementary to each other with enormous scope for learning from each other's experience. For example, the use of antiretroviral therapy as a part of HIV care is becoming a major priority for AIDS programmes due to the drastic reduction in the prices of drugs, and there are those who advocate the use of the DOTS approach for ART to ensure treatment adherence and follow-up. On the other hand, in order to enhance case detection rates, TB programmes have now identified community mobilisation through information and communication campaigns, and building partnerships with NGOs and the private sector as priority areas for attention.

Considerable progress is being made in a number of countries, namely, Thailand, Myanmar and to some extent India, in forging collaboration between the two programmes. The idea is simple—to try and strengthen each programme and then build collaboration by identifying areas where HIV programmes could contribute (VCT, ART, surveillance), where TB programmes could work (DOTS, intensified case finding), and areas where the two programmes could work together (joint planning, joint training, joint supervision and monitoring).

In carrying out HIV/TB collaborative activities at the country level, the following are some of the guiding principles that should drive the effort:

- establish functional collaboration between national AIDS and TB programmes and not programmatic integration;
- build on existing programmes, strengthening both AIDS and TB programmes in order that they complement each other better;
- identify and agree on responsibilities to be carried out by respective programmes and those that could be performed jointly; and
- recognise that the collaboration is a win–win situation, where the two programmes as well as the community could benefit.

A step-by-step approach is, therefore, necessary to implement the collaborative programme. In many countries the WHO in the South-East Asia region is presently advocating for piloting TB/HIV interventions at the district level and based on the experience gained to expand these in other geographic areas in a phased manner. The process could start with a situation analysis at the district level to review the HIV/TB epidemiological situation and risk factors; and services available, including what needs to be strengthened or introduced, that is, whether DOTS is being implemented or STD syndromic management is being practised or whether VCT services are available. The idea would be to identify the intervention gaps and also get to know the stakeholders active in the area and their relative strengths. Based on the situation analysis, a joint HIV/TB committee could prepare a plan of action. The resources needed to implement the plan could be mobilised primarily from the existing programme or from local resources. The programme could be reviewed periodically and the experience gained shared. Based on practical experience, the interventions could be extended to other districts. The WHO is presently funding pilot projects in selected districts in India, Bangladesh, Nepal, Indonesia and Myanmar.

Conclusions

HIV/TB is an important emerging crisis in Asia and the Pacific, as evidenced from the extent of both epidemics in the countries of the region and the high number of co-infected persons living in Cambodia, India, Myanmar and Thailand. The main strategies to successfully combat this deadly association, at least conceptually are: (a) preventing HIV through behaviour change in the context of sexual practices and injecting drug use; (b) preventing the progression of TB infection to clinical TB through preventive therapy; (c) effective case management of patients with HIV-associated TB or those with AIDS, thereby preventing further TB or HIV transmission; and (d) partnership building for surveillance, advocacy and programme management for the control of TB and HIV.

In order to mount a more meaningful response to the TB/HIV co-epidemic, many countries in the region have initiated efforts by establishing collaborative activities between TB and AIDS programmes. These experiences show that joint collaboration is possible, including sharing of resources. In addition, regional and national strategies are being developed to combat HIV/TB. However, the first and foremost priority should be to strengthen and build the capacities of both the national AIDS and TB programmes. Resource allocation for TB control, however, remains desperately inadequate, despite proof that measures like DOTS have been highly successful. In the absence of increased resources and commitment, the problem of HIV/TB will continue to cause human suffering and death, particularly in poor and vulnerable populations. It would be tragic if TB, particularly MDR TB, were allowed to spin out of control, when proven strategies and inexpensive efficacious drugs are available to contain the epidemic.

REFERENCES

Agarwal, A., P.S. Narendra, T.S. Dinamani and N.S. Devendra (1998). Survival of AIDS patients in Manipur, India. International Conference of AIDS, 12, 1015 (abstract 60078).

Fatkenheuer, G., H. Taelman, P. Lepage, A. Schwenk and R. Wenzel (1999). The return of tuberculosis. Diagnostic Microbiology and Infectious Diseases, 34(2), 139–46.

Kumarasamy, N., S. Solomon, R.E. Amalraj, B. Ravikumar, J. Biswas and S.P. Thyagarajan (1998). Correlation between CD4/CD8 and total lymphocyte cell counts to opportunistic infections in PHIV/AIDS in Chennai (Madras), India. International Conference of AIDS, 12, 810 (abstract no. 42189).

Kumarasamy, N., S. Solomon, S.A. Jayaker Patul, R. Venilla and R.E. Amalraj (1995). Spectrum of opportunistic infections among AIDS patients in Tamil Nadu, India. International Journal of STD and AIDS, 6(6), 447–49.

Mohanty, K.C. and P.M.M. Basheer (1995). Changing trend of HIV infection and tuberculosis in a Bombay area since 1988. Indian Journal of Tuberculosis, 42(2), 117–20.

Narain, J.P., M.C. Raviglione and O. Kochi (1992). HIV associated tuberculosis in developing countries: Epidemiology and strategy for prevention. *Tubercule and Lung Disease*, 73(6), 311–21.

Narain, J.P., S.P. Tripathy and E. Pontali (2002). Tuberculosis and HIV infection. In Jai P. Narain (ed.), *Tuberculosis: Epidemiology and control* (pp. 84–100). New Delhi: WHO, Regional Office for South-East Asia.

Paranjape, R.S., S.P. Tripathy, P.A. Menon, S.M. Mehendale, P. Khatavkar, D.R. Joshi, U. Patil, D.A. Gadkari and J.J. Rodrigues (1997). Increasing trend of HIV seroprevalence among pulmonary tuberculosis patients in Pune, India. *Indian Journal of Medical Research*, 106, 207–11.

Punnotok, J., N. Shaffer, T. Naiwatanakul, O. Pumprueg, P. Subhannachart, A. Iffiravivongs, C. Chuchotthaworn, P. Ponglertnapagorn, N. Chantarojwong, N.L. Young, K. Limpakarnjanarat and T.D. Mastro (2000). Human immunodeficiency virus-related tuberculosis and primary drug resistance in Bangkok, Thailand. *International Journal of Tubercule and Lung Disease*, 4(6), 537–4s3.

Rajasekaran, S., A. Uma, S. Kamakshi, D. Jeyaganesh, A. Senthamizhchelvan, S. Savithri and Gopinathan (2000). Trend of HIV infection in patients with tuberculosis in rural south India. *Indian Journal of Tuberculosis*, 47(4), 223–26.

Sacks, L.V., S. Pendle, D. Orlovic, L. Blumberg and C. Constantinou (1999). A comparison of outbreak- and nonoutbreak-related multidrug-resistant tuberculosis among human immunodeficiency virus-infected patients in a South African hospital. *Clinical Infectious Disease*, 29(1), 96–101.

Siriarayapon, P., H. Yanai, J.R. Glynn, S. Yanpaisarn and W. Uthaivoravit (2002). Links: The evolving epidemiology of HIV infection and tuberculosis in northern Thailand. *Journal of Acquired Immune Deficiency Syndrome*, 31(1), 80–89.

Solomon, S., S. Anuradha and S. Rajasekaran (1995). Trend of HIV infection in patients with pulmonary tuberculosis in south India. *Tubercule and Lung Disease*, 76(1), 17–19.

Sunderam, G., R.J. MacDonald, T. Maniatis, J. Oleske, R. Kapila and L.B. Reichman (1986). Tuberculosis as a manifestation of the acquired immunodeficiency syndrome (AIDS). *Journal of the American Medical Association*, 256(3), 362–66.

Supawitkul, S., T. Yoshima, D. Rienthong, P. Akarasewi, N. Kunyanone, S. Saisorn and H. Yanai (1998). Increasing burden of tuberculosis and high rate of drug resistance in an HIV epicenter in northern Thailand 1989–1997. *International Conference of AIDS*, 12(abstract no. 452/22131).

Tripathy, S.P., D.R. Joshi, P. Menon, R.S. Paranjape, S.M. Mehendale and P. Khatavkar (1996). Seroprevalence of HIV-1 infection in tuberculosis patients at Pune, India. Paper presented at the Ninth International Conference on AIDS, Vancouver, Canada, 7–12 July.

Vittinghoff, E., S. Scheer, P. O'Malley, G. Colfax, S.D. Holmberg and S.P. Buchbinder (1999). Combination antiretroviral therapy and recent declines in AIDS incidence and mortality. *Journal of Infectious Diseases*, 179(3), 717–20.

WHO (2001). *Global tuberculosis control*. WHO report, http://www.who.int/gtb/publications/globrep01/index.html.

WHO (2003). *Global tuberculosis control: Surveillance, planning, financing.* WHO report, http://www.who.int/gtb/publications/globrep03/index.html.

Yanai, H., W. Uthaivoravit, V. Panich, P. Sawanpanyalert, B. Chaimanee, P. Akarasewi, K. Limpakarnjanarat, P. Nieburg and **T.D. Mastro** (1996). Rapid increase in HIV-related tuberculosis, Chiang Rai, Thailand, 1990–1994. *AIDS*, 10(5), 527–31.

ANTIRETROVIRAL TREATMENT IN RESOURCE-LIMITED SETTINGS | 17

Emanuele Pontali, Basil Vareldzis, Jos Perriens and Ying-Ru Lo

The number of people affected by HIV is bound to increase all over the world, including Asia. It will require an additional effort to cope with the needs of those infected. Provision of care and support to people living with HIV/AIDS and to their families will become crucial in decreasing the burden on families and on communities, and consequently on the most affected countries. Provision of care will progressively include the use of antiretrovirals even in resource-limited settings, with support provided by local political commitment and by donors. Therefore, it is necessary that these drugs be properly and rationally used. In this regard the WHO—at all levels—continues to advocate for larger access to ARVs and to provide the necessary support to member countries for implementing HIV/AIDS care programmes that include the use of ARVs.

Providing care and support to those living with HIV/AIDS has become as important as preventing HIV/AIDS. The care concept includes voluntary counselling and testing, nursing care, elimination of stigma related to HIV/AIDS in the community, partnership building between various providers and clinical management of symptomatic HIV infection using effective ARV drugs. For a great majority of infected persons living in the developing world access to ARVs is an exception rather than the rule (Narain et al. 2000). The WHO estimates that the number of people needing ARV treatment in developing countries is about 6 million, but less than 5 per cent of them are currently receiving it. The WHO-led '3 by 5' Initiative envisages to put 3 million people living with HIV/AIDS in the developing world on antiretroviral therapy by 2005.

Progress in ARV Development

Within a decade of availability of antiretroviral drugs, new classes of drugs and their use in combination have dramatically changed the management of HIV infection. Although these treatments are not a cure and present new challenges of their own to people living with HIV/ AIDS (PLHA), they have considerably improved rates of mortality and morbidity, prolonged lives, improved quality of life, let people come back to work and to care of their household, relieved families from care of PLHA, revitalised communities and transformed perceptions of HIV/ AIDS from a plague to a manageable, chronic illness.

A rational approach to HIV therapy derives from the evolving understanding of disease pathogenesis. A continuous high level of replication of HIV is present from early stages of infection. At least 10^{10} particles are produced and destroyed each day (Perelson et al. 1996). Ongoing HIV replication leads to progressive immune system damage resulting in susceptibility to opportunistic infections (OI), malignancies, neurologic diseases, wasting and ultimately leading to death. Plasma HIV RNA levels indicate the magnitude of HIV replication and the associated rate of CD4+ T-cell destruction, whereas CD4+ T-cell count indicates the extent of HIV-induced damage already suffered by the immune system. The measures of concentration of viral load and of CD4+ T-cell count are very good predictors of the subsequent risk of disease progression and death (ibid.). Regular and periodic measurements of plasma HIV RNA levels and CD4+ T-cell count are useful in determining the risk for disease progression in HIV-infected persons and in identifying the moment to start or modify antiretroviral treatment.

The only regimens potent enough to drastically reduce viral replication, prevent the emergence of resistance and ultimately treatment failure are combinations of at least three antiretrovirals, usually belonging to at least two different classes (Jordan et al. 2002). Such regimens have been associated with immunologic restoration, slowed disease progression, durable therapeutic responses, improved quality of life and prevention of emergence of drug resistance (Matthews et al. 2002). The improvements in morbidity and mortality seen as a result of the introduction of potent antiretroviral therapy have been confirmed in all settings where it has been used, including developing countries (for example, Brazil, Thailand, Senegal and Uganda) (Piot and Coll Seck 2001).

The antiretroviral drugs currently employed belong to five different classes: nucleoside reverse transcriptase inhibitors (NRTI), nucleotide reverse transcriptase inhibitors (NtRTI), non-nucleoside reverse transcriptase inhibitors (NNRTI), protease inhibitors (PI) and fusion inhibitors (FI). Drugs included in each of these classes are indicated in Table 17.1.

Table 17.1
Antiretroviral Drugs*

Class	Generic name
Nucleoside reverse transcriptase inhibitors (NRTI)	Abacavir (ABC)
	Didanosine (DDI)
	Lamivudine (3TC)
	Stavudine (D4T)
	Zalcitabine (DDC)
	Zidovudine (AZT, ZDV)
Nucleotide reverse transcriptase inhibitors (NtRTI)	Tenofovir (TFV)
Non-nucleoside reverse transcriptase inhibitors (NNRTI)	Delavirdine (DLV)
	Efavirenz (EFV)
	Nevirapine (NVP)
Protease inhibitors (PI)	Amprenavir (APV)
	Indinavir (IDV)
	Lopinavir/Ritonavir (LPV/r)
	Nelfinavir (NFV)
	Ritonavir (RTV)
	Saquinavir (SQV)
Fusion inhibitors (FI)	Enfuvirtide (ENF)

Note: * Current formulations of certain ARVs are not routinely used in clinical practice due to high side effects (DDC, DLV) or complicated regimens requiring multiple pills several times a day (DLV). TFV and ENF are not widely available in developing countries due to high costs at this time.

ARVs act by inhibiting viral replication. Their targets in the viral replicating cycle are—with different mechanisms of action—the viral enzyme reverse transcriptase for NRTI, NtRTI and NNRTI, and the viral protease for PI. The mechanism of action for each of these classes is as follows:

1. NRTI and NtRTI act by incorporating themselves into the DNA of the virus (competing with natural nucleotides), thereby stopping the building process of transcription from RNA to DNA. The resulting DNA is incomplete and cannot create a new virus.

2. NNRTI act by stopping HIV production by binding directly onto reverse transcriptase (non-competitively) and preventing the conversion of RNA to DNA.
3. PI act by binding to the viral protease and preventing the correct cleavage of viral proteins. Thus, they prevent HIV from being successfully assembled and released from the infected cells.
4. FI block fusion of the HIV viron into susceptible cells.

Guiding Principles for Antiretroviral Treatment

In resource-limited settings the goals of ARV treatment are: reduction of HIV-related morbidity and mortality; improvement of quality of life; restoration and/or preservation of immunologic function; and maximal and sustained suppression of viral load.

Antiretroviral drugs used in combination therapy regimens should follow optimum schedules and dosages. Antiretroviral drugs are limited in number and mechanism of action, and cross-resistance between specific drugs has been documented. Frequent or unnecessary change in ARV therapy decreases future therapeutic options. Combination ARV therapy by suppressing HIV replication limits the potential for selection of antiretroviral-resistant HIV variants and delays disease progression. The same principles of antiretroviral therapy apply to HIV-infected children, adolescents and adults, although the treatment of HIV-infected children involves special considerations.

HIV-infected persons, even if under optimal and successful anti-retroviral treatment, should be considered infectious. Therefore, they should be counselled to avoid sexual and drug use behaviours that are associated with either transmission or acquisition of HIV and other infectious pathogens (Centres for Disease Control and Prevention 1998).

Introducing Antiretrovirals at Programme Level

Introduction of ARVs at programme level should be preceded by the preparation of a policy for introduction and use of ARVs, and national guidelines for the use of antiretrovirals and the estimates of the number of PLHA that are expected to benefit from the programme. These will enable rational use of standardised ARV regimen and obtain a better estimate of the precise needs of the programme in terms of drugs and other necessary resources. Furthermore, ARVs should be introduced in the context of an HIV/AIDS care strategy and programme. This will include support services, such as access to voluntary HIV counselling

Antiretroviral Treatment in Resource-limited Settings

and testing (VCT); follow-up counselling services to ensure continued psychosocial support and to enhance adherence to treatment; medical services capable of identifying and treating common HIV-related illnesses and opportunistic infections; reliable and uninterrupted access to quality antiretroviral drugs and drugs to treat opportunistic infections and other related illness; and reliable laboratory monitoring facilities capable of doing routine laboratory investigations. Laboratories to measure CD4 are crucial, but measurement of viral load is not recommended. Besides CD4 enumeration, antiretroviral treatment depends also on the WHO system as shown in Table 17.2.

Table 17.2
Interim Proposal for a WHO Staging System for
HIV Infection and Disease in Adults and Adolescents

Stage	Symptoms and signs
Clinical stage I	1. Asymptomatic
	2. Persistent generalised lymphadenopathy (PGL)
	Performance scale 1: asymptomatic, normal activity
Clinical stage II	3. Weight loss, <10% of body weight
	4. Minor mucocutaneous manifestations (seborrhoeic dermatitis, prurigo, fungal nail infections, recurrent oral ulcerations, angular cheilitis)
	5. Herpes zoster within the last five years
	6. Recurrent upper respiratory tract infections (i.e., bacterial sinusitis)
	And/or performance scale 2: symptomatic, normal activity
Clinical stage III	7. Weight loss, >10% of body weight
	8. Unexplained chronic diarrhoea, >1 month
	9. Unexplained prolonged fever (intermittent or constant), >1 month
	10. Oral candidiasis (thrush)
	11. Oral hairy leukoplakia
	12. Pulmonary tuberculosis within the past year
	13. Severe bacterial infections (i.e., pneumonia, pyomyositis)
	And/or performance scale 3: bed-ridden, <50% of the day during the last month
Clinical stage IV	14. HIV wasting syndrome, as defined by the CDC*
	15. *Pneumocystis carinii* pneumonia
	16. Toxoplasmosis of the brain
	17. Cryptosporidiosis with diarrhoea, >1 month
	18. Cryptococcosis, extra-pulmonary
	19. Cytomegalovirus (CMV) disease of an organ other than liver, spleen or lymph nodes

(Table 17.2 contd.)

(Table 17.2 contd.)

Stage	Symptoms and signs
Clinical stage IV	20. *Herpes simplex* virus (HSV) infection, mucocutaneous >1 month, or visceral any duration
	21. Progressive multifocal leukoencephalopathy (PML)
	22. Any disseminated endemic mycosis (i.e., histoplasmosis, coccidioidomycosis)
	23. Candidiasis of the oesophagus, trachea, bronchi or lungs
	24. Atypical mycobacteriosis, disseminated
	25. Non-typhoid salmonella septicaemia
	26. Extra-pulmonary tuberculosis
	27. Lymphoma
	28. Kaposi's sarcoma (KS)
	29. HIV encephalopathy, as defined by CDC** And/or performance scale 4: bed-ridden, >50% of the day during the last month

Notes: Both definitive and presumptive diagnoses are acceptable.

* HIV wasting syndrome: Weight loss of more than 10 per cent of body weight, plus either unexplained chronic diarrhoea (greater than 1 month) or chronic weakness and unexplained prolonged fever (greater than 1 month).

** HIV encephalopathy: Clinical findings of disabling cognitive and/or motor dysfunction interfering with activities of daily living, progressing over weeks to months, in the absence of a concurrent illness or condition other than HIV infection that could explain the findings.

Criteria for Starting ARV Therapy in Adults and Adolescents

The WHO recommends that in ARV treatment programmes in resource-limited settings should start therapy among HIV-infected adolescents and adults when they have confirmed HIV infection and one of the following conditions:

- Clinically advanced HIV disease:

    – WHO stage IV HIV disease irrespective of CD4 cell count; or
    – WHO stage III disease with consideration of using CD4 cell counts <350/mm^3 to assist in decision making.

- WHO stage I or II HIV disease with CD4 cell counts ≤200/mm^3 (see Table 17.3).

Table 17.3

Recommendations for Initiating Antiretroviral Therapy in Adults and Adolescents with Documented HIV Infection

CD4 testing	Disease stage
Available	• WHO stage IV disease irrespective of CD4 cell count • WHO stage III disease (including but not restricted to HIV wasting, chronic diarrhoea of unknown aetiology, prolonged fever of unknown aetiology, pulmonary tuberculosis, recurrent invasive bacterial infections or recurrent/persistent mucosal candidiasis) with consideration of using CD4 cell counts <350/mm³ to assist decision making★ • WHO stage I or II disease with CD4 cell counts ≤200/mm³★★
Unavailable	• WHO stage IV disease irrespective of total lymphocyte count • WHO stage III disease (including but not restricted to HIV wasting, chronic diarrhoea of unknown aetiology, prolonged fever of unknown aetiology, pulmonary tuberculosis, recurrent invasive bacterial infections or recurrent/persistent mucosal candidiasis) irrespective of total lymphocyte count • WHO stage II disease with a total lymphocyte count ≤1200/ mm³★★★

Notes: ★ CD4 count advisable to assist with determining need for immediate therapy. For example, pulmonary TB may occur at any CD4 level and other conditions may be mimicked by non-HIV aetiologies (e.g., chronic diarrhoea, prolonged fever).

★★ The precise CD4 level above 200/mm³ at which ARV treatment to start has not been established.

★★★ A total lymphocyte count of 1200/mm³ can be substituted for the CD4 count when the latter is unavailable and HIV-related symptoms (stage II or III) exist. It is not useful in the asymptomatic patient. Thus, in the absence of CD4 cell testing, asymptomatic HIV-infected patients (WHO stage I) should not be treated because there is currently no other reliable marker available in severely resource-constrained settings.

The rationale for these recommendations is as follows. Treatment of patients with WHO stage IV disease (clinical AIDS) should not be dependent on a CD4 cell count determination, but, where available, this test can be helpful in categorising patients with stage III conditions with respect to their need for immediate therapy. For example, pulmonary TB can occur at any CD4 count level and, if the CD4 cell count level is well maintained (for example, >350/mm³), it is reasonable to defer therapy and continue to monitor the patient. For stage III conditions, a threshold of 350/mm³ has been chosen as a level below which immune deficiency is clearly present such that patients will be eligible for treatment when their clinical condition portends rapid clinical progression. A level of 350/mm^3 is also in line with other consensus guideline documents. For patients with stage I or II HIV disease, the presence of a CD4 cell count <200/mm^3 is an indication for treatment. In cases where CD4 cell counts cannot be assessed, the presence of a total lymphocyte count of 1200/mm^3 or below may be used as a substitute indication for treatment in the presence of symptomatic HIV disease (that is, WHO stages II or III). While the total lymphocyte count correlates relatively poorly with CD4 cell count in asymptomatic persons, in combination with clinical staging it is a useful marker of prognosis and survival (Gebo et al. 1999). As indicated earlier, an assessment of viral load (for example, using plasma HIV-1 RNA levels) is not considered necessary to start therapy. Given the cost and complexity of viral load testing at the present time, the WHO does not currently recommend its use as a routine test to assist with the decision of when to start therapy in severely resource-constrained settings. It is hoped, however, that increasingly affordable methods to determine viral load will become available so that this adjunct to treatment monitoring can become more available.

Treatment Regimens

Countries should use a public health approach to facilitate the introduction and scale-up of ARV use in resource-limited settings. This means that antiretroviral treatment programmes should be developed in the context of a care strategy for PLHA.

Countries are encouraged to use a public health approach to facilitate the scale-up of ARV use in resource-limited settings as delineated in the WHO's '3 by 5' strategy. This means that antiretroviral treatment programmes should be developed that can reach as many people as possible in need of therapy and requires that ARV treatment be standardised. Use of standardised regimens is an essential component of the '3 by 5' plan and will facilitate the WHO's efforts to assist member states with achieving this goal. This is the approach to ARV regimen selection taken into consideration in new WHO treatment guidelines (WHO 2003). For large-scale use, countries should select a limited number of first-line and second-line regimens. This approach should also consider individuals who cannot tolerate or fail the first- and second-line regimens. In this case a referral system for individualised care by specialist physicians should be made available. The SEA regional guidelines are in press.

Considerations in the selection of ARV treatment regimens at both the programme level and at the level of an individual patient should include the potency, side effect profile, laboratory monitoring requirements, the potential for maintenance of future treatment options, anticipated patient adherence, coexistent conditions (for example, co-infections, metabolic abnormalities), pregnancy or the risk thereof, the use of concomitant medications (that is, potential drug interactions), the potential for infection with a virus strain with diminished susceptibility to one or more ARVs including that resulting from prior ARV exposure given as prophylaxis or treatment, and, very importantly, availability and cost.

The use of quality-assured antiretrovirals in fixed-dose combinations (FDCs) or as coblister packs is another important consideration as this promotes better adherence, which would in turn limit the emergence of drug resistance.[1] It would also facilitate ARV storage and distribution logistics. Additional considerations relevant to the developing world include access to a limited number of ARV drugs, limited health service infrastructure including human resource personnel, the need to deliver drugs to rural areas, a high incidence of tuberculosis and hepatitis B and/or C in the population, and the presence of varied HIV types, groups and sub-types.

In the previous (April 2002) version of these treatment guidelines the WHO recommended that countries should select a first-line treatment regimen, and identified regimens composed of two nucleosides plus either a non-nucleoside, or abacavir, or a protease inhibitor as possible choices (WHO 2002a). Since the April 2002 guidelines were published, many countries have started ARV treatment programmes and have chosen their first-line treatment regimens, taking into account how the above factors would come into play in their setting. The majority of treatment programmes in developing countries have opted for a regimen composed of two nucleosides and a non-nucleoside reverse transcriptase inhibitor, namely, d4T/3TC/NVP due to low cost and ease of use. Triple nucleoside regimens including abacavir were almost never selected because of cost and concerns over hypersensitivity reactions, and protease inhibitor containing regimens became secondary options, mainly because of cost despite price decreases. However, high pill counts, their side effects profile and more difficult logistics (some require a cold chain) were also likely considerations.

Examining non-nucleoside-based regimens, the WHO writing committee that drafted the present treatment guidelines considered taking into account clinical experience with the efficacy and toxicity of the NRTI and NNRTI components, the availability of fixed-dose combinations, lack of requirement of a cold chain, drug availability and cost, and concluded that the four regimens listed in Table 17.4 are appropriate first-line antiretroviral regimens in adults and adolescents.

These regimens consist of a thymidine analogue nucleoside reverse transcriptase inhibitor (NRTI) (stavudine [d4T] or zidovudine [ZDV]), a thiacytidine NRTI (lamivudine [3TC]) and on NNRTI (nevirapine [NVP] or efavirenz [EFV]).

The choice between d4T and ZDV should be made at the country level based on local considerations, but the WHO recommends that both drugs be available. D4T is initially better tolerated than ZDV and does not require haemoglobin monitoring. However, among NRTIs, it has been consistently most associated with lipoatrophy and other metabolic abnormalities including lactic acidosis (particularly when combined with didanosine [ddI]) in the developed world. It can also cause peripheral neuropathy and pancreatitis. ZDV has also been implicated in metabolic complications of therapy, but to a lesser extent than d4T. Initial drug-related side effects are more frequent with ZDV (headache, nausea) and the drug can cause severe anaemia and neutropaenia, which requires that, at the very least, haemoglobin should be monitored prior and during treatment with ZDV. D4T can be substituted for ZDV for intolerance to the latter and vice versa (except in cases of suspected lactic acidosis in which instance neither drug should be prescribed). However, the initial need for lesser laboratory monitoring might favour the use of d4T at this time as the recommended nucleoside for the majority of patients in ART programmes in settings with severe resource limitations that aim to scale up rapidly.

3TC is a potent NRTI with an excellent record of efficacy, safety and tolerability. It can be given once or twice daily and has been incorporated into a number of fixed-dose combinations. Emtricitabine (FTC) is a recently approved nucleoside analogue that is structurally related to 3TC, shares its resistance profile and can be administered once daily. It is currently undergoing testing as a co-formulated product with tenofovir disoproxil fumarate (TDF). Given the relatively recent approval of FTC in a limited number of countries, it is not included in the WHO's recommended first-line regimens, but this may change based on future experience with the drug and its availability and cost.

The dual nucleoside component of d4T/ddI and ddC are no longer recommended as part of first-line regimens because of their toxicity profile, the former particularly in pregnant women. It is also worth emphasising

Table 17.4

First-line ARV Regimens in Adults and Adolescents, and Characteristics that Can Influence Choice

ARV regimen	Major potential toxicities	Usage in women (of childbearing age or who are pregnant)	Usage in TB co-infection	Availability as three-drug fixed-dose combination	Laboratory monitoring requirements	Price for least developed countries (June 2003) (US$/year)
d4T/3TC/NVP	d4T-related neuropathy, pancreatitis and lipoatrophy; NVP-related hepatotoxicity and severe rash	Yes	Yes in rifampicin-free continuation phase of TB treatment. Use with caution in rifampicin-based regimens	Yes	No	281–358
ZDV/3TC/NVP	ZDV-related GI intolerance, anaemia, and neutropenia; NVP-related hepatotoxicity and severe rash	Yes	Yes in rifampicin-free continuation phase of TB treatment. Use with caution in rifampicin-based regimens	Yes*	Yes	383–418
d4T/3TC/EFV	d4T-related neuropathy, pancreatitis and lipoatrophy; EFV-related CNS toxicity and potential for teratogenicity	No	Yes, but EFV should not be given to pregnant women or women of childbearing potential unless effective contraception can be assured	No, EFV not available as part of FDC. However, partial FDC available for d4T/3TC.*	No	350–1,086

(Table 17.4 contd.)

(Table 17.4 contd.)

ARV regimen	Major potential toxicities	Usage in women (of childbearing age or who are pregnant)	Usage in TB co-infection	Availability as three-drug fixed-dose combination	Laboratory monitoring requirements	Price for least developed countries (June 2003) (US$/year)
ZDV/3TC/ EFV	ZDV-related GI intolerance, anaemia, and neutropenia; EFV-related CNS toxicity and potential for teratogenicity	No	Yes, but EFV should not be given to pregnant women or women of childbearing potential unless effective contraception can be assured	No, EFV not available as part of FDC. However, partial FDC available for ZDV/3TC	Yes	611–986

Source: Sources and prices of selected medicines and diagnostics for people living with HIV/AIDS, June 2003 (http://www.who.int/HIV_AIDS).

Note: ★ These combinations have been not pre-qualified by the WHO, but could be used if assured quality formulations of proven bio-equivalence are available.

that ZDV/d4T, TDF/ABC and SQV/IDV should never be used together because of proven antagonism between the two drugs.

Taking into account all of these considerations, member countries may decide on a preferred first-line antiretroviral regimen from among the options provided above. Most probably each country should go through this same process of selection of various regimens, also considering the experiences of other developing countries that implemented the use of ARVs before (WHO 2002a; WHO/SEARO 2002).

Monitoring ARV Resistance

Antiretroviral drug resistance is a major challenge for treatment programmes in both developed and developing countries. Currently approximately 10 per cent of new HIV-1 infections in the United States and Europe are with viral strains exhibiting resistance to at least one drug. Scale-up programmes in the developing world can take advantage of the lessons learned in developed countries through proper initiation of potent regimens, incorporation of culturally appropriate adherence training and maintenance programmes, and synchronisation with drug resistance surveillance and monitoring initiatives.

Drug resistance genotyping is not on the near- or mid-term horizon for individual patient management in resource-limited settings, but country programmes are encouraged to develop or participate in drug resistance surveillance and monitoring programmes to assist with planning at the population level. This may involve developing or expanding genotypic capabilities at regional or national centres of excellence. This capability can be considered an important public health tool, which can be used to inform national, regional and global ARV scale-up programmes concerning trends in prevalence of drug resistance so that decisions can be made to minimise its impact.

The WHO recommends that countries planning to implement ART programmes also concurrently implement an HIV drug resistance sentinel surveillance system. This will allow countries to detect potential drug resistance at the population level and modify recommended treatment regimens accordingly. As a start, the approach should be to survey treatment-naïve persons to establish prevalence rates of drug resistance in the infected population and to monitor treatment experienced persons, particularly those diagnosed with their first episode of treatment failure. A Global HIV Drug Resistance Surveillance and Monitoring

Network is being established by the WHO in collaboration with partner organisations to assist member states in this area.

Role of the WHO

Since the beginning of the HIV epidemic, the WHO has been intensely involved in improving access to care for PLHA in developing countries. The recent decrease in the cost of ARVs—due largely to competition from generic manufacturers—has provided new opportunities to improve current HIV/AIDS care programmes in many countries. Following declaration by WHO director-general LEE Jong-wook in September 2003 that failure to provide ARV treatment as a global emergency, the organisation has moved forward and developed a '3 by 5' strategy to provide technical and operational support to member countries in scaling up ART and achieving the global target. In the last few years the WHO has developed technical documents to support countries in preparing their new strategies on HIV/AIDS care and support.

During 2002 the WHO released new guidelines for the use of ARVs in developing countries (WHO 2002a), which has now been revised in light of the new developments (WHO 2003). They also released the first 'WHO list of pre-qualified products' for the treatment of HIV and of related infections (WHO 2002b) and, finally, antiretrovirals were included in the 'WHO model list of essential medicines' (WHO 2002c).

These new WHO guidelines are intended to support and facilitate the proper management and scale-up of ARV treatment in the years to come by proposing a public health approach to achieve these goals. The key tenets of this approach are:

1. scaling up of antiretroviral treatment programmes to meet the needs of people living with HIV/AIDS in resource-limited settings;
2. standardisation and simplification of ARV regimens to support the efficient implementation of treatment programmes; and
3. ensuring that ARV treatment programmes are based on the best scientific evidence in order to avoid the use of substandard treatment protocols that compromise the treatment outcome of individual clients and create the potential for emergence of drug-resistant virus.

The 'WHO list of pre-qualified products' is a quality assessment on a selected number of pharmaceutical products that are considered for purchase by UN agencies involved in the procurement of drugs and diagnostics. In the list are presently included drugs manufactured by three generic manufacturers from India, namely, Cipla, Ranbaxy and Hetero. Many more drugs and manufacturers are currently under evaluation and the list is being updated approximately every two months. The recent inclusion of 12 ARV drugs in the WHO list of essential medicines (Table 17.5) is a further step in the direction of increasing the accessibility of these drugs in developing countries.

Table 17.5
ARVs in the WHO Model List of Essential Medicines

ARVs	Dosage
6.4.2.1 Nucleoside reverse transcriptase inhibitors	
Abacavir (ABC)	Tablet, 300 mg (as sulfate)
	Oral solution, 100 mg/5 ml
Didanosine (ddI)	Buffered chewable, dispersible tablet, 25 mg, 50 mg, 100 mg, 150 mg, 200 mg
	Buffered powder for oral solution, 100 mg, 167 mg, 250 mg packets
	Unbuffered enteric coated capsule, 125 mg, 200 mg, 250 mg, 400 mg
Lamivudine (3TC)	Tablet, 150 mg, oral solution, 50 mg/5ml
Stavudine (d4T)	Capsule, 15 mg, 20 mg, 30 mg, 40 mg
	Powder for oral solution, 5 mg/5 ml
Zidovudine (ZDV or AZT)	Tablet, 300 mg
	Capsule, 100 mg, 250 mg
	Oral solution or syrup, 50 mg/5 ml
	Solution for IV infusion injection, 10 mg/ml in 20 ml vial
6.4.2.2 Non-nucleoside reverse transcriptase inhibitors	
Efavirenz (EFV or EFZ)	Capsule, 50 mg, 100 mg, 200 mg
	Oral solution, 150 mg/5 ml
Nevirapine (NVP)	Tablet, 200 mg
	Oral suspension, 50 mg/5 ml
6.4.2.3 Protease inhibitors	
Indinavir (IDV)	Capsule, 200 mg, 333 mg, 400 mg (as sulfate)
Ritonavir	Capsule, 100 mg
	Oral solution, 400 mg/5 ml
Lopinavir + ritonavir (LPV/r)	Capsule, 133.3 mg + 33.3 mg
	Oral solution, 400 mg + 100 mg/5 ml
Nelfinavir (NFV)	Tablet, 250 mg (as mesilate)
	Oral powder, 50 mg/g
Saquinavir (SQV)	Capsule, 200 mg

Source: WHO (2002c).

In the South-East Asia region the WHO continues to advocate for the introduction of comprehensive HIV/AIDS care programmes and for a rational use of ARVs in particular, and to provide technical support to countries on this aspect. In this regard, WHO/SEARO has developed specific guidelines for the use of ARVs in countries of the region (WHO/ SEARO 2002), which is currently being updated, and also prepared 'fact sheets on antiretroviral drugs' (Matthews et al. 2002; WHO 2002b, 2002c), which can be useful for the better use of these drugs in the day-to-day practice of physicians treating PLHA.

Unfortunately, given the present situation in terms of financial and health resources of most HIV-affected countries, a few issues have prevented generalised implementation of antiretroviral therapy at the present time, the most important of which is lack of budgetary support, particularly for ARV drugs, and the need for capacity building at the country level for ART delivery. One concern remains paramount in the minds of the national programmes regarding the possible shift of resources from prevention programmes to the simple purchase and distribution of drugs. Even if prevention programme budgets were not affected, it should be ensured that other care interventions are not compromised. A good balance between the different components of national programmes is essential.

N O T E

1. Quality-assured medicines assembled in fixed-dose combinations (FDCs), in the context of this document, include individual products that have been deemed to meet or exceed international standards for quality, safety and efficacy. In the case of drug combinations whose components are from different manufacturers, the international standards include a requirement for clinical bio-equivalence studies to establish therapeutic interchangeability of these components. For WHO's work on prequalification of ARVs see: http://www.who.int/medicines/.organization/qsm/activities/pilotproc/proc.shtml.

    FDCs are based on the principle of inclusion of two or more active pharmacological products in the same pill, capsule, tablet or solution. A co-blister pack is the inclusion of two or more pills, capsules or tablets in the same plastic or aluminum co-blister.

R EFERENCES

Centres for Disease Control and Prevention (1998). Report of the NIH panel to define principles of therapy of HIV infection. *Morbidity and Mortality Weekly Report*, 47(RR-5), 1–41.

Gebo, K.A., R.E. Chaisson, J.G. Folkemer, J.G. Bartlett and R.D. Moore (1999). Costs of HIV medical care in the era of highly active antiretroviral therapy. *AIDS*, 13(8), 963–69.

Jordan, R.G.L., C. Cummins and C. Hyde (2002). Systematic review and meta-analysis of evidence for increasing numbers of drugs in antiretroviral combination therapy. *British Medical Journal*, 324(7340), 757–60.

Matthews, G.V., C.A. Sabin, S. Mandalia, F. Lampe, A.N. Phillips, M.R. Nelson, M.A. Johnson and B. Gazzard (2002). Virological suppression at 6 months is related to choice of initial regimen in antiretroviral-naive patients: A cohort study. *AIDS*, 16(1), 53–61.

Narain, J.P., C. Chela and E. van Praag (2000). Planning and implementing HIV/AIDS care programmes: A step-by-step approach. SEA/AIDS/106, WHO, New Delhi.

Perelson, A.S., A.U. Neumann, M. Markowitz, J.M. Leonard and D.D. Ho (1996). HIV-1 dynamics in vivo: Virion clearance rate, infected cell life-span, and viral generation time. *Science*, 271(5255), 1582–86.

Piot, P. and A.M. Coll Seck (2001). International response to the HIV/AIDS epidemic: Planning for success. *Bulletin of the World Health Organization*, 79(2), 1106–12.

WHO (2002a). Scaling up antiretroviral therapy in resource-limited settings: Guidelines for a public health approach. WHO/HIV/2002.02, WHO.

——— (2002b). WHO list of pre-qualified products, http://www.who.int/medicines/organization/qsm/activities/pilotproc/pilotproc.shtml.

——— (2002c). WHO model list of essential medicines, http://www.who.int/medicines/organization/par/edl/expertcomm.shtml.

——— (2003). Scaling up antiretroviral therapy in resource-limited settings: Revision treatment guidelines for resource poor settings, http://www.who.int.

WHO/Regional Office for South-East Asia (SEARO) (2002). The use of anti-retroviral therapy: A simplified approach for resource-constrained countries. SEA/AIDS/133, WHO SEARO.

ENHANCING ACCESS TO ARV IN DEVELOPING COUNTRIES

Ranjit Roy Chaudhury

It is unfortunate that treatment of persons with HIV/AIDS in developing countries has not been seriously considered and provided until recently. Except in very few countries, national authorities accepted an unacceptable situation—that the new ARV therapies were too expensive for use by poor people in poor countries. Very few attempts were made to aggressively enhance the access of these populations to newer ARV therapies. Before the advent of these drugs there was no therapy available and the diagnosis of HIV was virtually a death sentence. There was nothing significant that the health provider could do to prolong life, and the attitude was of helpless resignation. The situation today is not the same. Diagnosis of HIV is not the death knell it once was and drugs are available to prolong life. Though it is not known how long life can be prolonged by judicious and regular use of these new drugs, we do know that it *can* be. However, in spite of a totally different scenario in the therapeutics of HIV/AIDS, the attitude of health providers, society and national governments has not changed. The feeling that death was inevitable and that nothing much could be done that existed when there were no drugs has been replaced by the feeling that since the available drugs are so expensive, their use in poor countries is not possible.

It is important that this attitude changes and that a strategy is worked out in developing countries so that people living with HIV/AIDS are able to prolong their life with dignity. It is not possible for government and society to ensure that all persons needing the drugs receive these. However, it is unethical and inequitous not to provide these therapies to as many persons as possible. It is hoped that this paper will provide some suggestions as to how this may be done. The examples are from

India, but could be applied to any developing country in Asia with a sizeable load of HIV/AIDS and with many poor people who cannot afford to pay much for drugs. It is not acceptable any more that only people living with HIV/AIDS in industrial countries should benefit from these treatments.

Availability of Drugs

The first step is to assess which drugs are available in the country—not in the so-called grey market but after having been approved for use. Table 18.1 lists the drugs available in India together with the name of the manufacturers. The list includes both the reverse transcriptase inhibitors as well as protease inhibitors. Research is in progress and more drugs in both these categories should become available in the future.

Table 18.1
Some Antiretroviral Drugs Available in India

Drugs	Local manufacturer (bulk & formulation)	Import & market (formulation)
Lamivudine (3TC)	Cipla, Sun Pharma, Hetero Drugs, Mepro Pharma, IPCA Labs	Glaxo (India)
Stavudine (d4T)	Cipla, Sun Pharma, Viron/Ranbaxy Labs, IPCA Labs, Hetro Drugs, Ranit Pharma, Aurobindo	
Zidovudine (AZT or ZDV)	Cipla, Hetero Drugs, Unichem	Burrough Welcome
Didanosine (ddI)	Cadila HC, Aurobindo, Ranit Pharma	Cipla (bulk)
Zalcitabine (ddC)	–	Roche (bulk)
Saquinavir (SQV)	–	Piramal Health Care
Ritonavir (r)	–	Abbott Laboratories
Indinavir (IDV)	Hetero Drugs, Unichem, Aurobindo	Cipla (bulk)
Efavirenz (EFZ)	Sun Pharma, Aurobindo, Ranit Cipla	Cipla (bulk)
Nelfinavir (NFV)	Aurobindo, Ranit Pharma	
Nevirapine (NVP)	Cipla, Viron/Ranbaxy, Unichem, Hetero Drugs, Ranit, Aurobindo Pharma	
3TC/AZT	Aurobindo	
ABC/3TC/ZDV	Ranbaxy	
3TC/d4T/NVP	Cipla	
AZT/3TC/NVP	Aurobindo	

The first drug to be given approval for use in India in April 1988 was zidovudine. There was a gap of five years when in July 1993 zalcitabine was approved for marketing. Two protease inhibitors, ritonavir and saquinavir, became available in 1997 while a third reverse transcriptase inhibitor, stavudine, also became available in 1997. Lamivudine was approved by the Drugs Controller General in 1998 and another drug of the same type—nevirapine—was approved in March 2000.

It is interesting to note that the time difference between obtaining US FDA approval and government of India approval is not much. The difference in years for the five reverse transcriptase drugs were one, three, one, three and four years for the drugs zidovudine, stavudine, zalcitabine, lamivudine and nevirapine respectively. The difference in the protease inhibiting drugs was one year for ritonavir and two years for saquinavir. These figures indicate that pharmaceutical houses that have developed ARV drugs do obtain approval for these drugs for use in developing countries. It is not correct to assume that they are not interested in selling these drugs in the Third World countries where the people are poor and the governments have little money to purchase drugs for use in the health care system.

The global pharmaceutical world is unlikely to be the same. In early 2001 an Indian firm, Cipla, made a dramatic offer to price a three-drug cocktail for AIDS treatment at US$ 350 only for an annual dose to Medicines San Frontieres (MSF, a prestigious NGO) for free distribution in the AIDS programme in Africa. This price was as little as one-thirtieth to one-fortieth the price (US$ 10,000 to 12,000 a year) at which the drug majors were selling these medicines in the Western market. Leading Western drug companies have recently negotiated discount deals with Senegal, Uganda and Rwanda, which bring the cost down by up to 90 per cent, but that still leaves their products at a premium to Cipla's offer. In a letter to a drug distributor of Ghana and the Indian generic drug maker Cipla, Glaxo said sales of a generic version of their drug Combivir would be illegal because they would be violating company patents. As a result, this Indian company stopped selling its low-cost versions in Ghana. However, officials at the multilaterial African agency that issued the Glaxo patent in question said these patents are either invalid in Ghana or do not apply. After pressure from Glaxo to withdraw its drugs from Ghana, Cipla wrote to five drug majors that owned the patents for antiretroviral drugs offering to pay 5 per cent as royalty in return for a licence to produce these drugs, citing a communication of US pharma association, Pharmaceutical and Research Manufacturers of America (PhRMA), which mentioned 5 per cent as the 'industry average' for a licence. The Cipla offer in early 2001 brought a global development in which the regime of high pharma prices and patents had been pushed on to the defensive by powerful political, ethical and economic arguments. Groups of senior citizens in the US have been lobbying the Congress to allow parallel imports of generic medicines to get around the high prices charged by local drug majors. Moreover, generic producers such as Cipla and Ranbaxy from India have successfully undergone the pre-qualification process of the WHO and are listed as 'quality drugs' producers from where the UN could procure at lower rates (WHO 2004). Thanks to the generic competition, the price of the ARV drugs has come down dramatically over the past two to three years, from US$ 10,000 to 12,000 per patient per year to less than US$ 300 per year now.

Strategy for Enhancing Access to ARV Drugs

Once programme managers and clinicians know which drugs are available in the country, the following seven steps need to be taken to enhance the access of ARV drugs to those in need in these countries:

1. Rational selection of drugs to be used and an alternative back-up regimen.
2. Attempt to bring down the prices of the selected drugs.
3. Selection of people to whom the drugs will be administered.
4. Steps to make available drugs not yet being imported into the country.
5. Training in rational prescribing of antiretroviral drugs.
6. Effective logistics for procurement and distribution of antiretroviral drugs.
7. Information and counselling to the patient about these drugs so that these may be used better and with enhanced compliance.

Each of these steps will be dealt with briefly.

Step I: Selection of Drugs

Selection depends on the availability of the drugs in the country, their relative efficacies, the side effects these induce and the cost of treatment.

The treatment of choice today for HIV/AIDS is to use at the same time two drugs that are reverse transcriptase inhibitors and one drug that is a protease inhibitor. This is known as 'triple combination therapy'. This combination is effective and reduces viral plasma loads to undetectable levels. There is also clinical improvement. However, although the viral plasma levels are below detectable levels the HIV still persists in 'sanctuary zones'. The treatment, therefore, has to continue for life just as treatment for hypertension, in most cases, and hypothyroidism do. It should be clearly mentioned that taking a large number of tablets throughout life is not easy, that many of the drugs have side effects, that other drugs for other ailments will also have to be taken from time to time and that routine monitoring for drug toxicity will also have to be done. What makes it even more difficult for a person living with HIV with no symptoms to accept is that his/her apparently healthy normal life is totally altered once he is put on therapy. In other words, therapy converts a healthy lifestyle into an unhealthy one, that of a person who has to take many medicines. This needs proper counselling.

Of the ARV drugs available in India, one could choose zidovudine as one of the reverse transcriptase inhibiting drugs. It is given at a dose of 200 mg three times a day. The second reverse transcriptase inhibiting drug could be zalcitabine at a dose of 0.75 mg three times a day. Although this is a weaker combination than, for example, zidovudine and lamivudine or stavudine and lamivudine, it is a much cheaper alternative. The protease inhibiting drug that could be combined with the administration of zidovudine and zalcitabine could be saquinavir at a dose of 2,400 mg three times a day. However, since ritonavir is also available in India, saquinavir (400 mg twice a day) and ritonavir (400 mg twice a day) would be preferable instead of saquinavir alone. However, the cost of the therapy would go up for a day's treatment. The total daily cost of using zidovudine, zalcitabine and saquinavir would be around Rs 318 per day. This could certainly be reduced further. If, however, a combination of nevirapine, lamivudine and ritonavir is used, the daily cost would go up to a little over Rs 1,000 per day. The costs are, however, coming down almost on a daily basis. The message that comes out loud and clear is that if access to ARV drugs is to be enhanced, careful selection has to be made regarding the drugs to be used as the first line of defence. Though this is not the place to discuss the side effects induced by each of the drugs mentioned, it should be stated that zidovudine should not be administered if the patient's haemoglobin is low. Saquinavir should not be administered to persons receiving rifampicin for treatment of tuberculosis as the latter reduces absorption of saquinavir.

Step 2: Bringing Down Prices of Selected Drugs

Once the drugs have been selected, it is possible to bring the cost of therapy to half of what it is now. Thus, the combination of zidovudine, zalcitabine and saquinavir could be brought down to Rs 150 per day instead of Rs 318. Negotiations should be initiated with the pharmaceuticals manufacturing the drugs. Already, social, national and international pressure from international agencies, non-governmental organisations and consumer organisations, particularly at the international conference on AIDS held in Durban in 2001, has led to pharmaceutical houses themselves slashing the cost of anti-HIV drugs. There have been several newspaper reports of drug prices being reduced and it is certain to continue.

Another reason for reduction in prices is the bulk pooled procurement of the selected drugs. It has already been demonstrated (Chaudhury 1999) that by resorting to pooled procurement the Delhi government obtained drugs at prices that were 35 per cent less than what others were paying for the same drugs. This has also been the experience of other states like Punjab and Tamil Nadu, which have also obtained drugs at much lower prices—without change in quality—after resorting to pooled procurement. A combination strategy of social and national pressure for equity, negotiations with individual pharmaceutical houses and the fact that the quantity of drugs being procured are much more needs to be initiated for reduction in prices of selected drugs. There is need for concerted coordinated action.

Step 3: Selection of HIV/AIDS Patients for Administration of Drugs

Once the national government and the public sector have funds, albeit limited, for ARV drugs to be provided free to those in need, a careful, well-reasoned, objective and unemotional decision has to be made as to which category of persons should be given the drugs.

The first category would be pregnant mothers who are HIV positive so as to prevent the newborn from having the infection. The mother-to-child transmission can be prevented in 51 per cent of cases with proper treatment (WHO ASD 1998b). Only one drug can be effective for such treatment. It has been clearly shown that zidovudine in either 'long' or 'short' regimen reduces the risk of mother-to-child transmission in non-breastfeeding mothers. There has been a significant reduction in the price of ARVs for such use. One report after the Durban meeting states that the earlier cost of zidovudine at approximately Rs 1,200 has now been reduced to Rs 200 after the fall in the price of nevirapine. Undoubtedly, these women would be provided the drug free.

It would not be feasible to provide treatment to all HIV-infected individuals in India. If funds are available it could be suggested that those who are developing some symptoms should be provided drug treatment. It has been accepted that 'a maximum benefit on the quality of life of patients is expected in patients with CD4 counts <200 mm^3 and/or a viral load more than 30,000–100,000 copies/ml plasma' (WHO ASD 1998a, 1998b). Such treatment should be continued for life unless remarkable progress is seen during monitoring.

Again, it would be neither feasible nor really much beneficial to the patient to start therapy with ARV drugs during the acute phase of the illness. Treatment, therefore, should be for pregnant mother and babies in the public sector where resources are limited and, if funds available, for HIV-positive persons who have started to show symptoms. These are most likely to benefit. In the private sector and in the case of affluent persons needing treatment and can afford to pay, ARV drugs can be given also to asymptomatic HIV carriers and to patients in the acute phase of the illness.

Step 4: Steps to Increase Availability of Antiretroviral Drugs

India is fortunate to have at least a number of anti-HIV drugs that could be used for treatment of the poor and needy in government hospitals. It also has the potential to produce these drugs. It is, however, possible that in some countries pharmaceutical houses who have discovered and patented these anti-HIV drugs are not interested in bringing them to these countries. This is unethical because it means persons with HIV/AIDS are being denied a treatment that exists and is being used in other richer countries.

There are ways to address this problem. One such mechanism available to countries is to request for compulsory licensing of the drug within the intellectual property provisions provided by TRIPS. The country has, however, to enact legislations within the country. The basis of this is that ARV drugs are a public good and the World Health Organisation supports countries to use TRIPS safeguards as provided, including exceptions what can promote generic competition, compulsory licensing, parallel imports and collection of evidence to support country applications for extension of the transitional period outlined in TRIPS (Velasquez and Perriens 2000). Compulsory licensing will also bring down the prices of these drugs. This mechanism should be used by countries to bring into the country antiretroviral drugs that may never have been seen. Generic prescribing of antiretroviral drugs and generic manufacture of such drugs should be looked at much more carefully than is being done at the moment. Already, generic drugs from Cipla and Ranbaxy have been pre-qualified by the WHO and UNAIDS as 'quality drugs'. The UN could now procure drugs from these manufacturers at much lower prices.

Step 5: Training in Rational Prescribing of Antiretroviral Drugs

To make the best use of resources available and to use drugs purchased with these resources rationally, it is important that they are prescribed according to a framework of standard treatment guidelines. The WHO has recently developed guidelines for use of ART, including for starting ART, regimens to use, when to switch therapy and so on (WHO 2002; WHO/SEARO 2002). These guidelines can be adapted for country use. Doctors should be provided such a framework or national guidelines on the standard treatment regimen to be used as has been developed and being used for the five categories of TB patients and taught how to use it. Otherwise the therapy may become irrational. Even now, for example, in addition to the triple therapy described earlier, some investigators use two protease inhibitors and one reverse transcriptase inhibitor while others use two drugs only in what is known as double therapy. They prefer to keep the third drug in abeyance to be used when the need arises. It is acceptable to use such regimens provided these have been discussed and find a place in the framework. Rational prescribing and training in rational prescribing is an important plank in the strategy for enhancing better use of anti-HIV drugs.

Step 6: Effective Logistics for Procurement and Distribution of ARV Drugs

It is important that the ARV drugs selected are procured, stored and distributed in an effective manner to ensure that these are always available when needed, that shortages do not occur and that drugs near their expiry dates do not accumulate. Together with procurement systems, a quality assurance system should be developed to make certain that the drugs being supplied are of good quality.

310 Ranjit Roy Chaudhury

Mechanisms to ensure this include careful technical screening of potential suppliers before accepting price bids from them, good manufacturing practices, inspections at pharmaceutical houses and random samples being sent for testing for quality and potency.

Step 7: Information and Counselling to the Patient

Earlier a patient had to take over 15 drugs for HIV/AIDS—some of which are potentially toxic. An exit interview carried out at a major hospital in New Delhi showed that only about 35 per cent of the patients had adequate knowledge about the drugs they were taking with them. The number of doses to be used now has come down, including those taken even twice a day. The issue with antiretroviral drugs assumes much more significance because these are powerful drugs and can cause serious side effects if not used in a rational manner. For example, zidovudine should not be given with stavudine because of viral antagonism; rapid resistance to lamivudine is seen when it is used alone; and rifampicin decreases nevirapine absorption. This information should not only be with doctors, but also with patients. Besides counselling, drug information sheets prepared in simple local languages should be provided to the patients. For example, patients on the drug indinavir must drink at least 1.5 litres of water every day to prevent the formation of kidney stones. Ritonavir reduces the effectiveness of the contraceptive pill. Patient compliance will undoubtedly be enhanced by providing counselling and information to the patients about the drugs they will use.

Conclusions

Antiretroviral drugs have to be provided rationally and in a systematic manner to patients of HIV infection and AIDS in developing countries. It is no more possible nor ethical to say that these drugs are too expensive for poor people in these countries and that they will have to go without them. To ensure maximum benefit with limited resources it is essential to develop a framework for action and develop a strategy around such a framework. Several components of such a framework have been identified and discussed. If concerted efforts are made, anti-HIV drugs can be made available to some segments of the society, particularly to prevent HIV transmission and as part of comprehensive HIV/AIDS care.

REFERENCES

Chaudhury, R.R. (1999). Rational use of drug: Change in policy changes lives. *Essential Drugs Monitor*, 27, 1–4.

Velasquez, G. and **J. Perriens** (2000). Access to HIV/AIDS-related drugs in Thailand. Report of a WHO/UNAIDS joint mission, Geneva, May.

WHO (2002). Scaling up antiretroviral therapy in resource-limited settings: Guidelines for a public health approval. WHO, WHO/HIV/2002.02, Geneva.

——— (2004). *WHO list of pre-qualified products*. Available at: http://www.who.int/ medicines/organization/qsm/activities/pilotproc/pilotprocoutcomes.shtml.

WHO AIDS and STD Department (ASD) (1998a). Safe and effective use of antiretrovirals. *Guidance Modules on Antiretroviral Treatments*, 4.

——— (1998b). The use of antiretroviral drugs to reduce mother-to-child transmission of HIV. *Guidance Modules on Antiretroviral Treatments*, 6.

WHO/SEARO (2002). The use of antiretroviral therapy: A simplified approach for resource-constrained countries. WHO/SEARO, SEA/AIDS/133, New Delhi.

DEVELOPING A NATIONAL ANTIRETROVIRAL PROGRAMME FOR PEOPLE WITH HIV/AIDS: THE EXPERIENCE OF THAILAND | 19

Sombat Thanprasertsuk, Cheewanan Lertpiriyasuwat and Sanchai Chasombat

Thailand was among the first countries in Asia to face the most serious epidemic of HIV/AIDS. The first case in Thailand was reported in 1984, about three years after the initial discovery of AIDS (Limsuwan et al. 1986). In 1988 an explosive HIV outbreak was identified among intravenous drug users in the country's capital, Bangkok (Wright et al. 1994). Subsequently, the virus spread widely in this group to other provinces across the country. The HIV prevalence among intravenous drug users has since then remained constant at about 40 to 50 per cent (Jittiwutikarn et al. 2000; Nelson 1994; Nelson et al. 2002).

Another outbreak of HIV was identified among female commercial sex workers and their customers (Limanonda et al. 1994; Limpakarnjanarat et al. 1999; Sawanpanyalert et al. 1994). It was observed that the national average HIV prevalence among female commercial sex workers in brothel settings increased from 3 per cent in 1989 to 28 per cent in the mid-1990s (Figure 19.1).

During the late 1980s and the early 1990s, HIV prevalence among 21-year-old male military recruits and pregnant women attending antenatal clinics showed an increasing trend (Mason et al. 1998; Saengwonloey et al. 2003; Sirisopana et al. 1996; Torugsa et al. 2003). The peak HIV prevalence among military recruits was 4 per cent in 1993; among pregnant women the peak prevalence was 2 per cent in 1995 (Figure 19.2).

Thailand's HIV epidemic continues to spread to various population groups. It is estimated that more than 1 million Thais have been infected

Figure 19.1
HIV Prevalence among Direct and
Indirect Sex Workers in Thailand: 1989–2002

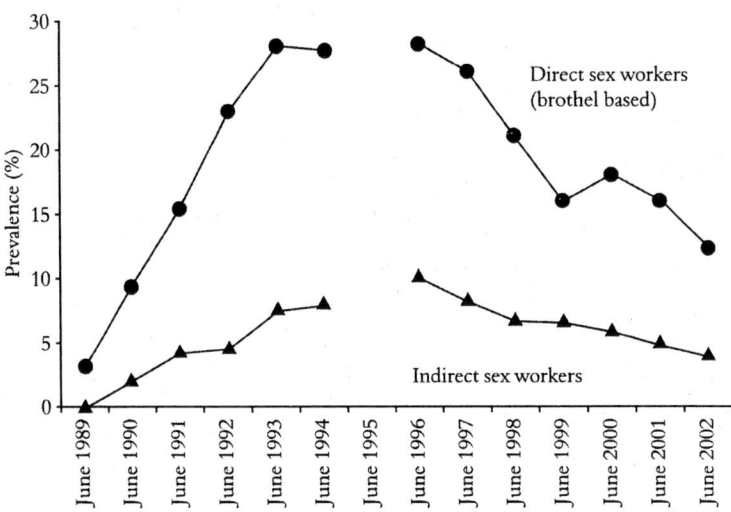

Source: Bureau of Epidemiology, Ministry of Public Health, Thailand.

Figure 19.2
HIV Prevalence among Men Aged 21 Years and
Pregnant Women in Thailand: 1989–2002

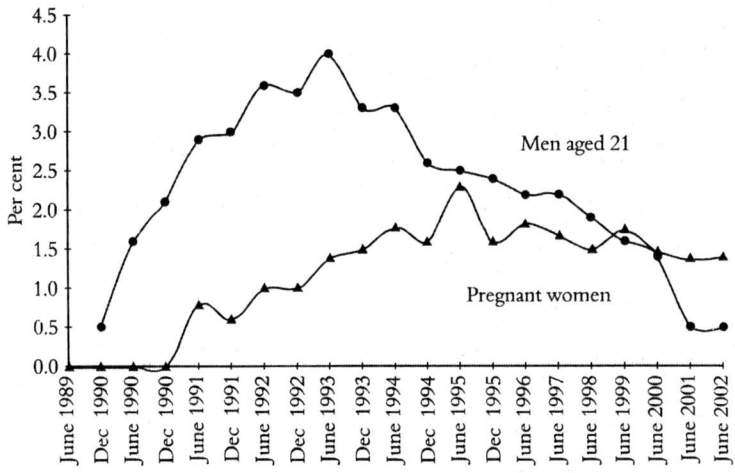

Source: Bureau of Epidemiology, Ministry of Public Health, Thailand.

with the virus during the past 20 years. Of these, more than 400,000 have died and about 600,000 are currently living with the virus.

The government of Thailand has made considerable efforts to interrupt the spread of HIV and to provide care and support for people living with HIV/AIDS (PLHAs). Under the policy guidelines of the National AIDS Committee chaired by the prime minister, numerous national and local programmes have been undertaken (Ainsworth et al. 2001; Ruxrungtham and Phanuphak 2001).

After several years of hardship in the implementation of programmes, both in the prevention of HIV transmission and in the provision of support and care for PLHAs, recent results show a declining trend in the number of new HIV infections. Coverage of AIDS patients with comprehensive care and support interventions has also expanded satisfactorily (AIDS Division, no date).

Despite the successful reduction of new HIV infections in recent years, the AIDS crisis in Thailand will continue to grow. This is because many PLHAs who were infected during the past 10 years or earlier are likely to develop AIDS during the coming years. This in turn will cause tremendous burden on the families of these patients as well as on the health system, and will affect the development of the country. It is projected that each year approximately 50,000 new AIDS cases will continue to occur in Thailand (Figure 19.3) (Thai Working Group on HIV/AIDS Projection 2001).

Figure 19.3
New HIV Infections and New AIDS Cases, Thailand: 1985–2010

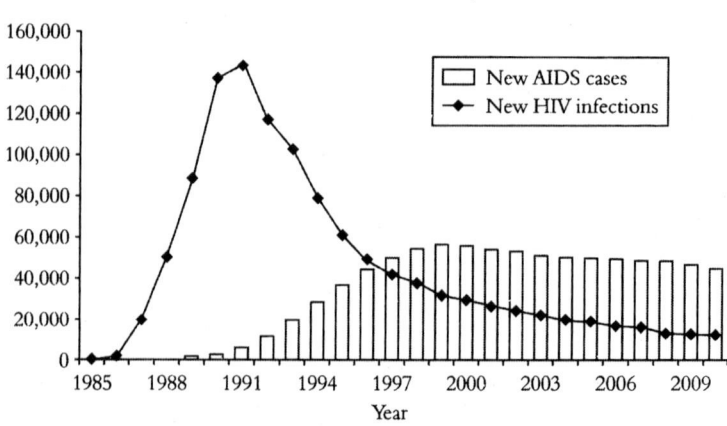

Source: Division of Epidemiology, Ministry of Public Health, Thailand.

Loss of lives due to AIDS and the impact on families and communities has become the primary driving force behind the initiation of the ARV programme in Thailand. It was started in 1992 and has been continuously evolving. Based on the past 12 years of experience, the development of the programme can be described in three phases.

The First Phase: Introduction of ARV

The first phase (1992–97) was the introductory phase, wherein an attempt to support AIDS patients with modern and expensive medicine was made. The programme was launched within the public health system based on a single-drug regimen, that is, zidovudine mono-therapy. Only a handful of referral and university hospitals participated in the programme. The number of patients enrolled in the programme was still very limited due to the high costs of ARV.

The objectives of the first phase were to assess the readiness of the health service system, particularly tertiary care settings, in using ARV and to identify the most appropriate mechanisms for providing treatment services to patients. The first phase of implementation had limited success, as expected, due to the use of a single-drug therapy that does not have long-lasting beneficial effects on clinical outcomes.

Based on an evaluation (Prescott 1995), it was recommended that the ARV programme be further developed with greater emphasis on strengthening the health service system for efficient delivery of ARV services to eligible patients. Thus, in the next phase, the ARV programme was remodelled and conceptualised as a clinical service system linked to research and development.

The Second Phase: Clinical and Public Health Research Network

The objectives during this second phase were to strengthen the clinical service centres through capacity building and networking, with a strategy to integrate ARV into a comprehensive care and support programme for PLHAs. It also focused on the monitoring aspects of long-term ARV treatment (WHO 2000).

Fifty-eight referral and university hospitals participated in the Clinical Research Network Programme. Mono-therapy was still used for a short period. However, in 1998 dual therapy with an appropriate combination of antiretroviral drugs was used as the standard line of treatment. It was estimated that the programme covered 1,200 patients during this phase using a two-drug combination.

At the end of this phase, highly active ART was introduced. However, the number of patients who had access to ART was still very limited.

In the second phase only a few thousand patients out of the more than 50,000 new AIDS patients needing treatment were enrolled in the programme each year. To address this limitation, the idea of co-payment was introduced and tested. However, it had limited success with just a few hundred patients participating in this scheme.

The Third Phase: National Access to ARV

The third phase, currently ongoing, focuses on ARV expansion with the ultimate goal of universal coverage. The factors that attributed to the development of this phase were based largely on the reduction of ARV drug prices and the local production of generic medicines.

Generic production of antiretroviral drugs by the Government Pharmaceutical Office has brought down the price of the ARV drugs, including the combination regimen, in which the price has decreased to an unbelievingly low level. The current price of a combined regimen called GPO-VIR® is US$ 30 or about 1,200 baht per month. The local generic production of ARV drugs is the key factor in increasing the access of patients to treatment.

In the third phase, which began in the year 2000, the programme was renamed Access to Care 1. Initially, eight highly active ART (HAART) regimens were listed in the treatment guidelines. Subsequently, when the generically manufactured GPO-VIR® became available, the guidelines were revised and the programme was upgraded to Access to Care 2 .

Later, with the adoption of the policy of expanding the programme to cover all patients needing ARV, the title of the programme was revised to National Access to Antiretroviral Programme for People with HIV/ AIDS (NAPHA). Sites to provide ARV were gradually expanded to identify a larger number of patients. Training for relevant health care professionals such as medical doctors, nurses, pharmacists, laboratory technicians and counsellors or social workers is an essential activity to build knowledge and skills of health personnel. In addition to increasing access to ARV drugs, there is also a need to acknowledge that a parallel development of capacity in CD4 laboratory service is necessary for expanding ARV programmes.

Ensuring adherence to treatment has been another important component of the programme. The programme has successfully engaged PLHAs, families and the civil society in improving adherence to ARV. It has been observed that with the support of close family members, friends, peers and others, patients can be empowered to take drugs continuously and regularly. Based on this experience, hospitals providing ARV are suggested to encourage and support civil society organisations as well as PLHA groups to participate in the ARV programme.

The number of hospitals participating in the programme has increased from 119 in 2001 to 491 in early 2003. During the past two years health staff from all the government hospitals, that is, more than 400 additional sites, have been trained and enrolled to provide ARV. The intention is to geographically expand ARV services to every corner of the country. This will ensure the availability of ARVs to all patients who need them, regardless of their location.

In commitment to the universal coverage of essential health services for all Thais, the government has recently decided to increase the budget for the ARV programme. US$ 25 million has been allocated to scale up access to ARVs. With this figure, the number of patients who have access to ARVs is likely to increase from 13,000 patients in 2003 to 50,000 patients in 2004, or a four-fold increase; this would indicate universal coverage for all who need the drugs. This is a very challenging task for the programme administration and civil society organisations who are actively involved in the planning and management of the programme.

Components of the Current National Access to ARV Programme

Components and characteristics of the present National Access to ARV Programme can be described as follows.

Protocol

Currently, the criteria to include adult patients in the programme are AIDS or asymptomatic HIV infection with CD4 < 200 cell/mm^3. A special scheme, the PMTCT+ Project, has been set up to follow up HIV-infected pregnant women with any CD4 count and their family.

Guidelines on ARV service provision and system have been developed. ART has been used as the standard regimen. Available ARV regimens in NAPHA include:

- D4T+3TC+NVP (GPO-VIR®) as a first-line regimen;
- D4T+3TC+EFV as the second line; and
- D4T+3TC+IDV/r as the third line.

The cost of the first-line regimen is around US$ 30 per month, while the second- and the third-line regimens cost US$ 75 and US$ 135 per month.

It is estimated that the proportion of patients taking the first-line regimen will be 80 to 85 per cent, while the remaining 15 to 20 per cent will have to shift to the second-line regimen. The programme optimistically forecasts that only 5 per cent of the patients will have to eventually take the third-line regimen.

Infrastructure Development and Capacity Building

As mentioned above, all hospitals belonging to the Ministry of Public Health have been trained in a core programme. Health personnel participating in the training programme are medical doctors, nurses, counsellors or social workers, laboratory technicians and pharmacists. Each professional has a responsibility in delivering ARV services in the system. In addition to the core training, additional special training courses for each of the professionals will be offered to improve their knowledge and skills.

Drug Procurement and Distribution

Presently, the estimated ARV requirement is planned centrally, based on the targets of the patients by region and province. Similarly, ARV procurement has also been done by the central office. ARVs are distributed to the participating hospitals through the Regional Office of Disease Prevention and Control.

Monitoring and Evaluation of the ARV Programme

A computerised system has been developed to record ARV service provision. Minimal data are entered to keep track of the number of patients receiving service, occurrence of opportunistic infection, clinical outcome and adherence. Each hospital is required to submit patients' individual reports to the Provincial Health Office and the Regional Office of Disease Prevention and Control, where a monthly summary report is further sent to the Bureau of AIDS, TB and STIs. Special attention will be given to the adherence aspects and to patients who interrupt treatment.

Laboratory Networks

The routine laboratory investigations for clinical assessment are performed at hospitals. In addition, CD4 count facilities for initiating and monitoring treatment are available in 19 regional centres. It is expected that CD4 machines will become more widely available in the near future with funding from the Global Fund.

Civil Society, PLHA and Family Caregiver Involvement

In several ARV demonstration projects, the involvement of the civil society, PLHAs and family caregivers have been shown to have a crucial role in supporting the patient both morally and emotionally to continue taking drugs. Each participating hospital is encouraged to enable and provide support to civil societies, PLHAs and family caregivers to participate in ARV programmes.

Outcomes of the ARV Programme

By September 2003 the cumulative number of AIDS patients having access to ARV was 14,677. Of these, 13,279 are still continuing to take ARVs. The distribution of patients receiving ARVs by type of project is listed in Table 19.1.

Table 19.1
Number of AIDS Patients in ARV Programmes
According to Projects, Thailand: September 2003

Projects	Total enrolment	Current receivers
Access to Care Project: Adults (phase 3)	11,086	10,081
Access to Care Project: Paediatrics (phase 3)	1,621	1,359
PMTCT+ (phase 3)	123	122
Research (continued from phase 2)	1,223	1,160
Co-payment (continued from phase 2)	624	557
Total	14,677	13,279

Future Direction and Challenges

As stated above, the government of Thailand has decided to expand the ARV programme to cover all AIDS patients. To ensure accessibility to all, the system to provide ARV will be developed continuously. The programme will be assessed for its readiness to be included in the benefit package of the Universal Health Assurance Programme. When this happens, the overall management of the ARV programme will be decentralised to the hospital level. The role of the central and regional office will then change to focus on monitoring, quality improvement and evaluation.

In terms of future sustainability, the programme will continue to build the necessary infrastructure, including human resource development, and strengthen partnerships among all stakeholders in the programme. It has been committed that resources will be allocated and funds mobilised for the ARV programme. Almost 80 per cent of all the cost of ARVs this year is coming from the government budget, while the remaining 20 per cent is provided by the Global Fund. Furthermore, ARV drugs have now been adopted as a part of the benefit package in the Social Security Fund, which covers more than 12 million people. It is clear that in future, the programme will move ahead in the direction of including ARV in the Universal Health Insurance.

It must be highlighted that the high costs associated with laboratory tests for the ARV programme must be addressed. While the cost of ARV has dramatically declined in the past five years, the cost for CD4 counts and viral load assessment has not reduced proportionately. As the demand for ARV will predictably increase, the demand for such tests will increase, too. The cost and availability of these tests may have a detrimental effect on the accessibility to ARV programmes.

Adherence to ARV is one of the most important issues in a programme. There is a need for the programme to do its best to maintain levels of adherence. In conjunction to monitoring treatment adherence, programmes must not ignore monitoring ARV drug resistance.

REFERENCES

AIDS Division (no date). Bureau of AIDS, TB and STIs, Department of Diseases Control, Ministry of Public Health, Thailand, http://www.aidsthai.org/aidsenglish.

Ainsworth, Martha, Chris Beyrer and **Agnes Soucat** (2001). AIDS and public policy: The lessons and challenges of 'success' in Thailand. Report, World Bank, Washington, DC.

Jittiwutikarn, J., P. Sawanpanyalert, N. Rangsiveroj and **P. Satitvipawee** (2000). HIV incidence rates among drug users in northern Thailand, 1993–7. *Epidemiological Infection*, 125(1), 153–58.

Limanonda, B., G.J. van Griensven, N. Chongvatana, P. Tirasawat, R.A. Coutinho, W. Auwanit, C. Nartpratarn, C. Likhityingvara and **V. Poshyachinda** (1994). Condom use and risk factors for HIV-1 infection among female commercial sex workers in Thailand. *American Journal of Public Health*, 84(12), 2026–27.

Limpakarnjanarat, K., T.D. Mastro, S. Saisorn, W. Uthaivoravit, J. Kaewkungwal, S. Korattana, N.L. Young, S.A. Morse, D.S. Schmid, B.G. Weniger and **P. Nieburg** (1999). HIV-1 and other sexually transmitted infections in a cohort of female sex workers in Chiang Rai, Thailand. *Sexually Transmitted Infections*, 75(1), 30–35.

Limsuwan, A., S. Kanapa and **Y. Siristonapun** (1986). Acquired immune deficiency syndrome in Thailand. A report of two cases. *Journal of the Medical Association of Thailand*, 69(3), 164–69.

Mason, C.J. et al. (1998). Nationwide surveillance of HIV-1 prevalence and subtype in young Thai men. *Journal of Acquired Immune Deficiency Syndrome and Human Retrovirology*, 19(2), 165–73.

Nelson, K.E. (1994). The epidemiology of HIV infection among injecting drug users and other risk populations in Thailand. *AIDS*, 8(10), 1443–50.

Nelson, K.E., S. Eiumtrakul, D.D. Celentano, C. Beyrer, N. Galai, S. Kawichai and **C. Khamboonruang** (2002). HIV infection in young men in northern Thailand, 1991–1998: Increasing role of injection drug use. *Journal of Acquired Immune Deficiency Syndrome*, 29(1), 62–68.

Prescott, Nicholas (1995). Economic analysis of antiretroviral policy options in Thailand. Paper presented at the Third International Conference on AIDS in Asia and the Pacific, Satellite Session on Regional Use of Antiretrovirals, Chiang Mai, Thailand.

Ruxrungtham, K. and **P. Phanuphak** (2001). Update on HIV/AIDS in Thailand. *Journal of the Medical Association of Thailand*, 84(Supplement 1), S1–17.

Saengwonloey, O., C. Jiraphongsa and **H. Foy** (2003). Thailand report: HIV/AIDS surveillance 1998. *Journal of Acquired Immune Deficiency Syndrome*, 32(Supplement 1), S63–67.

Sawanpanyalert, P., K. Ungchusak, S. Thanprasertsuk and **P. Akarasewi** (1994). HIV-1 seroconversion rates among female commercial sex workers, Chiang Mai, Thailand: A multi cross-sectional study. *AIDS*, 8(6), 825–29.

Sirisopana, N. et al. (1996). Correlates of HIV-1 seropositivity among young men in Thailand. *Journal of Acquired Immune Deficiency Syndrome and Human Retrovirology*, 11(5), 492–98.

Thai Working Group on HIV/AIDS Projection (2001). Projections for HIV/AIDS in Thailand: 2000–2020. Division of AIDS, Department of Communicable Disease Control, Ministry of Public Health, Nonthaburi.

Torugsa, K. et al. (2003). HIV epidemic among young Thai men, 1991–2000. *Emerging Infectious Diseases*, 9(7), http://www.cdc.gov/ncidod/EID/vol9no7/02-0653.htm.

WHO (2000). Evaluation of the HIV/AIDS clinical research network (CRN), coordinated by the Ministry of Public Health, Thailand. Mission report, Office of the WHO Representative to Thailand, July 24–28, 2000.

Wright, N.H., S. Vanichseni, P. Akarasewi, C. Wasi and **K. Choopanya** (1994). Was the 1988 HIV epidemic among Bangkok's injecting drug users a common source outbreak? *AIDS*, 8(4), 529–32.

20

SOCIAL AND CULTURAL DIMENSIONS OF HIV/AIDS

Waranya Teokul

HIV/AIDS has profound effects on individuals and the society. Several researchers have measured the social impact of HIV/AIDS at the individual, family and community levels in terms of socio-demographic indices, morbidity and mortality. The way the impact is measured and reported helps shape the public response to the HIV/AIDS problem. For example, reports on the stigma and discrimination suffered by people living with HIV/AIDS and their families have drawn attention to 'human rights' issues even in societies such as the Thai one, which once valued community rights over individual rights. Barnett et al. (2000) reviewed several studies on the social and economic impact of HIV/AIDS in poor countries and concluded that most of the social impact can be observed at micro and macro levels. While numerous studies have investigated the social impact of HIV/AIDS in Africa, there are few similar studies in South and South-East Asia. This paper unfolds the social impact of HIV/AIDS in selected countries of South and South-East Asia and summarises lessons learned and the potential challenges in shaping future responses.

Impact on People Living with HIV/AIDS and Their Families

Many social and economic determinants such as poverty and societal marginalisation render groups of individuals and their families susceptible and vulnerable to HIV infection. Stigma, discrimination and collective denial associated with HIV infection makes the life of the individual and that of family members agonising. A study on the forms, determinants and outcomes of HIV/AIDS-related discrimination, stigmatisation and denial in India showed that people living with HIV/AIDS (PLHA) were sometimes denied the right to health services or discriminated against in health settings. Examples of such discrimination include:

> refusal to provide treatment for HIV/AIDS-related illness; refusal to hospitalise for care/treatment; refusal to operate or assist in clinical procedures; restricted access to facilities like toilets and common utensils; physical isolation in the ward (e.g., separate arrangements for a bed outside the ward in a gallery or corridor); cessation of on-going treatment; early discharge from hospital; mandatory testing for HIV before surgery and during pregnancy; restrictions on movement around the ward or in the room; over precaution by health care staff; refusal to lift or touch the dead body of an HIV-positive person; use of plastic sheets to wrap the dead body; and reluctance to provide transport for the body. (UNAIDS 2001)

Even in their daily lives PLHAs are faced with 'severed relationships, desertion and separation from family members or relatives, even physical isolation at home, e.g., separate sleeping arrangements' (ibid.). Similar practices were also observed in Thailand during the early stages of the epidemic in the mid-1990s. Various activities of hospital staff led indirectly to breach of confidentiality, resulting in patient's sero-status becoming known to persons other than their direct health care providers. A recent survey conducted in Thailand during 1999–2001, however, reported a positive change: among the 85 survey sites in the country, 82 per cent of respondents reported either positive or neutral overall community reaction, and 87 per cent reported a trend towards more tolerance. Areas without NGOs actively working on AIDS had fewer AIDS families treated the same way they were before their misfortune. Negative community reaction towards PLHAs arises from questionable character of the PLHAs themselves rather than because of their sero-status. Meanwhile, negative community reactions towards affected families were more pronounced during illness than after their death (VanLandingham et al. 2002).

On Orphans

Children of PLHAs, regardless of their HIV status, face social exclusion such as not being able to play with other children or being forced to drop out of school due to irrational fears among parents of other children. The situation causes these children psychological trauma (Kulkarni and Shukla 2001). Anecdotal reports of similar instances have been made from few provinces of Thailand. The children eventually become orphans after the death of one or both parents. Some of them are themselves living with HIV, thereby subjecting them to daily hardships. According to UNAIDS, by the end of 2001, there were 325,000 orphans aged 0 to 14 years living in South-East Asia countries except in India (UNAIDS et al. 2002). It should be noted that in terms of absolute numbers Asia has a higher number of both orphans and AIDS orphans than Africa. While the percentage of AIDS orphan to total number of children in Asia is steady over years at approximately 3 per cent throughout the period, Africa shows an alarming increase from 0.4 per cent in 1990 to an estimated level of 5.8 per cent in 2010 (Figure 20.1). These projections render the problem of AIDS orphans in Asia 'invisible', though its magnitude deserves 'global' attention.

Figure 20.1
Percentage of AIDS Orphans to Total Number of
Children Aged 0–14 Years in Asia and Africa: 1990–2010

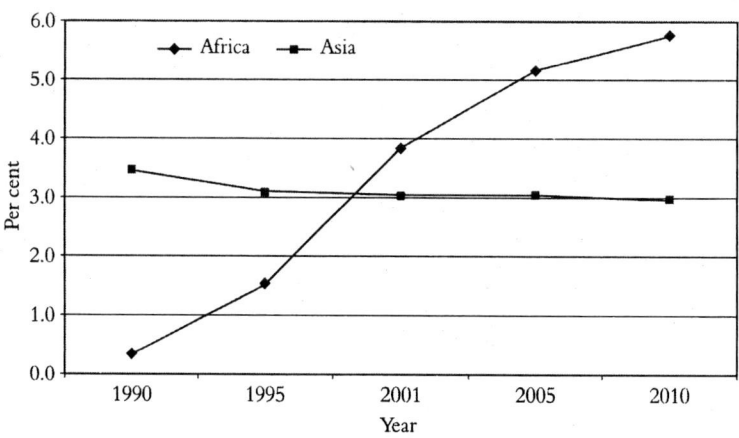

Source: UNAIDS et al. (2002).

On Widows

Besides emotional stress and the burden of caregiving, women in India face difficulties in maintaining their share of matrimonial or joint family property. After their husband's death, most Indian women were denied shelter in their own home by their in-laws and are not welcomed in their maternal home (Ghosh 2001; Johari and Divan 2001; Johari and Parmar 2001).

On the Elderly

In Thailand aged parents are a source of refuge and safety net for PLHAs. A study in the upper northern part of Thailand among 963 adult cases—who either died of AIDS or were currently symptomatic—showed that, regardless of their gender, two-thirds of PLHAs move back to their communities to live near their parents during the terminal stages of their illness. The parents are actively involved in caregiving and in providing financial and material support for people with HIV. In most cases, when PLHAs die, the aged parents, besides grieving for the untimely death of their sons or daughters, also bear the burden of bringing up their grandchildren. Some face negative reactions from the community, but not after the death of the family member with HIV (Knodel et al. 2000a, 2000b; Knodel and Saengtienchai 2002; Knodel and VanLandingham 2001; VanLandingham et al. 2002).

On the Community

In the South-East Asian community the social impact of HIV/AIDS range from expressions of shock and disbelief to social disintegration due to irrational fear, discrimination and stigmatisation; changes in community life, cultural, norms and practices; and demographic change due to excessive deaths among the adult population. Furthermore, increasing evidence that efforts to counter such social consequences resulting from the HIV/AIDS epidemic often lead to the formation of community-based organisations and fostering of civil society.

In most communities the very first groups that experienced the impact of HIV/AIDS were those who were socially disadvantaged and those who engaged in risk behaviour. As an initial response, usually the community tended to disassociate itself from HIV/AIDS with denial, discrimination and stigmatisation. Hence, most studies highlight the role of the community in mitigating negative attitudes and in creating a supportive environment. While communities have not been systematically assessed for sociocultural change after the impact of HIV/AIDS, empirical evidence suggests that some communities in Thailand changed their cultural practices regarding the 'purification' of the body (ritually observed for one who has passed away) in order to prevent the spread of HIV (Songwattana 2001). One-fifth of families in the upper north and one-third elsewhere with a family member living with AIDS have reported negative community reactions or being isolated, but few report such negative experiences after death of an adult member (Knodel et al. 2000b).

In the upper north of Thailand, where half of the total AIDS deaths in the country have been reported since the beginning of the HIV/AIDS epidemic, most rural communities have experienced adult illness or death due to HIV/AIDS (Im-emm and Phuangsaichai 1999). On an average, 20 persons in each village of Sanpatong, a district with the highest prevalence of AIDS in Chiang Mai province, had died of AIDS since 1992. This certainly affected community resource management (Thangphet 2001). Most studies at the community level usually focus on the economic impact rather than social change. Therefore, it cannot be concluded that such phenomena would lead to demographic change, although a different demographic profile was observed in the six upper northern provinces hardest hit with HIV. Census figures of 1990 and 2000, when compared, showed that there were fewer people between 20 and 34 years of age in 2000 than 10 years ago.

Generally, community is referred to as a group of people living in the same geographical location or administrative boundary such as a village or a sub-district. The HIV/AIDS epidemic, together with international and national support, has created a new definition of community. It binds together a group of individuals who share a common interest across the boundaries of their residential area to respond to HIV/AIDS. These groups of people may come together for counselling services as self-help groups. According to the AIDS Division, Ministry of Public Health, Thailand, the number of AIDS NGOs increased from 23 to 184 between 1992 and 1997. Similarly, the number of PLHA groups increased from 11 in 1994 to 108 in 1997. A survey among 304 PLHA groups in Thailand, between August 1999 and January 2000 found that most of them were established during 1996–99 and almost half were based in the upper north (Smitakestrin 2001).

Collective Responses to the HIV/AIDS Problem

Generally, the social impact of HIV/AIDS at the national level is always understood to mean impact in terms of the increasing burden in delivery of social services such as health, education and welfare, rather than observing changes in the social context. In any country, including those that are resource limited, financial resources to mitigate social impact is often skewed towards health and medical care for people living with HIV/AIDS. As a consequence, limited resources are provided for the increasing demand for social services, either for PLHAs or for their dependents. Table 20.1 provides examples of the social impact on each group affected by HIV/AIDS and the potential response. However, it should be noted that none of social impact studies document long-term impact on families and children of PLHAs, though some countries, including Thailand, have experienced AIDS deaths for more than two decades.

In the health sector, knowledge and experiences have been widely shared, both at international and national levels, for improving or inducing changes in regular health practices to respond to the HIV/AIDS problem. For example, health personnel who directly provide treatment and care for PLHAs must keep patients' HIV status confidential. They are repeatedly trained to improve their capabilities in the area of HIV/AIDS care and familiarised with the latest medical technology. For example, even in the midst of an economic crisis, the Thai government's spending for expansion of health facilities and improving health care for AIDS and related illness accounted to almost one-fifth (19.2 per cent) of the total government spending on HIV/AIDS prevention and control programme in 1997.

The HIV/AIDS problem also highlights deficiencies in the existing social protection systems in developing countries. Most empirical studies describe the social impact and tragedy suffered by those afflicted and affected by HIV/AIDS. But it is hard to find well-documented systematic responses for any country in the South-East Asia region. A common intervention to mitigate social impact is psychosocial support through provision of counselling services. While most persons affected by HIV/ AIDS face difficulties in living their daily lives, responses to meet such needs, from the government and NGOs are neither comprehensive nor wide in coverage, and are considered marginal and fragmented.

Table 20.1
Examples of Social Impact in Particular Groups
Affected by HIV/AIDS and Potential Responses

Population group	Nature of social impact	Results	
		Emerging problems	Preventive measures
Babies/children	• Psychological trauma due to stigmatisation and discrimination • Forced to leave school • Forced into orphanage	• Limited availability of orphanage homes • Providing foster families • Family members, relatives help taking care after death of parents	• Preventing mother-to-child transmission by providing ARV and formula milk
Wives/widows	• Psychological trauma due to stigmatisation and discrimination • Inheritance rights	• Counselling services • Temporary shelters	• None
Parents/elderly	• Psychological trauma due to stigmatisation and discrimination	• None	• None
People living with HIV/ AIDS	• Psychological trauma due to stigmatisation and discrimination • Loss of job	• Counselling services • Social support by groups of PLHAs • Occupational retraining • Financial support for head start of self-employed businesses	• None

For example, in 2001, an administrative report by the Ministry of Interior, Thailand, indicated that in rural areas there were 54,604 orphans and 11,674 children affected by HIV/AIDS. The UNAIDS estimates for the number of AIDS orphans in Thailand in the year 2001 is 289,000, which is over five times higher than the government's figures. Even the public response to this problem is strikingly marginal. The Department of Social Welfare, as of August 2003, has been able to care for only 285 orphans, 1,206 abandoned children and 291 children affected by HIV/AIDS, out of the 4,214 children in their custody. In addition, the agency also provides child allowance to a limited number of poor families. A scheme covers 11,117 children in the Bangkok metropolitan area and 50,000 children in the rest of the country, compared to 2.9 million children living below poverty level. However, with limited resources, such financial support is equivalent to 286 baht per child per year (or US$ 75 a year), which is barely adequate for raising a child in decent conditions. Although the government has mobilised additional resource from non-budgetary sources, such as education scholarship for children from poor families, including children affected by HIV/AIDS, this new source of money can only support up to 75,000 children per year.

The situation reflects the enormous gap in responding to the HIV/AIDS problem, both in terms of sufficiency and adequacy. It is likely that these children are trapped in the vicious cycle of poverty. The key questions are: Why are concerned parties complacent with such a situation? Why are none of the AIDS NGOs vigorously campaigning for mobilising more financial support to children affected by HIV/AIDS as they have been doing for antiretroviral treatment for PLHAs? A possible explanation is that there is a social welfare system put in place to provide social support to those affected with HIV/AIDS, regardless of its limited availability. ARV treatment, despite being expensive for per capita financing, is not very well in place and cannot be claimed as a success story in fighting against HIV/AIDS. HIV/AIDS programmes around the world are biased towards care for PLHAs and not enough concern is being shown to secure the future of the dependents of PLHAs. There is still lack of innovative mechanisms and financial resources from the public or private sector to adequately respond to this social aspect of the HIV/AIDS epidemic.

Despite the gloomy situation, as in the case of Thailand, the HIV/AIDS problem has induced positive social changes. HIV/AIDS demands multi-sectoral collaboration from public sectors, both health and non-health, and from private sectors such as NGOs, CBOs and private businesses. All these stakeholders actively participate in the whole process of HIV/AIDS management at both the local and national levels. It also stimulates formation of community-based organisations to fight against the spread of HIV/AIDS and to provide psychosocial support for PLHAs. It makes the concerned authorities recognise the necessity of engaging civic groups in the overall process of development, which had never been done earlier. Though these NGOs and CBOs seem to confine their response only to specific interests and for the benefit of their constituency, that is, PLHAs, they occasionally elevate their response for public interest—this helps foster social capital in any society.

Future Challenges

Published literature on the social impact of HIV/AIDS describes the suffering of individuals and families, often without providing the magnitude of the problem. It is considerably difficult to find any documentation on the systematic responses being made to combat the social impact associated with HIV/AIDS. The interventions to address adverse consequences of HIV/AIDS mainly consist of counselling services (either institutional service or promoting formation of self-help groups), preventing mother-to-child transmission through antiretroviral treatment and providing milk substitute, home visits, financial assistance to the family, occupational training and financial support for education. These fragmented interventions serve PLHAs while they are alive. Interventions targeting the group of individuals affected by HIV/AIDS are extremely limited. These target groups include orphans caused by HIV/AIDS, widows and the elderly, who are an integral part of social services. Currently there is a huge gap relative to the demand of these target groups. How come we have failed to mobilise substantial support for mitigating adverse consequences of HIV/AIDS to our society? This may be in part due to competing priorities. When the public and PLHAs place more emphasis on one intervention, there will be less resource to finance other interventions.

Ironically, though we can anticipate the magnitude of social impact experienced by each population group and know what types of response are needed, there is still a huge gap between actual demand and availability of public response. Future challenges include allocating limited resources appropriately between health care interventions for people living with HIV/AIDS and social support interventions for those affected by HIV/AIDS, and mobilising additional resources that sufficiently respond to current unmet needs. In addition, there is a need for studying the long-term social impact of HIV/AIDS on families of people living with HIV/AIDS.

R EFERENCES

Barnett, T., A. Whiteside and **C. Desmond** (2000). The social and economic impact of HIV/AIDS in poor countries: A review of studies and lessons. Draft report, UNAIDS, Geneva.

Ghosh, M. (2001). HIV positive widows trapped between the dilemma of social inequality and disease. Poster presentation at the Sixth International Congress on AIDS in Asia and the Pacific, Melbourne , 5–10 October.

Im-emm, W. and **S. Phuangsaichai** (1999). Household resources allocation and responses toward AIDS-related illnesses. Paper, Institute for Population and Social Research, Mahidol University, Nakhon Pathom, Thailand.

Johari, V. and **V. Divan** (2001). The legal system: Breaking the silence and social barriers. Abstract presentation at the Sixth International Congress on AIDS in Asia and the Pacific, Melbourne, 5–10 October.

Johari, V. and **S. Parmar** (2001). Gender bias in personal laws relating to property, inheritance, maintenance and residence. Poster presentation at the Sixth International Congress on AIDS in Asia and the Pacific, Melbourne, 5–10 October.

Knodel, J. and **C. Saengtienchai** (2002). Older aged parents: The final safety net for adults sons and daughters with AIDS in Thailand. Paper presented at IUSSP Regional Population Conference, Bangkok, 10–12 June.

Knodel, J. and **M. VanLandingham** (2001). Return migration in the context of parental assistance in the AIDS epidemic: The Thai experience. Paper presented at the Twenty-fourth General Population Conference of the IUSSP, Salvador, Brazil, 18–24 August.

Knodel, J. M., M. VanLandingham, C. Saengtienchai and **W. Im-emm** (2000a). Older people and AIDS: Quantitative evidence of the impact in Thailand. Report no. 00-443, Population Studies Centre, Institute for Social Research, University of Michigan, Michigan.

———— (2000b). The impact of Thailand's AIDS epidemic on older persons: Quantitative evidence from a survey of key informants. Report no. 00-448, Population Studies Centre, Institute for Social Research, University of Michigan, Michigan.

Kulkarni, S. and **A.D. Shukla** (2001). Are we the reason for their social death? A HIV positive children's dilemma. Poster presentation at the Sixth International Congress on AIDS in Asia and the Pacific, Melbourne, 5–10 October.

Smitakestrin, S. (2001). Characteristics of people living with HIV/AIDS groups in Thailand, 1999–2000. Poster presentation at the Sixth International Congress on AIDS in Asia and the Pacific, Melbourne, 5–10 October.

Songwattana, P. (2001). Role of faith based organizations in HIV/AIDS care in southern communities. Paper presented at the Eighth Thailand National AIDS Conference, 11–13 July.

Thangphet, S. (2001). The impact of HIV/AIDS on community-based resource management: A case study of an indigenous irrigation system in northern Thailand. Mimeograph, Mahidol University, Bangkok, http://www.cbnrm.net/pdf/Thangphet_s_001_hivaidsirrigation.pdf.

UNAIDS (2001). *India: HIV and AIDS-related Discrimination, Stigmatization and Denial.* UNAIDS.

UNAIDS, UNICEF and USAID (2002). Children on the brink 2002: A joint report on orphans estimate and program strategies. 16–30 July.

VanLandingham, M., W. Im-Emm and C. Saengtienchai (2002). Community reaction to persons with HIV/AIDS and their parents in Thailand. Report no. 02-530, Population Studies Centre, Institute for Social Research, University of Michigan, Michigan.

21

NGOs in Asia: Key Partners in the Fight against AIDS

Teresita Marie P. Bagasao

When AIDS started gaining public attention in the 1980s, amongst the first to take action to provide support and care were close friends, family members and other individuals who came from the same interest groups as people living with HIV and AIDS (PLHAs). Several community-based organisations and non-governmental organisations have since emerged from these groups hardest hit by HIV. Despite reluctance and slow action from many governments, these NGOs, particularly AIDS service organisations (ASOs), came forward to provide the critical care and support to HIV-affected people mainly because they were closer to the problem and enjoyed the trust of people on the ground. Beyond this personal support, many of these organisations have evolved into effective advocates who helped put issues squarely on to national agendas (Bagasao 1998). Even up to the present time, these NGOs push the boundaries and open debates on a range of sensitive issues like sex, gender, illness, human rights, mobility and drug use, while at the same time they have pioneered in carrying out innovative action to make prevention, care and treatment available.

NGO Involvement: Beyond Mere Service Provision

Reviewing developments around involvement of civil society[1] until the mid-1990s, Söderholm (1997) confirmed the critical role of NGOs as social advocates. In his observation, the innovative ways to reach civil society essentially had boiled down to advocating for NGO and PWA participation in national AIDS programmes, providing resources earmarked for NGO activities and stimulating networks and consortia with an eye to the development of joint policy formulations among the heterogeneous NGOs, and lastly, representation on decision making at all levels by PWA and NGO representatives. He likewise noted that even in the broader field of development, NGOs were brought in primarily at the last level of the process, that is, as providers of services and contractors. Despite the insistence of NGOs to participate in the entire process—from policy development to implementation and evaluation—this remained a major challenge, especially at the country level as governments were perceived by ASOs to be very hesitant to enter into shared decision making.

AIDS Successes in the Region and Civil Society Participation

Updates on the regional situation seem to indicate that the Asia Pacific continues to be characterised by multiple AIDS epidemics with equally diverse modes of HIV transmission, the populations and communities affected, and policy and programme responses (Kaldor et al. 1998). Within this context, NGOs have been unrelenting in facing up to the challenge, and they continue to push for their place in the policy and decision-making arenas, from local to national and regional. From a review of a number of prevention, care and support programmes in the region, it can be concluded that effective programmes were those that:

- Involve and grow out of the community whose behaviours they seek to change. Only when those engaging in risk behaviour are involved in the design and implementation of prevention efforts are those efforts likely to adequately reflect an understanding of the local environment and context of risk and vulnerability.
- Involve multiple partners and multiple prevention components to address the multitude of environmental and contextual factors influencing risk and vulnerability. That is, they must be multisectoral in nature and involve multiple components working at multiple levels.

Growing Out of the Community

Well over two decades into the epidemic, the responses to AIDS continue to grow out of direct actions taken by diverse affected communities.

336 Teresita Marie P. Bagasao

A more recent example of such action among a marginalised group involves a local Indonesian CBO that set up a programme for trans-gender (*waria*) sex workers. As part of coming together in their efforts at building their community, the *warias* included the dissemination of information on HIV and appropriate safer behaviours. While the longer-term impact is yet to be seen, this has led *warias* to reach an agreement amongst them not to have unprotected sex and monitor each other in the parks when they meet their clients.

Another example involves a network of women sex workers from Sonagachi, the largest red-light area in Kolkata existing for over a century. The network has evolved into Durbar Mahila Samanaya Committee (DMSC) with about 60,000 sex workers in West Bengal. The peer education programme initiated in the early 1990s led to empowerment of these sex workers. This peer-to-peer interaction elicited a more open and accepting response from the sex workers. Today these peer educators also include men who interact with customers, mostly in getting them to agree to condom use. One of Sonagachi's most documented successes is the reported dramatic increase in overall condom use from 2.7 per cent in 1992 to over 90 per cent in 1998 among female sex workers. Besides promoting behaviour change related to safer sexual practices, Sonagachi developed a self-run cooperative called Usha Cooperative Society. This society offers loans to women to purchase daily needs from reasonably priced stories, especially in times of need. This has freed them from dependence on their pimps and madams. The success of Sonagachi has been promoted as a model in other areas. In New Delhi female sex workers called a meeting with the theme *Meri Awaz Suno* (Listen to My Voice) and protested with one voice against social injustice and demanded attention from the state government, particularly on police harassment, poor health care and forced HIV testing. This was the first time that sex workers met on the same platform with government officials and health workers. This resulted in Delhi's chief minister ordering a survey of the city's brothel conditions to identify problems needed to be addressed by policy.

The story of Mae Chan in northern Thailand further demonstrates how action that grows out of and also involves different sectors of the community can lead to desired outcomes. The community has succeeded in bringing together unlikely partners—monks, students, sex workers, people living with HIV and AIDS, and health providers. For example, monks deliver prevention messages as part of their sermons and visit people living with HIV and AIDS in their homes. Another key feature is that groups normally excluded, such as sex workers and PLHAs, are invited to take active part in the village meetings. The acceptance and visibility of these groups is said to help decrease the alienation among marginalised groups. Working together, these different community groups have contributed to the decline in new infections and the 'stabilisation' of the epidemic (Hart 2001).

Shalom, an NGO in Manipur, India, has received international recognition for its work on injecting drug use and HIV. From a pilot needle and syringe project set up in 1995, it has evolved into a state-wide programme involving 12 other NGOs under the Manipur State AIDS Control Society, and receives support from national and international agencies. From a single organisational action initially regarded as controversial by authorities who perceived the project to be a blatant endorsement of drug use, evidence showed that the intervention actually helped reduce the rampant practice of needle sharing among drug users and subsequently helped decrease HIV transmission. While the programme still faces its share of problems, it continues to be used in the state.

In a decentralised political environment, NGOs in the Philippines working with their local governments demonstrated positive outcomes of collaboration. In the island province of Palawan, south-west of Manila, despite no reported HIV cases, the NGO IHAIN managed to get the provincial government to launch education programmes as a major prevention effort. In Olongapo City, located in a province north of Manila, the scenario was different, since the city reported many HIV infections. In this setting, the NGO OCAFI managed to work well with the city government to launch initiatives that protected the rights of PLHAs and provide them with appropriate support. These initiatives included sensitising the community and raising their awareness and understanding of HIV/AIDS-related issues, providing counselling services and referral for health care as well as support for livelihood opportunities for PLHAs.

Strengthening National Response through Collaboration

The impact of NGO involvement is not only manifest in local action. Over the last two decades NGOs and even governments realised the need and value of coordination and joint action. A lesson learned across the following examples is that NGO umbrella bodies can enhance proper coordination and networking amongst AIDS NGOs and at the same time provide a mechanism for NGOs to work with their own government and other sectors.

When everyone was still grappling with difficulties of breaking the silence around AIDS, Australia provided a model of how many organisations representing a diverse range of interests growing out of the epidemic from all over the country can come together to support each other as well as help inform government policy. The peak body for such groups is the Australian Federation of AIDS Organisations (AFAO). It also pioneered in reaching out to its neighbours throughout the Asia and the Pacific, to share lessons learned from its own expertise that evolved from experience primarily with marginalised groups—sex workers, gay men and IDUs. The AFAO's position gives it a unique role in developing partnerships with such groups. The responses, which are based on capacity building and emphasising peer education as a central process in promoting safe sex, appear to have been relatively successful.

In Malaysia the seed of coordination among NGOs in the country was sown in the early 1990s when the Ministry of Health (MOH) called for an informal meeting with a handful of NGOs working on HIV/AIDS (Hussein 1996). The MOH hoped that through this meeting a national NGO umbrella body to increase networking between NGOs and the different government ministries would result. Two years later the umbrella body known as the Malaysian AIDS Council (MAC) was born with eight affiliated organisations and at the turn of the century included more than 30 affiliates. This growth in membership is proof enough of MAC's strength and capacity to respond to its memberships needs—ranging from HIV/AIDS education, care and treatment to advocacy and outreach, and fund raising to sustain their efforts. One of its notable achievements is the setting up of a PLHA Business Assistance Fund in 2002 to provide loans to PLHAs and their families with no interest. The example set by MAC 'strengthens the position of NGOs, giving them one voice, making for easier interaction with government'. It should come as no surprise, therefore, that MAC continues to be the avenue for government and NGO interaction and liaison on HIV/AIDS work as well as the government's conduit for financial support to NGOs in the country.

In Cambodia the Khmer HIV/AIDS NGO Alliance (KHANA) was set up in 1996 as a project of the UK-based International HIV/AIDS Alliance. KHANA gradually evolved and registered as a local NGO in 1999 with a mission to support and strengthen local NGO and CBO responses to HIV/AIDS. From a modest start of seven local partner

NGOs within a year of its establishment, KHANA has increased its reach and provides up to '39 local NGOs and CBOs in 2002 to implement 53 HIV/AIDS projects in 14 provinces and three municipalities across Cambodia. As a result, KHANA is now recognised nationally as a key player in the national response to the epidemic in Cambodia' (KHANA 2003). KHANA works in close collaboration with the government to strengthen services that improve quality of care for PLHAs. It has managed to expand geographical reach as well as 'scaling out'[2] to support development of new groups in 2002 with a strategic focus in increasing the involvement of key vulnerable populations such as young people, sex workers and men who have sex with men as well as people living with HIV and AIDS. At the same time, KHANA participates actively in the national NGO coordinating mechanism, the HIV/AIDS Coordinating Council (HACC). Sopheap, coordinator of the HACC, attests that both technical and financial support from KHANA since 2000 has helped the HACC to strengthen the capacities of NGOs working on the issue as well as the coordination of common activities, allowing the HACC to increase the number of NGOs participating in the network from 30 to 80.

The Indian Network of People Living with HIV/AIDS (INP+), formed in February 1997 by 12 people living with HIV, has developed into a national network of, for and by people living with HIV/AIDS in India. Through several capacity building programmes ranging from organisational and network development, leadership, skills building in public speaking, women's workshops, communications and public relations, INP+ has managed to set up state-level networks in at least 12 states, including Tamil Nadu, Maharashtra, Karnataka, Goa, Kerala and Manipur. Its efforts at unifying and providing a voice for PLHAs is slowly being recognised. In practical terms, it participates as a new member, providing the PLHA perspective to the UN theme group on AIDS, a forum that forges links between UN agencies and local government ministries around AIDS policy and programme development.

Advocating for Responsive Policy and Action

Bringing about responsive policies and action does not always readily result from collaboration with policy makers. Often groups most affected come together to advocate for these changes to take place on the basis of universal human rights or evidence of what works (Quan 2003).

In the case of Thailand, two national coalitions came together to work on a common issue related to access to treatment. For three years the Thai NGO Coalition on AIDS (TNCA) worked with the Thai Network of People Living with HIV/AIDS (TNP+) to encourage its government to provide ARV drugs under its national health insurance scheme. Another global network, the International Gay and Lesbian Human Rights Commission (IGLHRC) also helped in the letter campaign addressed to the prime minister and the minister of health, containing the Thai coalitions' position on universal access to ARV. On World AIDS Day 2001 (following the UN General Assembly Special Session on HIV/AIDS [UNGASS]), the MOH formally announced its decision to extend its 30-baht health care scheme to cover ARVs and created a panel to oversee the implementation, which includes representatives from TNP+. Moreover, further campaigning of both national coalitions to improve access played a key role in pushing for compulsory licensing of generic drugs. Reports state that this helped to reduce the time it took to license generic brands from three months to one month (Lockhart et al. 2001).

In the meantime, similar outcomes were documented in India around the issue of drug use. Through joint advocacy of NGOs like Sharan, the Lawyers Collective and other voluntary organisations, the harsh Narcotics Drugs and Psychotropic Substances Act (NDPS) of 1995 was reviewed and amended in 2001, 'making the code related to drug use more realistic, including making needle exchange and buprenorphine substitution services legitimate in the country' (Samson and Batra 2003).

Moving Beyond Borders

From individual organisational responses, NGOs have realised the value of strength in numbers and the advantage of cooperation. In recent years civil society has put more efforts into building capacities to forge alliances and coalitions, moving beyond one interest group to include other groups, in communities, at all levels from local, national and across borders. In the case of AIDS, one of the factors that facilitated the groundswell of community response is when more experienced and resourced coalitions reach out to NGOs in neighbouring countries. Soon enough, even under-resourced organisations started to form alliances based on common interests and tried to strategise advocating changes in country through cooperation reached in regional and international arenas.

Moving from their own in-country experience, the AFAO began to reach out to local NGOs from its Asia Pacific neighbours. The series of study tours it initiated in 1990 brought together NGOs from across the region to share and learn about effective prevention and care strategies. Further strengthening its international programme, it supported work with Wednesday's Friends, a fledgling group of PLHAs in the early 1990s involved in care, support and peer education in Thailand. The project aimed to provide a venue for Wednesday's Friends to plan and carry out activities by out-of-town PLHAs when they came for hospital visits. In this way, the development of Wednesday's Friends from a group of committed people to a well-run, self-help community organisation was facilitated (Marshall and Hunt 1997).

Also, in late 1990, the Asia Pacific Council of AIDS Service Organisations (APCASO) grew out of the need for NGOs and CBOs to come together in safe spaces, and share experience and strategies to strengthen community responses in an environment of widespread denial about HIV and its threat to communities and societies. Seizing opportunities in conferences and other forums, it facilitated spaces and support that gave birth to or led to strengthening of regional networks, for example, the Asia Pacific Network of People Living with HIV/AIDS (APN+) and the Coordination for Action Research on AIDS and Mobility (CARAM) network. Even with the emergence of strong interest-based networks, APCASO still finds itself very much playing the role of a facilitator and promoting civil society spaces where voices of different constituencies can be presented. In the mid-1990s it carried out a number of sub-regional skill-building workshops on HIV and human rights in South-East and South Asia as well as with the network of PLHAs. This has led to the adoption of frameworks of action on HIV founded on universal human rights at both country and regional levels such as in Cambodia, Malaysia and the Philippines.

Using the Declaration of Commitment as framework, APCASO is moving in two areas of action. The first relates to the newly created Global Fund to Fight AIDS, TB and Malaria (Global Fund), which clearly supports civil society participation in the country coordinating mechanisms it set up to develop and implement proposals. As a new mechanism, it was not clear how NGOs could actually participate and ensure that their issues are reflected in the proposals submitted by governments. A review of NGO participation in this new financing mechanism indicated that NGOs felt that there was 'a complete lack of information flow to NGOs from the Global Fund and the government, even to those of us who are members of the CCM' (Daly 2002). In September 2002 APCASO organised an NGO consultation for the region, bringing together more than 35 participants in over 13 countries. The consultation helped NGOs at the country level to understand Global Fund processes, and provided an opportunity to share experiences regarding their participation in the country coordinating mechanisms set up the Global Fund.

APCASO also saw the opportunity to increase the profile and capacities of civil society to be involved by using the 2001 UNGASS on AIDS Declaration of Commitment, which embodied language that supports civil society participation in all aspects of the response to the epidemic (APCASO 2002). From feedback in several forums, APCASO recognised that NGOs at the country level, even those that work in coalitions, were grappling with how to move on the commitments contained in the Declaration. Two advocacy workshops have so far been carried out. The Philippine workshop brought together 21 NGOs in 2002 and resulted in concrete recommendations to the Philippine National Council on the country's progress report and led to the formation of a forum to explore how NGOs can further participate in monitoring and accounting for progress. In Bangladesh the STI/AIDS Network managed to bring together over 40 participants, including the government, in 2003. As a direct result, separate working groups with links to the government AIDS programme were created to address the following key issues identified in the advocacy workshop: prevention among vulnerable groups, prevention among young people, and care and support, with the issue of stigma and discrimination as a cross-cutting issue to be dealt with by all groups.

Central to any response to HIV/AIDS is the role that PLHAs play. In 1994 the APN+ was born when 40 PLHAs from self-help groups in eight different countries within the region met in Kuala Lumpur, Malaysia. At its inception many PLHAs reported experiencing tremendous pressure both from their governments and society as well as feeling neglected in terms of treatment and care. It tried to foster the development of local and national PLHA organisations, for example, Spiritia in Indonesia or CPN+ in Cambodia, through supporting information exchange and skills building on a number of issues. It also developed a manual called 'Lifting the Burden of Secrecy', a tool to help PLHAs strengthen their skills to speak out on their issues, and put not only a face but, more importantly, the voice of PLHAs in the national response. The APN+ also undertook a human rights pilot monitoring project in India, Indonesia, the Philippines and Thailand. The project empowered PLHAs in these countries to gather and analyse information related to their conditions. The information has been used to foster dialogue not only within the respective PLHA organisations that participated, but also with governments and other sectors to try and address the needs identified in the study. In relation to the issue of access to treatment, it has initiated a regional buyers' club to explore ways of bringing much-needed treatment to its members. To date, the APN+ works with local PLHA groups in at least 13 countries, including the TNP+ and INP+, featured in other sections of this paper.

Coordinated Action and Networks on Specific Issues

To address issues related to migration and HIV, the CARAM network traces its beginnings to a consultation workshop on migration and HIV/AIDS in 1991. However, the network was formally born in 1997 in seven countries and is now working in 11 countries. CARAM examines issues from two sides of the coin—from the perspective of both the sending and host countries. While sending countries provide some support for their migrant labour, much needed services in receiving or host countries are often inadequate or non-existent. Programmes are developed through participatory action research that involves the communities. As a result, some of the innovative programmes the members of the network have initiated include: pre-departure programmes on reproductive health for domestic workers in Cambodia, reintegration programme for returnees and peer educators' development in Bangladesh; seafarers' spouse programme in the Philippines; development of legal support and rights education in Malaysia; and radio programmes and violence against women programmes for Burmese migrants in Thailand. Besides these concrete support programmes, the network also engages in policy development. One success story is how through its work in this area it helped get the government in Bangladesh to include in its 1997 strategic plan document a policy on non-mandatory HIV testing for HIV.

Another regional network that has grown out of modest beginnings of 49 individual pioneers in pushing effective programmes dealing with the difficult issue of drug and HIV in the region is the Asian Harm Reduction Network (AHRN). Having turned seven in early 2003, the

AHRN has grown immensely to a network of over 2,500 members. It links as well as provides support services and technical assistance from its internal pool of experts and contacts to promote activities to prevent HIV and other harm associated with injecting drug use. Proof of its effective promotion of partnerships between communities and experts who provide law makers with evidence of harm reduction as a solution is the reported recent turn of events in Indonesia, where a needle and syringe exchange is being considered as a ministerial decree by the health ministry.

Sex workers have also shown solidarity across borders. In South Asia reaching out to its neighbours in Bangladesh and Nepal, the DMSC's latest action involves a campaign to raise awareness of tuberculosis among its members and to get them to seek treatment. Moreover, in the last couple of years, the network has put together three large conferences, inviting other international bodies to participate. Among the demands that came from these conference include the right to self-governance, restriction of under-age girls to be forced into sex work, regular health checks and recognition under the government's labour laws.

The DMSC links with other organisations of sex workers beyond South Asia, through the Asia Pacific Network of Sex Workers (ASPNSW). Bringing together lessons learned and experiences of what works for sex workers in prevention, care and support, the network came together early in 2003 and in collaboration with an international NGO is currently producing a multimedia pack entitled *Making Sex Work Safe* borne out of their own strategies that work. The tool, when completed, will be made available throughout the region in language that sex workers can understand.

Connecting Communities through Technology

One of the major factors that lead to change is access to information. In this age of digital technology, this is made possible through electronic communications. An NGO that has pioneered in using this medium to bridge communities on a range of issues is the Health and Development Network (HDNet 2001). The use of electronic networking and communications technology allows it to operate virtually to act on its vision of moving more effective responses by strengthening the sharing of information, communication and improving the quality of debate.

Besides bringing issues discussed on various regional and international platforms on health and development, including AIDS, it moderates feedback received from NGOs, CBOs and other sectors to feed back into this debate. The thematic forums on AIDS it currently runs include: SEA-AIDS a forum for Asia Pacific, GENDER-AIDS, PWHA-Net on people living with HIV and AIDS, SEX-WORK, STIGMA and TREATMENT-ACCESS. These forums bridge not only NGOs and CBOs within the region, but have enabled the exchange of updated information and resources. More recently, other NGOs and PLHA organisations who attended a first ever round-table consultation on access to treatment in Asia Pacific in Canberra in 2002 and also a global consultation organised by treatment activists in South Africa in early 2003 have used e-mail lists to provide feedback on meetings and for important follow-up action that has happened since. In particular, drawing inspiration from the Canberra round table, several NGOs in Indonesia organised a second regional round table in September 2003 in Jogjakarta. It brought together more than 80 participants from 12 countries from the region, namely, Australia, Brunei Darussalam, Cambodia, India, Indonesia, Japan, Lao PDR, Malaysia, Papua New Guinea, Philippines, Singapore and Vietnam as well as two from across the Pacific, Cuba and the USA. These participants included PLHAs, health care workers, CBOs activists, NGOs, journalists, and research-based and generic AIDS drug manufacturers. While this second round table still echoed the small successes shared in the first in Canberra, it has showed movement and has given participants reason for hope. In addition, it moved a number of attending mediapeople to try and broadcast more stories on access to treatment over the radio.

Conclusion

As the epidemic in the region continues to unfold in many different ways, so do the responses and the roles played by NGOs and CBOs manifest themselves in diverse forms. A common thread that weaves through these diversities is that wherever it is possible, there will be grassroots responses to the epidemic, and governments and international agencies need to find ways to cooperate with and support such responses. Placing AIDS on the agenda of state and international organisations not only strengthens state authority, but also provides space for community movements and the empowerment of those most affected (Altman 1995).

While marginalised populations have come forward to educate, advocate and mobilise, the experiences shared herein also shows the positive spin-off that joining forces with other sectors leads to changes in respective communities and societies. The examples serve as inspiration and bring forth processes and principles that could be shared and applied elsewhere with as much success. Though initially limited in coverage, working with other groups through networks and coalitions and engaging with the government at all levels, NGOs and CBOs were able to scale up and scale out their response. In many other cases the support of international NGOs and other bilateral and multilateral organisations, including the UN, have helped create opportunities for communities to be empowered and claim their rightful place in the discussion table. That is yet another story.

Compared to the early 1980s and even the 1990s, political commitment to support civil society engagement include vulnerable populations and promote the participation and inclusion particularly of people living with HIV and AIDS. All that was expressed globally by 189 governments through the UNGASS Declaration of Commitment (June 2001) and finds an echo regionally in the ministerial statement reached by 28 Asia Pacific countries in October 2001. In his status report on the progress made regarding the commitments in the UNGASS Declaration, Secretary-General Kofi Annan (2003) stated:

> The value of engaging civil society in the national response to HIV/AIDS is now universally recognized and organizations representing people living with HIV/AIDS, faith based groups, workers' organizations and the business sector have extended the reach of essential HIV/AIDS programmes and services. However, such engagement remains inadequate.

NGOs are part of the solution. Their role and capacity building needs require support. The task is far from over, as many more NGOs and CBOs, including mainstream organisations such as cooperatives and other development bodies, are brought in to complete the picture. Likewise, as the epidemic and responses evolve, so should spaces be kept open for emerging responses that may not yet be in place. One thing is certain, if we look at history to provide an answer, it will be the fire and passion of NGOs and CBOs on the ground that will ensure that political commitments from the top are galvanised into action.

N OTES

1. The term civil society refers to non-government and not-for-profit entities, including NGOs and CBOs.
2. It has been pointed out that the need to look at how strategic alliances can be formed among organisations with different values and interests.

R EFERENCES

Altman, D. (1995). Change, co-option and the community sector. *AIDS*, 9(Supplement A), S239–43.

Annan, K. (2003). Progress towards implementation of the Declaration of Commitment on HIV/AIDS: Report of the Secretary General. Document no. GA/58/184, United Nations General Assembly, New York, 25 July.

APCASO (2002). Executive summary: United Nations General Assembly Special Session in the Philippines workshop. Manila, 22–24 October.

Bagasao, T.M.P. (1998). Moving forward through community response: Lessons learned from HIV prevention in Asia and the Pacific. In S. Gruskin, J. Mann and D. Tarantola (eds.), *Health and human rights* (pp. 8–19). Boston: Harvard School of Public Health.

Brown, T., B. Franklin, J. MacNeil and **S. Mills** (2001). *Effective prevention strategies in low HIV prevalence settings* (UNAIDS Best Practice Key Materials) Family Health International and Impact, with contribution from USAID.

Daly, Kieran (2002). NGO participation in the Global Fund. Unpublished review paper, International HIV/AIDS Alliance, UK.

Hart, C. (2001). Confronting HIV/AIDS: Working together in Thailand. *Choices*, December, 14–15.

HDNet (2001). Treatment victory for Thai people living with HIV/AIDS (PWAs). Fifth International Conference on Home and Community Care for Persons Living with HIV/AIDS, *CARE Conference News*, 1–4.

Hussein, H.B. (1996). Formation of a national non-governmental organisation (NGO) umbrella body: The Malaysian AIDS Council. In abstract book of International Conference on AIDS, 7–12 July.

Kaldor, J.M., T. Brown, S. Bharat, R. Chan and **Z. Kong-Lai** (1998). HIV/AIDS in the Asia-Pacific region: The road remains long. In J.M. Kaldor, T. Brown,

S. Bharat, R. Chan and Z. Kong-Lai (eds.), *AIDS in Asia and the Pacific* (pp. 2–3) Philadelphia: Lippincott-Raven.

KHANA (2003). Participation, hope, action: Mobilising communities to respond to HIV/AIDS. In Khmer HIV/AIDS NGO Alliance, *Annual report for 2002*. Pnom Penh, Cambodia: KHANA.

Lockhart, Maureen, Susan Chaplin and Tom Seddon (eds.) (2001). Treatment advocacy and partnership building. Congress report of the Sixth International Congress on AIDS in Asia and the Pacific, Melbourne, 5–10 October.

Marshall, Phil and Janet Hunt (1997). Non government organisations: Imperatives and pitfalls. In Godfrey Linge and Doug Porter (eds.), *No place for borders: The HIV/ AIDS epidemic and development in Asia and the Pacific* (pp. 70–78). St. Edwards: Allen-Unwin.

Quan, Andy (2003). Access to HIV/AIDS treatment and care: New inspiration, New friendships. Available at http://www.dgroups.com, 30 September.

Samson, Luke and Sunil Batra (2003). Drug policy reforms in India. *AHRNewsletter*, issue no. 32–33, 9.

Söderholm, Peter (1997). *Global governance of AIDS: Partnerships with civil society*. Lund: Lund University Press.

22

CURRENT ISSUES IN
HIV VACCINE DEVELOPMENT

José Esparza and Saladin Osmanov

Introduction

An HIV preventive vaccine constitutes the best long-term hope to control the HIV/AIDS pandemic. A number of scientific challenges must be addressed before a vaccine is developed. An important issue to be solved relates to the significance of the HIV genetic variability in terms of potential vaccine-induced protection. Since 1987 more than 30 different candidate vaccines have been tested in more than 6,000 healthy human volunteers. Most of these trials have been conducted in the United States and Europe, and also in developing countries. The first phase-III efficacy trials were initiated in 1998 and 1999 in the United States and Thailand. Although the results of these trials have been disappointing and did not show vaccine efficacy, they have provided valuable experience in conducting phase-III vaccine trials. To continue and further accelerate vaccine development, it is important to conduct multiple trials to simultaneously evaluate several types of vaccines against different HIV sub-types in diverse populations. Developing countries must strengthen their infrastructure to be able to conduct trials to the highest scientific and ethical standards.

A safe, highly effective and affordable preventive vaccine offers the most hope for the HIV/AIDS pandemic, especially in developing countries. But a future HIV vaccine should not be seen as a replacement for other HIV prevention strategies. Those preventive vaccines, when available, will have to be delivered as part of comprehensive HIV prevention programmes, including other behavioural and health promotion interventions, which may have to be redesigned around strategies for vaccine delivery. For this reason the development of an HIV vaccine will probably increase the future costs of HIV/AIDS prevention programmes, although it is expected that it would be more effective than current interventions, finally leading to the definitive control of the HIV/AIDS pandemic.

Scientific Challenges

Ever since HIV was identified in 1983–84 as the aetiological agent of AIDS, the goal of developing a preventive vaccine has been one of the priorities of the scientific community. But several scientific challenges will have to be solved before we have such a vaccine.

What Type of Immune Response?

Preventive vaccines are designed to induce the type of immune responses that individuals develop after natural infection with viral or bacterial pathogens, which are responsible for disease recovery, also conferring protection against reinfection by the same agent. But HIV/AIDS may be different from other vaccine-preventable diseases in that HIV infection persists and disease develops even in the presence of strong anti-HIV immune response from the host, which includes neutralising antibodies and cell-mediated immunity (CMI). This lack of information on 'immunological correlates of protection' has been the major conceptual problem for the rational development of HIV vaccines. After years of debating if vaccines should induce antibodies or CMI (or mucosal immunity), the scientific community began to accept the idea that protection against HIV/AIDS may be the result of a combination of different immune responses that, as a whole, can act as immunological barriers to infection or disease.

Candidate (Experimental) Vaccines

The traditional approaches for viral vaccine development are based on the use of whole inactivated viruses (as is the case with the Salk's polio vaccine) or, more effectively, on the use of attenuated strains of the virus (as with the Sabin's polio vaccine, the yellow fever vaccine and many others). However, in the case of HIV vaccines these two 'classical' approaches are considered too risky to be considered for human use.

Consequently, all HIV candidate vaccines being developed for testing and future use in humans are based on pieces of the virus produced by genetic engineering techniques so as to ensure that vaccine recipients never get infected from the vaccine. The first generation of candidate vaccines were based on the HIV envelope glycoproteins gp120 or gp160, and they were designed to induce neutralising antibodies. Other candidate vaccines, also designed to induce neutralising antibodies, were based on synthetic peptides, representing important antigenic regions of the envelope glycoprotein. Other types of candidate vaccines are designed to induce CMI, and most of them use viral or bacterial vectors to deliver selected HIV proteins. In these cases a non-pathogenic micro-organism is genetically modified to carry specific HIV genes that are expressed after inoculation into the appropriate host. The Vaccinia virus, the poxvirus that was used as the vaccine to eradicate smallpox, has been extensively studied as a vector for HIV antigens although there are some safety concerns regarding potential side effects if given to an already immunodeficient individual. To obviate that problem, safer poxvirus vectors are being developed, including canarypox and fowlpox (both of which are avian poxviruses incapable of fully replicating in mammalian cells) and the modified (highly attenuated) Ankara strain of the Vaccinia virus (known as MVA). Other live vectors are being explored, including the Venezuelan Equine Encephalitis (VEE) replicon, BCG and *Salmonella*. Another approach for HIV vaccine development is by genetic immunisation using DNA (or RNA) representing selected HIV genes, which after expression in the host result in antigen production and induction of immune responses. Finally, combinations of different vaccine concepts are also being explored in prime-boost regimes, such as in Thailand.

Animal Models

Three experimental animal models have been extensively used in HIV vaccine research: HIV infection of chimpanzees, infection of monkeys with simian immunodeficiency viruses (SIV) and infection of monkeys with chimeric viruses containing HIV and SIV genes (SHIVs). Chimpanzees have been protected from HIV infection after vaccination with gp120 vaccines and, to some extent, also with nucleic acid vaccines. On the other hand, SIV-challenged monkeys are very difficult to protect with experimental vaccines, and SHIVs experiments have given different results depending on the challenge virus used. The bottom line emanating from multiple animal protection experiments is that some experimental vaccines can induce varying levels of protection in different primate models, although how relevant that information is in relation to protection in humans is unknown and remains to be validated by human trials. An interesting finding has been that although most vaccines fail to confer absolute protection against SIV infection in monkeys (so-called 'sterilising immunity'), many are capable of decreasing virus loads in the infected animals who show slower progression to disease. That information may be relevant for human trials with vaccines not necessarily protecting against infection but preventing disease. In addition, if virus loads are significantly decreased (to less than 1,500 copies of HIV RNA per millilitre of plasma), virus transmission would probably be reduced, resulting in an interruption in the chain of virus transmission, with important epidemiological implications.

Virus Variability

Another potential obstacle for HIV vaccine development is related to the extensive genetic variability of HIV. HIV-1 strains are classified within a major (M) group and two minor (O, N) groups, as defined by their genetic relationships. Strains from the M group, the most prevalent ones, are subclassified into 10 genetic sub-types (clades A through J) according to the nucleotide sequence of the gene coding for the envelope proteins (Table 22.1 and Figure 22.1). The most frequent genetic sub-type is C, which accounted for approximately 56 per cent of all HIV infections in 1999, and which is prevalent in southern Africa and in India. Three genetic sub-types are prevalent in Africa (C, A and D) and sub-type E is the one prevalent in Thailand and other South-East Asian countries. Sub-type B, which accounted for only 8 per cent of all HIV infections in 1999, is the one prevalent in the Americas, Western Europe, Japan, Australia and New Zealand. In addition, it is increasingly recognised that genetic sub-types recombine among themselves and several 'circulating recombinant forms' are already associated with emerging epidemics in China (C/B), Thailand (E/A), West Africa (A/G) and Eastern Europe (A/B).

What is not clear at the present time is the potential relevance of HIV genetic variability in terms of vaccine-induced protection. It is clear that genetic sub-types do not strictly correspond to immuno-types, as defined by immunological relationships. It is entirely possible that more than one genetic sub-type could constitute a single immuno-type

Table 22.1
Incidence of HIV-1 M Envelope (Env) Genetic Sub-types per Region

HIV-1 env sub-type	Global infections in 1999 (%)	Geographic distribution
A	23	East, Central and West Africa. In West Africa the predominant virus is an A/G recombinant. A and A/B recombinant are prevalent in Eastern Europe.
B	8	The Americas, Western Europe, Japan, Australia and New Zealand.
C	56	Southern Africa, Ethiopia and India. The predominant virus in China is a C/B recombinant.
D	5	East and Central Africa.
E	6	Thailand and other South-East Asian countries. The E virus is actually an E/A recombinant.
Others (F, G, H, J, not typed)	2	Present with low prevalence in all continents. Sub-type F may be relatively frequent in South America.

Source: WHO/UNAIDS.

and, conversely, that more than one immuno-type could be contained within a single genetic sub-type. The vaccine relevance of genetic sub-types could also depend on the type of vaccines. Envelope-based vaccines, aimed at inducing neutralising antibodies, are likely to be more strain specific than vaccines aimed at inducing cytotoxic T-cells (CTL), which already have been shown to cross-react between different clades.

Most existing candidate vaccines are based on the B sub-type of HIV, but candidate vaccines have also been developed based on sub-type E, and these are being tested in Thailand. New candidate vaccines are also being developed based on sub-types C, A and D for testing in Africa and elsewhere. To optimise the chances of success, the initial efficacy trials of HIV candidate vaccines must try to match the sub-type in the vaccine with that prevalent in the population. However, in future, we will have to explore the potential for cross-clade protection, either designing efficacy trials with an unmatched vaccine arm not corresponding to the prevalent clade in the testing population, or testing monovalent candidate vaccines in populations where different clades are circulating.

The other aspect of HIV variability that could be relevant for vaccine development is in relation to different co-receptor use by strains of HIV. All HIV strains use CD4 as their main receptor in target cells, but

Figure 22.1
Genetic Sub-types of HIV

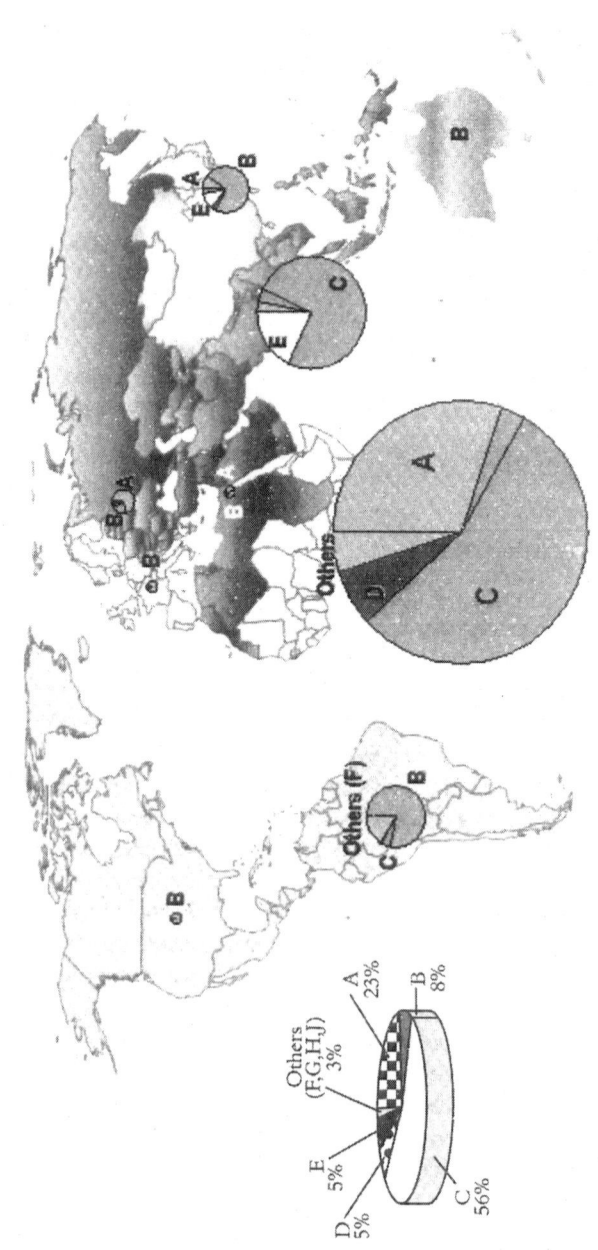

clinical isolates of HIV (those freshly isolated from patients) use CCR5 as its second receptor, while laboratory-adapted strains use the CXCR4 molecule. The potential importance of this second receptor usage lies in the fact that vaccines based on laboratory strains of HIV induce neutralising antibodies that only neutralise the infectivity of laboratory isolates but fail to neutralise the most relevant clinical isolates. We must accept, however, that the relevance of those in vitro observations in terms of potential vaccine protection in humans is not clear.

Clinical Trials in Humans

After extensive animal experimentation, candidate vaccines are tested in human volunteers in three sequential phases: Phase-I trials are conducted to obtain initial information on the safety and immunogenicity (ability to induce relevant immune responses) in a small number (30 to 50) of HIV-negative human volunteers. Phase-II trials are conducted in larger number of healthy volunteers (in hundreds) to obtain additional information on vaccine safety and immunogenicity. Depending on the results, candidate vaccines move to phase-III trials, which are large-scale field trials designed to assess the efficacy of the candidate vaccine in protecting against infection or disease. These are complex, double-blind-controlled trials, involving thousands of healthy volunteers at higher risk of HIV infection. Table 22.2 presents a summary of the different HIV vaccines tested in clinical trials.

Phase-I/II Trials

The first HIV vaccine trial was conducted in 1987 in the United States using a baculovirus-derived gp160 candidate vaccine. Since then more than 30 candidate vaccines have been tested in some 60 phase-I/II trials involving a total of 6,000 healthy HIV-negative volunteers. Most of these trials have been conducted in the United States and in Europe, but some have also been conducted in developing countries. The first trial in a developing country was done in 1993 in the Yunnan province of China, using a synthetic envelope peptide. Thailand had its first HIV vaccine trial in 1994 and since then has conducted eight out of the 12 HIV vaccine trials that have been implemented in developing countries, including a phase-III trial. The other three developing country trials were conducted in Brazil, Cuba and Uganda.

Table 22.2
Main HIV Candidate Vaccines in Clinical Trials

Vaccine concept	Main products	Trials
Recombinant envelope subunits	Rgp120, rgp160	Multiple phase-I/II trials have been conducted with monomeric gp120s. The only ongoing phase-III HIV vaccine trials are being conducted with monomeric bivalent gp120 candidate vaccines (BB and BE). Several rgp120 candidate vaccines have been tested in Thailand, including in an ongoing phase-III trail.
Synthetic peptides	V3-MAPS, V3PPD conjugates, HGP30(p17), rV3 peptides, rp24	Multiple phase-I/II trials, including trials in China, Thailand, Brazil, and Cuba.
Live vectors	Vaccinia-HIV, canarypox-HIV	Different versions of canarypox-HIV recombinant vaccines have been extensively tested, including one phase-I/II trial in Uganda. Other live vectors, including the MVA and the VEE replicon are been developed as HIV candidate vaccines.
Naked DNA	Different DNA constructs including gag, env and regulatory genes	Initial DNA-based candidate vaccines tested in phase-I/II trials were not very immunogenic. Vaccines are being redesigned with better promoters and humanising codon use.
Prime-boost combinations	Priming with canarypox-HIV and boosting with gp120, or priming with DNA and boosting with MVA-HIV vectors	Canarypox-HIV/gp120 boosting is being actively explored and may move to phase-IIb or -III trials in the near future. DNA/MVA-HIV prime boost has shown promise in animal models and is moving to phase-I trials in the UK and Kenya.

Source: WHO/UNAIDS HIV Vaccine Initiative.

These multiple phase-I/II trials have shown that candidate vaccines are safe and that some of them induce HIV-specific immune responses. To sum up, envelope-based candidate vaccines have been shown to induce neutralising antibodies in a majority of volunteers, but these antibodies are mainly directed against homologous laboratory strains of HIV. On the other hand, candidate vaccines aimed at inducing CMI, notably the canarypox-HIV vectors, have been shown to induce little neutralising antibodies and inconsistent CTL in approximately 30 to 50 per cent of the volunteers. These results suggest that better antigens (or combination of antigens) may have to be developed to induce consistently high levels of humoral and CMI responses in a majority of volunteers. In addition, it is clear that better laboratory techniques will have to be developed for a more accurate determination of vaccine-induced immune responses.

Phase-III Efficacy Trials

The first phase-III trials of an HIV vaccine were initiated in the United States in 1998 and in Thailand in 1999, using two different versions of bivalent gp120s based on locally prevalent sub-types (BB and BE respectively). The bivalent candidate vaccines also include a laboratory (CXCR4-user) and a clinical (CCR5-user) version of the gp120 molecule. The trial in the United States had 5,500 HIV-negative volunteers, mostly male homosexuals. The Thai trial enrolled 2,500 volunteers in Bangkok, mostly recovering intravenous drug users. The results showed vaccine efficacy of 4 per cent and 0 per cent respectively, indicating that the vaccine did not offer any protection against HIV (Vaxgen, Inc. 2003a, 2003b).

Discussions are already under way to decide how to use a vaccine according to different scenarios of efficacy. A cause for concern is that even if the candidate vaccine with B sub-types had showed some degree of efficacy (and the phase-III trials would have the last word!), those candidate vaccines would not be appropriate for areas of the world where the epidemic is worse, including Southern Africa and India, where sub-type C is the prevalent virus. An alternative would be to start manufacturing equivalent gp120 candidate vaccines now based on the most prevalent A, C and D clades. Even if gp120 alone shows little efficacy, it could still be used as a protein boost for other vaccine concepts. We must concede, however, that our scientific knowledge is still incomplete and that any policy decision would have to be taken with a considerable degree of uncertainty. We could make a big mistake by prematurely invsesting funds and efforts in a still unproven candidate vaccine. But we could also be making a mistake by not anticipating a possible success, with the consequent delay in making a vaccine available.

Conclusions

The most rational strategy to accelerate the future availability of an urgently needed HIV vaccine is to pursue in parallel the development and field evaluation of multiple candidate vaccines. Multiple trials will be needed to evaluate several types of candidate vaccines, against different HIV sub-types and in diverse populations. The next candidate vaccine that may move to an efficacy evaluation is a prime-boost combination using a canarypox-HIV recombinant vector followed by gp120. This trial, sponsored by the National Institutes of Health of the United States, could be initiated soon in the United States and in other countries in the Americas, including Brazil, Haiti, and Trinidad and Tobago. Other developing countries that are gearing up to conduct HIV vaccine research and trials include (but are not limited to) China, Ethiopia, India, South Africa, Tanzania and Zambia.

The conduct of trials in developing countries call for the full participation of local scientists and institutions, which need to build capacity for the long-term effort required to conduct trials to the highest scientific and ethical standards.

Since 1989 the WHO has been collaborating with developing countries in HIV vaccine development activities, including the provision of technical and financial support for the development of national AIDS vaccine plans. The WHO/UNAIDS HIV Vaccine Initiative, established in January 2000, will continue to expand those activities in response to the recent request from WHO member states.

It is recognised, however, that no single organisation or country can address the multiple scientific, economic, ethical and logistical challenges confronted in the search for an HIV vaccine. Fulfilling its international mandate, WHO/UNAIDS acts as a neutral broker, collaborating with other agencies and institutions in the private and public sector, in industrialised and in developing countries, to ensure that a true international effort accelerates the development and future availability of safe and effective HIV vaccines.

REFERENCES

VaxGen, Inc. (2003a). Initial results of VaxGen phase-III AIDS vaccine trial (24 February 2003), http://www.newscom.com/cgi-bin/prnh/19991112/VAXGEN LOGO or http://www.vaxgen.com.

———— (2003b). Results from first phase-III AIDS vaccine trial in Thailand: Vaxgen news (12 November 2003). Press release, Brisbane, California, http://www.vaxgen.com.

FURTHER READING

Esparza, J. and N. Bhamarapravati (2000). Accelerating the development and future availability of HIV-1 vaccines: Why, when, where and how? Lancet, 355(9226), 2061–66.

Esparza, J., W.L. Heyward and S. Osmanov (1996). HIV vaccine development: From basic research to clinical trials. AIDS, 10(Supplement A), S123–32.

Osmanov, S. and J. Esparza (1998). Development and evaluation of preventive HIV-1 vaccines. In N. Saksena (ed.), Human immunodeficiency viruses: Biologic, immunology and molecular biology (pp. 501–55). Genoa: Medical Systems.

UNAIDS (2000). Ethical considerations in HIV preventive vaccine research. Document UNAIDS/00.07E, UNAIDS, Geneva, http://www.unaids.org/publications documents/vaccines/ethicsresearch.doc.

UNAIDS/WHO/NIID (1999). AIDS vaccine research in Asia: Needs and opportunities—Report from a UNAIDS/WHO/NIID meeting, Tokyo, 28–30 October 1998. AIDS, 13(11), 1–13.

23

HIV Vaccine Development in South-East Asia

Jean-Louis Excler

The fight against HIV/AIDS poses enormous challenges worldwide, even generating fears that success may be too difficult or even impossible to attain (Okware et al. 2001). Conventionally, vaccines are considered most effective tools to combat a communicable disease. However, no HIV vaccine is currently available. Multiple factors are responsible for this situation.

The global public and private expenditure on research related to HIV vaccines in 1999 was estimated at less than $300 million globally, two-thirds of which was provided by the US National Institute of Health (NIH). Although impressive, it represents only a tenth of the expenditure for drugs to treat HIV infection and AIDS, which was about $3 billion in the USA and Europe alone in 1999. Additional financial support is required not only to develop new vaccine candidates, but also to strengthen appropriate infrastructure in less developed countries, where many vaccine trials will be carried out and where future effective vaccines will have to be used as a matter of emergency. Goals for an HIV vaccine have been shown in Box 23.1.

Outstanding Scientific and Strategic Difficulties

HIV is characterised by its genetic diversity and hyper-variability, especially in the envelope domain, to a lesser extent in core and regulatory genes. In addition, the genetic sequence of the full genome has allowed determining recombination between sub-types, now well established (McCutchan 2000; Piyasirisilp et al. 2000; Tovanabutra et al. 2001).

Box 23.1
Goals for an HIV Vaccine

- Protect against HIV infection (sterilising immunity):
  √ Against all routes of transmission
  √ Against intravenous transmission only
  √ Against mucosal transmission, including breastfeeding
- Protect against progression to disease (reduction of the viral load)
- Protect against progression of disease (immunotherapy)
- Reduce transmission (infectiousness)—infected vaccines with lower viral load expected to be low or non-transmitters

---

In Asia the HIV group M sub-type A/E (E envelope, A gag/pol) is predominant (>75 per cent) in Thailand (McCutchan et al. 2000) and Myanmar, followed by sub-type B (close to the North American and European B), essentially found in IDUs, and sub-type C in northern Thailand. In Indonesia sub-types B (predominant) and E are both circulating (Porter et al. 1997). In India HIV-1 sub-type C is predominant (78.4 per cent) (sub-type C accounts for 47.2 per cent of all HIV infections worldwide [Osmanov et al. 2002]), followed by sub-type B (8.8 per cent), sub-type A (2.4 per cent) and sub-type E (1.6 per cent) (Gadkari et al. 1998; Halani et al. 2001; Sahni et al. 2002; Tripathy et al. 1996). Recombinants (A/C, B'/C) have also now been described in India (Lole et al. 1999). HIV-2 is also circulating. This may have tremendous implications for the design of HIV vaccines. A vaccine protecting against a sub-type may not be protective or only partially protective against another sub-type or recombinant. The immune correlates of protection are still unknown (Nathanson and Mathieson 2000). Both arms of the immune system (humoral and cell-mediated) are thought to be important for protection. Efforts aim at developing vaccines that would induce both neutralising antibodies and cytotoxic T-lymphocytes (CTL) against primary HIV isolates (Letvin 1998; Peiperl 2001). Relevant animal models are lacking. The validity of animal models for protection will be resolved only when comparison of these animal results with the results of efficacy trials in humans are made possible.

The implementation and conduct of HIV vaccine clinical trials is difficult, long and costly. Recruitment of lower-risk volunteers for phases I and II, and of high-risk volunteers for phase-III efficacy trials is rendered more difficult in less-educated populations exposed to rumours and media opinion. Safeguarding the rights and welfare of individuals participating as research subjects in developing countries is a priority.

In September 1997 the Joint United Nations Programme on HIV/AIDS (UNAIDS) embarked on a process of international consultation; its purpose was further to define the important ethical issues and to formulate guidance that might facilitate the ethical design and conduct of HIV vaccine trials in international contexts (Guenter et al. 2000). The difficulties of implementing HIV vaccine efficacy trials in developing countries have been reviewed elsewhere (Esparza and Burke 2001; Excler and Beyrer 2000).

Reasons for the Success of HIV Vaccine Development in Thailand

Thailand was one of the four countries identified in 1991 by the World Health Organisation as an HIV vaccine evaluation site (Heyward et al. 1996, 1998). It has an optimal set of circumstances for carrying out HIV vaccine efficacy trials that will benefit both the nation and the world. These include solid medical and logistical infrastructure, and national commitment to HIV vaccine development in the face of a severe epidemic associated with viral strains of relatively narrow diversity. The Thai government is committed to active participation in the global effort to develop and evaluate HIV vaccines. It believes that a vaccine is a needed and complementary part of its total programme for prevention and control of the HIV epidemic. Also, it is expected that involvement in vaccine research will further develop the nation's scientific infrastructure. These circumstances prompted the establishment of several collaborations between Thailand and foreign agencies and institutions aiming at HIV vaccine trial preparedness and implementation. Thailand has played and is still playing a major role of leadership in Asia, as also among developing countries worldwide for HIV prevention, care and treatment, and HIV vaccine development. The reasons for such success are examined later (see Box 23.2).

The Thai Policy for HIV Vaccine Development and Evaluation

The National AIDS Prevention and Control Committee (NAC) of the Thai government, chaired by the prime minister, has designated the Ministry of Public Health (MOPH) as responsible for planning, co-ordinating and overseeing all HIV vaccine trials in Thailand. The NAC

> **Box 23.2**
> **Elements of Success for HIV Vaccine Development in Thailand**
> - Strong and long-term political commitment against HIV/AIDS
> - Multi-sectorial approach to fight against the HIV epidemic
> - National prevention, care and support programme
> - Open spirit to international scientific collaboration
> - Multi-disciplinary HIV research activities
> - National capacity building through constant training of all categories of staff involved in HIV vaccine development, participation at workshops and international conferences, exchanges with foreign research laboratories, national and academic institutions
> - Technology transfer
> - Excellent infrastructure (laboratory equipment and storage facilities)
> - National data management capacity
> - Well-defined approval process for clinical trials
> - Highest ethical requirements

has also appointed a scientific subcommittee to be responsible for scientific aspects of HIV vaccine research. A national plan for HIV vaccine research, development and evaluation was developed in 1992 with assistance from the WHO (MOPH 1993). This plan provided for coordination of HIV vaccine activities, including guidelines and regulations for HIV vaccine protocol review and approval. The plan required that prior to testing in Thailand all HIV vaccines undergo human testing in the country of manufacture. This requirement was modified by NAC in 1994. Human testing of new candidate HIV vaccines in the country of manufacture was no longer a prerequisite to approval trials in Thailand as long as the vaccine construct was specifically designed to match the prevalent sub-type of the Thai epidemic.

Thailand has developed a review and approval process of clinical protocols. These procedures cover diverse aspects of HIV vaccine research, including socio-ethical and scientific issues (Kilmarx et al. 2001; Nitayaphan and Brown 1998). The status of HIV vaccine trials in Thailand is presented in Table 23.1.

Thailand–US National Institute of Health Collaboration

One of the first major collaborative initiatives in moving towards HIV-1 field trials was the US National Institute of Allergy and Infectious Diseases (NIAID)-sponsored Preparations for AIDS Vaccine Evaluation (PAVE) programme launched in 1992. The PAVE programme supported

Table 23.1
HIV Vaccine Clinical Trials in Thailand

Year	Candidate vaccine	Sub-type	Number of volunteers	Pharmaceutical company
1994	Octameric peptide MN-V3	B	24	UBI
1995	Monomeric gp120	B	54	Chiron/Biocine
1995	Monomeric gp120	B	52	Genentech
1997	Monomeric gp120	B, E, B/E	383	Genentech
1998	Monomeric gp120	B/E	90	VaxGen
1999	Monomeric gp120	B/E	2,500	VaxGen
2000	Canarypox + gp120 or gp160	E/A+E	133	Aventis Pasteur Chiron
2000	Canarypox + gp120	E/A+B/E	128	Aventis Pasteur VaxGen
2000	Booster dose of gp120	B/E	24	Chiron Vaccines
2003	Canarypox + gp120	E/A+B/E	16,000	Aventis Pasteur VaxGen

several US research groups (Johns Hopkins University for Thailand and India) and their developing country partners in cohort development initiatives aimed at generating measures of HIV-1 incidence, sub-types, rates of cohort retention, behavioural aspects and interest in vaccine trial participation. The PAVE programme was clearly a preparatory study. It measured HIV vaccine trial interest through questionnaires to study participants (and perhaps 25 per cent of all 2,230 cohort subjects reported willingness to participate), but in the absence of a readily available vaccine (Celentano et al. 1995). The exercise was in one sense an abstract one: *if* there were a vaccine that might prevent HIV infection, *would* you be interested in participating in its testing? Answers to these kinds of questions may or may not provide the basis on which to measure potential trial interest. Second, all subjects in the five cohorts investigated (female sex workers, male STD patients, two groups of military recruits and one of recent military dischargees) were offered individual pre- and post-test HIV counselling throughout the study. All were offered STD testing and treatment, risk-reduction education, free condoms and the opportunity to enrol in several related prevention programmes (Nelson et al. 1994). Following the launch of the national '100 per cent condom campaign' (Rojanapithayakorn and Hanenberg 1996), HIV incidence fell dramatically through the 18- to 24-month periods of these cohorts (Nelson et al. 1996). Had an appropriate antigen been ready for testing in any of these cohorts, the initial incidence estimates and the first six-month incidence rates would have grossly overestimated the infection rate and grossly underpowered any trial. In the short PAVE mechanism in which initial funding was for two years, these sample size issues could not be addressed and four of the five cohorts were shut down by the investigators. The experience shows that while preparing to conduct a trial, longer follow-up times and much more flexible funding arrangements may be essential to success.

A new structure of collaboration has now been established with the National Institute of Allergy and Infectious Diseases, National Institute of Health (NIH) and US academic institutions through the HIV Vaccine Trial Network (HVTN). The Thai HVTN site is located in Chiang Mai, a collaborative effort between Johns Hopkins University School of Public Health and Chiang Mai University. The group continues to investigate HIV prevalence and incidence in cohorts of IDUs and commercial sex workers in northern Thailand, while offering prevention services through the HIV Prevention Trial Network (HPTN). Unfortunately, no vaccine candidate has been made available to be tested in this region at the moment.

Thailand–US Centres for Disease Control Collaboration

The first efficacy trial in a developing country (AIDSVAX gp 120 B/E from VaxGen) was conducted in Thai IDUs. The trial, now completed, unfortunately showed no vaccine efficacy. The preparedness and implementation of this trial are the result of a collaborative effort, the HIV/AIDS Collaboration (HAC), between the US Centres for Disease Control (CDC) and the Thai MOPH, established in 1990. The HAC conducted studies on epidemiology and prevention, including the molecular epidemiology of HIV-1 in Thailand, and began working with the Bangkok Metropolitan Administration (BMA) on studies on IDUs in 1991. In a cohort of 1,209 HIV-negative IDUs, HIV-1 incidence was estimated at 5.8/100 person-years. The HIV-1 sub-types were 80 per cent E and 20 per cent B (Vanichseni 2001). Willingness to participate in an HIV recombinant gp120 bivalent sub-types B/E candidate vaccine efficacy trial was assessed among 193 IDUs attending drug treatment clinics in Bangkok. At baseline 51 per cent were definitely willing to participate, and at follow-up 54 per cent; only 3 per cent were not willing to participate at either time. Comprehension was high at baseline and improved at follow-up. Participants who viewed altruism, regular HIV tests and family support for participation as important were more willing to volunteer. Frequency of incarceration and concerns about the length of the trial, possible vaccine-induced accelerated disease progression and lack of family support were negatively associated with willingness (MacQueen et al. 1999). Details about IDU population, trial enrolment and procedures are provided elsewhere.

Thailand–US Department of Defence Collaboration (Walter Reed Army Institute of Research)

The second efficacy trial will follow a series of phase-I/II trials conducted in Thailand. It is also the result of a strong, well-established collaboration between the Walter Reed Army Institute of Research (WRAIR) and the Thai Armed Forces Research Institute of Medical Sciences (AFRIMS), Bangkok.

Late in 1994 the Research Institute of Health Sciences (RIHES) at Chiang Mai University initiated collaboration with the HIV Research Programme, AFRIMS, to form the ARVEG (AFRIMS–RIHES Vaccine Evaluation Group). In 1997 two Mahidol University sites joined the collaboration, Siriraj Hospital and the Vaccine Trial Centre within the Faculty of Tropical Medicine. The four-site collaboration was named the Thai AIDS Vaccine Evaluation Group (TAVEG). The Joint Collaborative Research Committee (JCRC) has played an important role in the transfer of clinical trial expertise to new sites, helping build capacity in these academic centres. The JCRC has also facilitated exchanges of investigators between Thailand and other developing countries interested in HIV vaccine development.

The design and approach of the second planned efficacy trial that started in September 2003 are entirely different. The prime-boost vaccine consists of canarypox E gp140 env, B gag/pol priming (Aventis Pasteur) and AIDSVAX gp120 B/E boosting (VaxGen). The trial is community based. Volunteers are currently recruited in the Rayong and Chonburi provinces, south-east of Bangkok, where cohort studies have been conducted since 1997. This trial will explore the vaccine efficacy in the context of heterosexual transmission within the community.

Other HIV Vaccine Approaches Planned in Thailand

The Thai–Australian Collaboration

HIVNAT is a joint collaborative effort for HIV research between Thailand and Australia (University of New South Wales Consortium supported by a US NIH contract). A new HIV vaccine approach developed in

Australia is expected to be tested in a phase-I trial in Thai volunteers. A preliminary phase-I trial was to proceed mid-2002 in Australia. The vaccine approach is based on the prime-boost strategy using DNA priming and recombinant live fowlpox vector boosting. This recombinant construct expresses not only HIV genes (gag, pol, nef, tat) but also a Th-1 cytokine (INF-γ) supported to enhance the vaccine-induced cell-mediated immune responses including HIV-specific T-cell lymphoproliferation and CTL. This prime-boost strategy has been successfully tested in animals in the SIV model, showing a significant reduction in viral load in immunised and challenged animals (Kent et al. 1998, 2000).

The Thai–Japanese Collaboration

The Thai–Japanese HIV sub-type E prophylactic vaccine cooperative project was established between the Department of Medical Sciences, Ministry of Public Health, Thailand, and the National Institute of Infectious Diseases, Japan, supported by the Japan Science and Technology Corporation, the Japan Foundation of AIDS Prevention, the Japan International Cooperation Agency and the Sasakawa Memorial Health Foundation, and the Thai government. Thai researchers are staff of the Thai National Institute of Health as well as Mahidol (Vaccine Research Centre), Chulalongkorn and Chiang Mai Universities. Japanese researchers belong to the National Institute of Infectious Diseases and to the Japan Science and Technology Corporation. The research is simultaneously conducted in Thailand and in Japan.

Two live vector vaccine constructs have been prepared. The first is a recombinant BCG (Tokyo strain) vaccine. The second vaccine candidate is a recombinant non-replicative vaccinia or rDIS, very close to the Modified Vaccinia Ankara or MVA. The vaccine concept consists in a prime-boost regimen with rBCG priming and rDIS boosting. The preclinical phase started in 1998 and will terminate in 2003. The first experiments were conducted using HIV sub-type B gag constructs in mice and SIV gag constructs in monkeys. The prime-boost regimen significantly enhanced CTL activity in immunised mice. In monkeys this regimen induced strong immunity as measured by ELISPOT and conferred protection against mucosal challenge with pathogenic SHIV. Animals showed a decline in their HIV set point levels and HIV viral load was undetectable in two of three immunised monkeys. CD4 + cell count decline was also significantly reduced. In February 2002 an

International Advisory Committee meeting held in Bangkok with the participation of the WHO recommended proceeding with clinical trials. Pilot production plants are being set up in Bangkok (Thai Red Cross) for the GMP production of the two vaccine preparations: the Royal Thai Red Cross for rBCG-HIV vaccine and the Department of Medical Sciences for rDIS vaccinia-HIV vaccine. It is anticipated that a phase-I clinical trial could be initiated soon. Both vaccine constructs for clinical trials express HIV-1 gag from a Thai isolate. Various vaccine approaches in the pipeline are summarised in Box 23.3.

Box 23.3
HIV Preventive Vaccine Approaches in the Pipeline in Thailand

Advanced planning
- DNA + recombinant fowlpox, sub-type E/A genes with or w/o INF-y
- Recombinant BCG, gag sub-type E/A
- Recombinant live attenuated vaccinia virus (DIS), gag E/A
- Recombinant MVA, sub-type E/A genes (pending)
- Recombinant adenovirus

R&D and preclinical stages
- Recombinant live vectors
  - √ Venezuelan Equine Encephalitis virus, env/gag/pol sub-type C
  - √ Semliki Forest virus, gp120/gp160
  - √ Mengovirus, nef/V3/V4/C4 MN, multiple
  - √ Rhinovirus V3
  - √ Poliovirus, env/gag/pol LAI
  - √ Vesicular stomatitis virus, gp160
  - √ Influenza virus, V3/gp41
  - √ Moloney murine leukemia virus, env/rev LAI
  - √ Salmonella typhi, V3/gp120/p24/nef MN, LAI
  - √ Brucella abortus, V3
  - √ Listeria monocytogenes, gag
- DNA
  - √ gp160/rev/tat/nef (LAI)
  - √ DNA env/rev (IIIB)
  - √ DNA gp120/gp160 (IIIB, SF2, CM235, MN)
- Recombinant proteins
  - √ tat, RT/cholera toxin
- Synthetic
  - √ V4/p24/PPD/toxin A/p18/HA/CD4 binding
  - √ Gag, pol, nef, tat, env peptides linked to HBc antigen

Vaccine Development in India

The Indian HIV Vaccine Development Programme has not yet entered clinical development. At the moment this initiative is exclusively the domain of the Indian Council of Medical Research (ICMR) and the Department of Biotechnology, both governmental institutions, and the All India Institute of Medical Sciences. The private sector may be involved later on at the production level of HIV vaccines in India. Indian public research institutions and universities still require substantive inflows of cash to modernise existing facilities and to catch up with biotechnological advances. The Pharmaceutical Research and Development Committee of the Council of Scientific and Industrial Research has completed a report detailing the strengths and weaknesses of the Indian infrastructure and identifying where new investments are needed in order to bring the clinical trial research and approval phases up to internationally competitive standards (Kettler and Modi 2001).

Indian Institutions Involved in HIV Vaccine Research and Development

The ICMR's capabilities in HIV vaccine R&D are being expressed in partnership with the National AIDS Control Organisation (NACO), Ministry of Health and Family Welfare, Government of India. The National AIDS Research Institute (NARI), Pune, is an ICMR institute that undertakes studies on cohort, immunology, virology, molecular biology, vaccine development, vaccine testing, study design and behavioural studies, and is also the national HIV repository. HIV isolates have been collected from various states in India. There are more than 140 isolates in virus bank: 120 HIV-1 and 20 HIV-2.

The role of NACO is to facilitate granting of permissions and permits for persons to work on this initiative, transfer biological materials and products to and from India, and assure harmonisation of goals among its agencies. The role of the ICMR is to select appropriate HIV strains, provide technical expertise in India, receive technology, perform preclinical studies, provide facilities and laboratory support, and conduct clinical trials. The specific scientific expertise offered by the ICMR includes the performance of virus isolation, sub-type determination, genotyping and phenotyping, CTL assays (ELISPOT) lymphoproliferation assays, binding and neutralising antibody assays, clinical trial methodology and epidemiological characterisation of HIV infection (prevalence, incidence, biological and behavioural determinants). Most HIV in India are due to HIV-1 sub-type C (see Box 23.4).

NARI in collaboration with Johns Hopkins School of Public Health and Hygiene, Johns Hopkins University (Robert Bollinger, Baltimore,

Box 23.4
HIV-1 Sub-types in India

Sub-type C	91%
Sub-type A	3%
Sub-type B	3%
Sub-types D, E, Thai B	3%

MD), has been from the beginning of the epidemic in India the key player in HIV epidemiological and behavioural cohort studies with the establishment of a PAVE site at NARI, Pune, now a US NIH-funded Vaccine Trial Network as well as a Prevention Trial Networks site. New infrastructure (clinical centre and GCCP immunology laboratory) entirely dedicated to HIV vaccine trials have recently been developed at NARI in close collaboration with the International AIDS Vaccine Initiative (IAVI). A similar collaboration has recently been initiated between IAVI and the Tuberculosis Research Centre (TRC), Chennai.

HIV Vaccine Approaches Pursued in India

Four HIV vaccine approaches are currently being developed, all based on the induction of a specific cell-mediated T-cell response, especially CTL (Lubaki et al. 1999; Paranjape et al. 1998; Sharma 2001). All approaches are based on recombinant vectors: the MVA, either by using full-length HIV gene insertions or multi-epitope sequences from dominant CTL domains, the modified BCG; adeno-associated virus (AAV), adenovirus, alpha viruses (for example, Semliki Forest Virus (SFV) (Box 23.5).

Box 23.5
HIV Vaccine Approaches in India

HIV Sub-type C vaccine approaches in India
Modified Vaccinia Ankara
DNA
Multiple epitope
BCG
Semliki Forest Virus

The development of a multigenic recombinant MVA is a more advanced project in collaboration between the IAVI, NICED, NARI and a US-based biotechnology company Therion Biologics. Another

MVA-based vaccine approach is under consideration between the DBT, Emory University, Atlanta, GeoVax (US-based biotechnology company) and an Indian manufacturer. Another more recent and very promising vaccine approach, AAV, will soon enter into clinical trial at the NARI. AAV was developed by Targeted Genetics, Seattle, and the Columbus Children Research Institute, Columbus, Ohio, in collaboration with the IAVI. The BCG approach involves collaboration between TRC, Anna University, Indian Institute of Science and the NARI.

Difficulties Foreseen in Implementing HIV Vaccine Trials in India

The difficulties foreseen in the process of implementing HIV vaccine clinical trials in India are inherent to the young and little experienced HIV Vaccine Development Programme in India. The same difficulties were met earlier in Thailand—such as defining the scientific and ethical approval process, constituting advisory boards, committees and project teams, reinforcing national infrastructure and updating technical tools, and training staff for specific activities. These difficulties, although critical, can be easily overcome by strong political commitment, spirit of international collaboration and a well-defined work plan. India has the benefit of a large pool of experts and highly skilled medical scientists as well as a long tradition and experience of clinical trials. In addition, as for Thailand, India is implementing a national plan for HIV prevention, care and treatment, the necessary condition for initiating HIV vaccine research. Because of the strong Indian cultural heritage, current beliefs and behaviours, the fear of stigma and discrimination, major difficulty may certainly be the recruitment of volunteers needed for different clinical trials, especially for women. Recruitment of high-risk volunteers may be much easier for further steps of clinical development (efficacy trials). Mechanisms of retention of volunteers in clinical trials in particular phase-II and efficacy trials will be key factors for success. Past experiences in cohort development in Pune had shown low retention rates, at a time where limited intervention package was offered to participants. Efficacy trials in heterosexual community-based cohorts may well be difficult, but not impossible, whereas recruitment of IDUs may be easier although a more unstable population to follow-up.

R EFERENCES

Celentano, D.D. et al. (1995). Willingness to participate in AIDS vaccine trials among high-risk populations in northern Thailand. *AIDS*, 9(9), 1079–83.

Esparza, J. and **D. Burke** (2001). Epidemiological considerations in planning HIV preventive vaccine trials. *AIDS*, 15(Supplement 5), S49–57.

Excler, J.L. and **C. Beyrer** (2000). Human immunodeficiency virus vaccine development in developing countries: Are efficacy trials feasible? *Journal of Human Virology*, 3(4), 193–214.

Gadkari, D.A. et al. (1998). Transmission of genetically diverse strains of HIV-1 in Pune, India. *Indian Journal of Medical Research*, 107(January), 1–9.

Guenter, D., J. Esparza and **R. Macklin** (2000). Ethical considerations in international HIV vaccine trials: Summary of a consultative process conducted by the joint United Nations programme on HIV/AIDS (UNAIDS). *Journal of Medical Ethics*, 26(1), 37–43.

Halani, N., B. Wang, Y.C. Ge, H. Ghapure, S. Hira and **N.K. Saksena** (2001). Changing epidemiology of HIV type 1 infections in India: Evidence of subtype B introduction in Bombay from a common source. *AIDS Research and Human Retroviruses*, 17(7), 637–42.

Heyward, W.L., K.M. MacQueen and **K.L. Goldenthal** (1998). HIV vaccine development and evaluation: Realistic expectations. *AIDS Research and Human Retroviruses*, 14(Supplement 3), S205–10.

Heyward, W.L., S. Osmanov and **J. Esparza** (1996). Establishment of WHO-sponsored field sites for HIV vaccine evaluation in developing countries. *Antibiotica et Chemotherapia*, 48, 139–44.

Kent, S.J., A. Zhao, S.J. Best, J.D. Chandler, D.B. Boyle and **I.A. Ramshaw** (1998). Enhanced T-cell immunogenicity and protective efficacy of a human immunodeficiency virus type 1 vaccine regimen consisting of consecutive priming with DNA and boosting with recombinant fowlpox virus. *Journal of Virology*, 72(12), 10180–88.

Kent, S.J., A. Zhao, C.J. Dale, S. Land, D.B. Boyle and **I.A. Ramshaw** (2000). A recombinant avipoxvirus HIV-1 vaccine expressing interferon-gamma is safe and immunogenic in macaques. *Vaccine*, 18, 2250–56.

Kettler, H.E. and **R. Modi** (2001). Building local research and development capacity for the prevention and cure of neglected diseases: The case of India. *Bulletin of WHO*, 79(8), 742–47.

Kilmarx, P.H., G. Ramjee, D. Kitayaporn and **P. Kunasol** (2001). Protection of human subjects' rights in HIV-preventive clinical trials in Africa and Asia: Experiences and recommendations. *AIDS*, 15(Supplement 5), S73–79.

Letvin, N.L. (1998). Progress in the development of an HIV-1 vaccine. *Science*, 280(5371), 1875–80.

Lole, K.S. et al. (1999). Full-length human immunodeficiency virus type 1 genomes from subtype C-infected seroconverters in India, with evidence of intersubtype recombination. *Journal of Virology*, 73(1), 152–60.

Lubaki, N.M. et al. (1999). HIV-1-specific cytotoxic T-lymphocyte activity correlates with lower viral load, higher CD4 count, and CD8+CD38-DR-phenotype: Comparison of statistical methods for measurement. *Journal of AIDS*, 22(1), 10–30.

MacQueen, K.M. et al. (1999). Willingness of injection drug users to participate in an HIV vaccine efficacy trial in Bangkok, Thailand. *Journal of AIDS*, 21(3), 243–51.

McCutchan, F.E. (2000). Understanding the genetic diversity of HIV-1. *AIDS*, 14(Supplement 3), S31–44.

McCutchan, F.E. et al. (2000). Diversity of envelope glycoprotein from human immunodeficiency virus type 1 of recent seroconverters in Thailand. *AIDS Research and Human Retroviruses*, 16(8), 801–5.

Ministry of Public Health (MOPH) (1993). *Thailand National Plan for HIV/AIDS vaccine development and evaluation.* Bangkok: MOPH.

Nathanson, N. and **B.J. Mathieson** (2000). Biological considerations in the development of human immunodeficiency virus vaccine. *Journal of Infectious Diseases*, 182(2), 579–89.

Nelson, K.E. et al. (1994). Preparatory studies for possible HIV vaccine trials in northern Thailand. *AIDS Research and Human Retroviruses*, 10 (Supplement 2), S243–46.

——— (1996). Changes in sexual behaviour and a decline in HIV infection among young men in Thailand. *New England Journal of Medicine*, 335(5), 277–303.

Nitayaphan, S. and **A.E. Brown** (1998). Preventive HIV vaccine development in Thailand. *AIDS*, 12(Supplement B), S155–61.

Okware, S., A. Opio, J. Musinguzi and **P. Waibale** (2001). Fighting HIV/AIDS: Is success possible? *Bulletin of World Health Organization*, 79(12), 1113–20.

Osmanov, S., C. Pattou, N. Walker, B. Schwardlander and **J. Esparza** (2002). WHO–UNAIDS network for HIV isolation and characterisation. Estimated global distribution and regional spread of HIV-1 genetic sub-types in the year 2000. *Journal of AIDS*, 29(2), 184–90.

Paranjape, R.S., D.A. Gadkari, M. Lubaki, T.C. Quinn and **R.C. Bollinger** (1998). Cross-reactive HIV-1 specific CTL in recent seroconverters from Pune, India. *Indian Journal of Medical Research*, 108(August), 35–41.

Peiperl, L. (2001). Progress toward an AIDS vaccine: Prospects for protective immunity. *AIDScience*, 1(13).

Piyasirisilp, S. et al. (2000). A recent outbreak of human immunodeficiency virus type 1 infection in southern China was initiated by two highly homogeneous, geographically separated strains, circulating recombinant form AE and a novel BC recombinant. *Journal of Virology*, 74(23), 11286–95.

Porter, K.R. et al. (1997). Genetic, antigenic and serologic characterisation of human immunodeficiency virus type 1 from Indonesia. *Journal of AIDS*, 14(1), 1–6.

Rojanapithayakorn, W. and **R. Hanenberg** (1996). The 100% condom program in Thailand. *AIDS*, 10(1), 1–7.

Sahni, A.K., V.V. Prasad and **P. Seth** (2002). Genomic diversity of human immunodeficiency virus type-1 in India. *International Journal of STD and AIDS*, 13(2), 115–18.

Sharma, D.C. (2001). India to develop an AIDS vaccine. *Lancet*, 357(9261), 1024.

Tovanabutra, S. et al. (2001). First CRF01_AE/B recombinant of HIV-1 is found in Thailand. *AIDS*, 15(8), 1063–65.

Tripathy, S. et al. (1996). Envelope glycoprotein 120 sequences of primary HIV type 1 isolates from Pune and New Delhi, India. *AIDS Research and Human Retroviruses*, 12(12), 1199–1202.

Vanichseni, S. (2001). Continued high HIV-1 incidence in a vaccine trial preparatory cohort of injection drug users in Bangkok, Thailand. *AIDS*, 15(3), 397–405.

ABOUT THE EDITOR AND CONTRIBUTORS

Editor

Jai P. Narain is Coordinator/Regional Adviser on HIV/AIDS and TB programmes at WHO's Regional Office for South-East Asia (SEARO), New Delhi. He has an MBBS and an MD from the All India Institute of Medical Sciences (AIIMS), New Delhi, and a master's in public health and in epidemiology from Harvard University, Boston. Associated with HIV/AIDS and TB prevention and control programmes since 1988, he has held positions at PAHO/AMRO Caribbean Epidemiology Centre (1988–90) and WHO, Geneva (1990–91). He has been with SEARO since 1991 where he has also served as Team Leader, Global Programme on AIDS (1991–95). Dr. Narain has also worked at prestigious institutions like the National Institute of Communicable Diseases, AIIMS, the Indian Council of Medical Research and Centers for Disease Control, Atlanta. He has published extensively and has edited/authored several books on various aspects of communicable diseases, mainly HIV/AIDS and TB.

Contributors

Iyanthi Abeyewickreme is Director, National STD/AIDS Control Programme, Department of Health, Sri Lanka, providing leadership and technical direction for the national response to HIV by various stakeholders. She has been for 12 years a senior consultant venereologist in Sri Lanka, and is Chairman, Board of Study in Venereology in the University of Colombo. She has helped the WHO in the area of sexually-transmitted diseases. Dr. Abeyewickreme has a medical degree from the University of Ceylon, a Diploma in Venereology from London and a postgraduate degree in Community Medicine from University of Colombo.

Teresita Marie P. Bagasao is Chief of the Partnership Unit of Social Mobilisation and Information in the Joint United Nations Programme on HIV/AIDS (UNAIDS), Geneva. From 1996 to 2001, she was UNAIDS Programme Development Officer for Asia and the Pacific. Prior to joining UNAIDS, she worked for over 10 years in Manila as head of a health and development NGO, which worked with other NGOs, the private sector and government, including bilateral and multilateral organisations. Under this capacity, she facilitated the development and support of a number of regional NGO network working on HIV/AIDS and their participation in national and regional policy-making bodies. She has B.Sc. in social work and a masters degree in psychology.

Anne Bergenström is currently based in Vietnam as project director, coordinating a randomised controlled HIV/STD prevention intervention trial implemented by the Department of Epidemiology, Johns Hopkins University, Bloomberg School of Public Health, USA. A graduate in psychology from City University, London, she obtained a Ph.D. from the Royal Free and University College Medical School, London, where she worked for several years as a researcher on HIV/AIDS. During 1999 and 2002 she worked in the UN system, first at the Asia Pacific Desk in the Department of Country Planning and Programme Development, UNAIDS headquarters in Geneva, followed by the UNAIDS South Asia Regional Office and UNICEF in Indonesia.

Sanchai Chasombat has been working since 2001 at the Bureau of AIDS, TB and STIs, Department of Disease Control, Ministry of Public Health, Thailand, as Chief of Social Services and Research Section and Medical Services Section. In these positions, Dr. Chasombat has been responsible for the development of antiretroviral and the comprehensive and continuum of care for HIV/AIDS programmes in Thailand. He obtained his medical degree in 1996 and postgraduate degree in clinical sciences from Chulalongkorn University in 1998.

Anindya Chatterjee is Senior Adviser of Prevention and Public Policy at the Joint United Nations Programme on HIV/AIDS (UNAIDS) headquarters in Geneva. He graduated in medicine and subsequently obtained a doctoral degree in psychiatry and post-doctoral training in public health. He has worked with government authorities, NGOs, and research and international agencies in India, Bangladesh, Nepal and Iran. He was previously based in the UNAIDS regional team in Thailand and has worked extensively in countries of South-East and East Asia, particularly Myanmar, China and Indonesia.

Ranjit Roy Chaudhury is at present Emeritus Scientist at the National Institute of Immunology (NII), New Delhi, and UNESCO Professor in Rational Use of Drugs at Chulalongkorn University, Thailand. He is President of the Delhi Medical Council and Coordinator of the India–WHO Essential Drugs Programme. One of the leading clinical pharmacologists of India, he was Head of the Department of Pharmacology and Dean at the Postgraduate Institute of Medical Education and Research, Chandigarh, where he initiated the D.M. course in clinical pharmacology. He has held important positions in the WHO for 15 years. He has recently taken over as Chair of the International Clinical Epidemiology Network (INCLEN).

Anupong Chitwarakorn graduated from Siriraj Medical School, Mahidol University, in 1978. Since then, he has been working with the Department of Communicable Disease Control, Ministry of Public Health. He was appointed Director of the Venereal Disease Division in 1993. In 2000 he became Director of the AIDS Division and served as National Programme Manager for two years. Currently, he is Senior Expert in Preventive Medicine for HIV/AIDS/STI for the Department of Disease Control. As a technical expert, he has also assisted the WHO on many occasions.

José Esparza obtained his MD degree in Venezuela. He also has a Ph.D. in virology and epidemiology from Baylor College of Medicine, in the United States. From 1974 to 1985 he worked at the Venezuelan Institute for Scientific Research, where he was Full Professor and Head of the Laboratory of Biology of Viruses, and Chairman of the Department of Microbiology and Cell Biology. From 1980 to 1982 he was also a Visiting Professor at Duke University Medical Centre, in Durham, North Carolina. In 1986 he joined the WHO in Geneva, where he is currently Coordinator of the WHO–UNAIDS HIV Vaccine Initiative.

Jean-Louis Excler is currently Medical Director for the International AIDS Vaccine Initiative in India. A French citizen, Dr. Excler is a paediatrician, epidemiologist and tropical medicine specialist by training. He has been working on AIDS vaccines since 1991 successively for the pharmaceutical industry (Aventis Pasteur), the US government as

Scientific Director for the Henry M. Jackson Foundation (Walter Reed Army Institute of Research—US Army HIV Research Programme). He has also worked as a consultant for UNICEF in South-East Asia and for the WHO on vaccine research and development.

Charles F. Gilks is Director of the '3 by 5' initiative, working in the HIV department of the WHO in Geneva. He is on secondment from Imperial College, London, where he is Professor of International Health. He has worked on HIV/AIDS care issues in developing countries since 1988. His group in Kenya was the first to identify the importance of invasive bacterial infections (pneumococcus and non-typhi salmonellae) in adults immunosuppressed with HIV. He is the Principal Investigator of the DART trial, the largest multicentre trial of ART in Africa and has been closely working with DFID UK on care and support of people living with HIV/AIDS.

Heiner Grosskurth is a clinical epidemiologist based in Uganda where he leads the Research Programme on AIDS of the UK Medical Research Council, a collaborative programme of the MRC and the Uganda Virus Research Institute. A Reader in Epidemiology and International Health at the London School of Hygiene and Tropical Medicine (University of London), he has been focusing on the epidemiology and control of HIV infection and other sexually-transmitted diseases, and on primary health care and efforts to improve health care delivery in developing countries. From 2001 to 2003, he was seconded to the Population Council in India to help establish its HIV/STI research programme in the subcontinent.

Han Mengjie is at the National Centre for STD/AIDS Prevention and Control in China.

Subhash K. Hira is an infectious diseases specialist and Professor at the University of Texas, Houston, having served for a decade as Director of AIDS Research & Control Centre (ARCON) with the government of Maharashtra and Sir J. J. Hospital in Mumbai, India. He was appointed Technical Adviser to National AIDS Control Organisation (NACO) in India for design of its second national programme and launch of its prevention of parent-to-child transmission programme. For a decade in the 1980s, he served as the National Programme Manager for STD (later to include AIDS) for the Ministry of Health of Zambia. He is currently Programme Leader and Senior HIV/AIDS Specialist at the World Bank HQ supporting a 41-country portfolio.

Ahmed S. Latif is a Professor of Medicine, specialist physician and formerly Dean of Faculty of Medicine, University of Zimbabwe College of Health Sciences, Harare. Currently, he is Medical Officer (Public Health) in the Tristate STI/HIV Project, Alice Springs, Northern Territory, Australia, and Professor, Centre for Remote Health, Flinders University, Adelaide, Australia. He has extensive international experience with the WHO in the area of STI/HIV Prevention and Control, and in training health workers. His research experience encompass biomedical, behavioural and operations areas. Professor Latif has numerous publications in peer-reviewed international scientific journals. He has an M.B.Ch.B. degree from Zimbabwe and F.C.P. (from South Africa) and F.R.C.P. from England.

Cheewanan Lertpiriyasuwat is now working at the Medical Services Section of the Bureau of AIDS, TB and STIs, Department of Disease Control, Ministry of Public Health, Thailand. She has been actively involved in the development of the National Access to Antiretroviral Programmes for PWHA (NAPHA) in Thailand. Dr. Lertpiriyasuwat obtained her medical degree from Chulalongkorn University in 1996 and the Certificate of Field Epidemiology Training Programme in 2002.

Liu Kangmai is currently working as Division Secretary of the Chinese Communist Party in National HIV/AIDS Prevention and Control. He is also a member of the National Expert Consultation Committee on AIDS Prevention and Control, Vice Secretary General of the Chinese Association for STD/AIDS Prevention and Control, and a member of Editorial Committee of Journal affiliated to Chinese Association for STD/AIDS Prevention and Control as well as the journal *China Health Education*. He is former Director of the Department of Health Education and Information, and Director Assistant of the National Centre for AIDS Prevention and Control, Chinese Centre for Disease Control and Prevention. Dr. Liu Kangmai possesses extensive experience of more than a decade in AIDS health education, information and communication.

Bjorn Melgaard is currently WHO Representative to Thailand and to the Economic and Social Commission for Asia and the Pacific. He joined the WHO in 1995 as Chief of the Expanded Programme on Immunisation and was appointed Director of the Department of Vaccines and Biologicals at the WHO headquarters in Geneva in 1998. In this capacity he was responsible for all the WHO's work on vaccines and immunisation. Before joining the WHO, Dr. Melgaard worked for more than

10 years for the Danish Development Agency, DANIDA, in various positions in developing countries. He is a medical doctor and a public health expert, and has authored more than 50 papers on health topics.

Jette Nielsen was recently with the UNAIDS South-East Asia Intercountry Team in Bangkok where she worked for three years. She is presently in her home country, Denmark, as a freelance consultant and trying to settle there. Her educational background is in political science.

Saladin Osmanov was born in Russia and graduated as a physician from the 2nd Pirogov Medical Institute of Moscow and obtained Ph.D. in microbiology at the Metchnikov Research Institute of Vaccines and Sera in Moscow. From 1989 to 1996, he worked as a scientist at the Global Programme on AIDS (GPA) of the WHO in Geneva, Switzerland. From 1996 to 2000, he worked at the Joint United Nations Programme on HIV/AIDS (UNAIDS) as a virologist/vaccine specialist. Since January 2000, Dr. Osmanov has been working at a newly-created WHO–UNAIDS HIV Vaccine Initiative, as part of the Viral Vaccines Team of the WHO Initiative for Vaccine Research.

Salil Panakadan is Joint Director, NACO, India, and a public health specialist with the National AIDS Control Programme (NACP) in India. His special interests are in the fields of epidemiology and monitoring and evaluation of programmes. He is currently responsible for monitoring and evaluation of blood safety components of the NACP in NACO. A medical doctor with a postgraduate degree in community medicine, he has been in HIV/AIDS control efforts at the national level for over 12 years.

Jos Perriens is presently Director of Care and Support, HIV/AIDS Department, WHO, in Geneva. Before moving to WHO in 2002, Dr. Perriens was with the UNAIDS Secretariat in Geneva, responsible for HIV/AIDS care issues. He has wide-ranging experience, particularly in the area of HIV/AIDS care and support.

Emanuele Pontali graduated as an M.D. at the University of Genoa, Italy. He is a specialist in infectious diseases and has been associated with HIV/AIDS care and clinical research in paediatric HIV infection, immunological aspects of HIV infection and adherence to antiretroviral therapy at the Department of Infectious Diseases of the University of Genoa, Italy. Earlier he was Associate Professional Officer in WHO

South-East Asia Regional Office working on epidemiology and control of tuberculosis, HIV/AIDS and TB-HIV co-infection (January 2001– January 2003) in New Delhi, India. Trained in epidemiology in 2001 at CDC and Emory University, Atlanta, USA he is presently Senior Consultant in Infectious Diseases at the Health Department of the Prison of Genoa, Italy; WHO consultant and consultant in Infectious Diseases for the University of Genoa.

Gurumurthy Rangaiyan is presently working as a Project Director, HIV/STI Prevention and Care Research Programme in the Population Council. Prior to that, he served as a faculty member at the International Institute for Population Sciences (IIPS), Mumbai. In these positions, he has been actively involved in designing, implementing and evaluating a number of innovative HIV/STI projects. Dr. Rangaiyan obtained his doctorate degree from IIPS, Mumbai.

Wiwat Rojanapithayakorn is currently working at WHO Mongolia. He worked in the Ministry of Public Health in Thailand for over 20 years in the areas of STI, HIV/AIDS and other communicable disease control. Before joining WHO Mongolia, he was the Team Leader of the South-East Asia and the Pacific Inter-country Team of UNAIDS based in Bangkok. He is the founder of the 100 per cent Condom Use Programme in Thailand, and an active advocate of this approach in many Asian countries.

Naqibullah Safi is currently working as National Programme Manager of HIV/AIDS/STI in the Ministry of Health (MOH), Afghanistan. He is also working for the UNICEF Afghanistan country office as HIV/AIDS Focal Person. He has been in the field of public health for the last 10 years and has served as Director General of PHC/Preventive Affairs, Director of the National Infectious Disease Hospital, Provincial Health Director and Senior Adviser to the MOH, Afghanistan. He obtained his medical degree from Kabul University, a masters degree in community health from the Liverpool School of Tropical Medicine, and is currently a student of a postgraduate diploma in HIV/AIDS management with Stellenbosch University, South Africa.

Swarup Sarkar is an epidemiologist working in Bangkok with UNAIDS Inter-country Team for South-East Asia and the Pacific. Prior to that, he was Team Leader for the South Asia Inter-country Team based in New Delhi. He has considerable experience in HIV/AIDS epidemiology, prevention and care, and has travelled extensively to countries of the region. His work in the north-east Indian state of Manipur where injecting drug use the most important route of HIV transmission has been noteworthy. Dr. Sarkar has a medical degree from Kolkata and an M.P.H. from UCLA. He has contributed many scientific papers, including those pertaining to injecting drug use vulnerability and HIV.

Mohammed Shaukat is a public health specialist working in the Ministry of Health and Family Welfare, Government of India, with 18 years experience in public health management. Presently, as Joint Director (Technical) in NACO, he is responsible for planning and implementation of various activities related to surveillance under the NACP. He is an expert on HIV sentinel surveillance and has tracked the evolution of HIV epidemic in India since 1997.

Shen Jie is Director, National Centre for AIDS/STD Prevention and Control, Chinese Centre for Diseases Control and Prevention in Beijing. As Deputy Director, Chinese Centre for Disease Control and Prevention, she has been involved in AIDS prevention and control at the national level for almost 10 years. Prior to that Dr. Shen Jie occupied the post of Deputy Director, Division of Parasitic Diseases Control, Department of Disease Control, Ministry of Health and Director, Division II of Communicable Diseases Control, Department of Disease Control, Ministry of Health, in the People Republic of China.

B.K. Suvedi is formerly Director, National Centre for AIDS and STI Control in Kathmandu, Nepal (2002–3) and a Deputy Director (1993–98). Dr. Suvedi has been working in health services in Nepal for the last 20 years and his core areas of expertise include HIV/AIDS, STI, expanded programme of immunisation, research and training. He has a master's degree in anthropology (from Tribhuvan University, Kathmandu) as well as a medical degree (from USSR) and M.P.H. from John Hopkins University (Baltimore, USA).

Waranya Teokul, an economist, works for Office of National Economic and Social Development Board, Thailand's national planning agency. She has been closely involved in managing the HIV/AIDS problem in Thailand since 1991. Currently, she is heavily engaged with Thailand's poverty reduction programme, which includes solving problems of impoverished children, and children affected and afflicted with HIV.

Sombat Thanprasertsuk is Director of the Bureau of AIDS, TB and STIs, Department of Disease Control, Ministry of Public Health in

Thailand. He has more than 20 years of experience in HIV/AIDS in Thailand. Before assuming this post, he was Chief of Technical Unit of the AIDS Division, Director of Epidemiology Division and has served as the Adjunct Director of the Ministry of Public Health, Thailand, and US CDC HIV/AIDS Collaboration Programme. Dr. Thanprasertsuk is one of the key resource persons participating in HIV/AIDS programme planning and evaluation of many countries in the Asia Pacific region.

Basil Vareldzis is a public health physician trained in the USA and Canada with advanced degrees in medicine and public health. He has worked as clinical director of the largest HIV/AIDS clinic in the United States for three years and has also served as Medical Officer with the WHO's Tuberculosis Programme and HIV/AIDS Department as well as a Senior Technical Adviser for TB/HIV for the United States Agency for International Development (USAID) in Washington. He is currently a consultant in International Health and Development, based in Geneva, Switzerland.

Ying-Ru Lo is currently working as Medical Officer (AIDS) in the World Health Organization Regional Office for South-East Asia, New Delhi. Earlier, she worked in the WHO country office in Thailand for nearly five years. Prior to joining WHO, she served in the Department of Infectious Diseases (including HIV/AIDS) and Tropical Medicine, Bernhard-Nocht Institute of Nautical and Tropical Medicine, Hamburg. She has wide clinical and public health experience, particularly in the area of prevention of mother-to-child transmission and antiretroviral treatment. She obtained her Masters degree and doctoral thesis from the University of Hamburg and a postgraduate degree in tropical medicine and hygiene from the Bernhard-Nocht Institute of Nautical and Tropical Medicine, Hamburg.

Myint Zaw obtained his medical degree and master's degree in medical sciences (public health) from University of California at Los Angeles (UCLA). From 1998 till 2003, he was a national AIDS programme manager in Myanmar. He has worked in Timor Leste as WHO Short-term Consultant on HIV/AIDS and as HIV/AIDS Research Activity Coordinator with Family Health International. Dr. Myint Zaw has a broad experience in public health.

Zhang Fujie is with the Ministry of Health in China.

INDEX